The Complete Patient History

Second Edition

NOTICE

Medicine is an ever-changing science. As new research and clinical experience broaden our knowledge, changes in treatment and drug therapy are required. The editors and publisher of this work have checked with sources believed to be reliable in their efforts to provide information that is complete and generally in accord with the standards accepted at the time of publication. However, in view of the possibility of human error or changes in medical sciences, neither the editors, the publisher, or any other party who has been involved in the preparation or publication of this work warrants that the information contained herein is in every respect accurate or complete. Readers are encouraged to confirm the information contained herein with other sources. For example and in particular, readers are advised to check the product information sheet included in the package of each drug they plan to administer to be certain that the information contained in this book is accurate and that changes have not been made in the recommended dose or in the contraindications for administration. This recommendation is of particular importance in connection with new or infrequently used drugs.

The Complete Patient History

Second Edition

MAURICE KRAYTMAN, M.D.

Clinical Professor of Medicine
University of Brussels
Brussels, Belgium

McGraw-Hill, Inc.
Health Professions Division

New York   St. Louis   San Francisco   Auckland   Bogotá
Caracas   Lisbon   London   Madrid   Mexico City   Milan
Montreal   New Delhi   San Juan   Singapore
Sydney   Tokyo   Toronto

THE COMPLETE PATIENT HISTORY

Copyright © 1991, 1979 by McGraw-Hill, Inc. All rights reserved. Printed in the United States of America. Except as permitted under the United States Copyright Act of 1976, no part of this publication may be reproduced or distributed in any form or by any means, or stored in a data base or retrieval system, without the prior written permission of the publisher.

2 3 4 5 6 7 8 9 10 11 12 13 14 BKMBKM 9 9 8 7 6 5 4

ISBN 0-07-035614-9

This book was set in Meridian and Eras by Kachina Typesetting. The editor was William Day; the designer was Judith Michael; the production supervisor was Annette Mayeski. The project was supervised by Spectrum Publisher Services, Inc.

Library of Congress Cataloging in Publication Data

Kraytman, Maurice.
    The complete patient history.

    Includes bibliographical references.
    Includes index.
    1. Medical history taking. I. Title. [DNLM:
1. Medical History Taking—handbooks. WB 39 K91e]
RC65.K73 1991   616.07'51   90-6266
ISBN 0-07-035614-9

CONTENTS

PREFACE

History taking is undoubtedly the most important and difficult part of the clinical examination. This book is intended as an aid to medical personnel (medical students, residents, general practitioners, physician assistants, and nurse practitioners) in the taking of a patient's history. Because it is designed to establish and reinforce good habits in history taking, this book should also be useful to students taking courses in physical diagnosis, introduction to clinical medicine, or patient interviewing. It is divided into two parts and sixty chapters.

Chapter 1 delineates the sequential steps in history taking, stressing possible technical and psychological pitfalls and their avoidance. This chapter also emphasizes the respective places of nondirective and leading questions in the interview.

Part One contains fifty-one chapters devoted to specific complaints. Each chapter includes six sections: (1) introduction, with the definition and pathophysiology of the complaint to be investigated; (2) etiology, with tables of differential diagnosis, including the iatrogenic causes of the complaint; (3) a series of questions centered around the complaint, with the possible clinical and/or pathophysiological meanings of a positive response; (4) physical signs pertinent to the complaint and their possible clinical interpretation; (5) laboratory tests relevant to the complaint with the diagnostic possibilities of the results; (6) selected references.

Part Two deals with inquiries which apply to every patient regardless of his or her particular problem: obtaining an occupational, alcohol-use, and sexual history; evolution of the illness; its effects on the patient; complete personal and family medical history; review of systems; and personal and social profile.

It is technically impossible to present open-ended questions in lay language that could apply to every patient and be accompanied by their possible meanings. Therefore, the questions had to be put in a directive form. They should be considered as being addressed to the reader as reminders of what information must be collected in order to explore and understand the patient's illness. It is up to the reader to adapt the questions to the actual patient being interrogated and to rephrase them first in a nondirective form or, if necessary, in a directive form.

For each question, the most likely meanings of the positive response are given. It is evident, however, that a positive answer to a question could have several meanings and suggest several possibilities. The adjective "possible," which appears in the heading "Possible meaning of a positive response," reminds the reader that the suggested diagnoses are not exclusive of other clinical entities.

The tables of differential diagnosis are arranged, whenever possible, according to pathophysiological mechanisms. Common causes of complaints and/or urgent conditions are indicated in the lists of diseases. No attempt has been made to cite all drugs capable of causing a given complaint. Instead, the most frequently used medications have been mentioned. The sections "Physical Signs Pertaining to the Complaint" and "Laboratory Tests Pertaining to the Complaint" are intended to complement the clinical information derived from the history taking. Laboratory investigations have been limited to the most common and useful ones, and some of them are tagged with an asterisk (*) footnote (*When indicated) to remind the reader that diagnostic procedures should be ordered discriminately and economically. Problem-centered history taking inevitably results in the fragmentation of the various components of clinical syndromes under separate headings. The Glossary of Clinical Manifestations reassembles the main symptoms and signs making up disease entities, which are thus reconstructed according to their classical description.

Crucial differentiating questions and characteristic clinical features are *italicized*. Potentially life-threatening or urgent conditions are in **boldface** type.

The aim of this book is not to propose branching diagnoses or algorithms. Rather it attempts to help the interviewer gather clinical information and correlate the patient's responses with possible disease entities.

It is the author's hope that readers of this book will find it useful in their daily medical practice.

ACKNOWLEDGMENTS

I wish to thank Mr. W. Day and Mr. P. McCurdy of the McGraw-Hill Book Company for their helpful and skillful editorial guidance.

Maurice Kraytman

1
The Sequential Steps in History Taking

The importance of history taking in the process of making a differential diagnosis cannot be overemphasized. It has been estimated that the history allows a correct diagnosis in over 50 percent of internal diseases. However, history taking is not just a process of collecting information on the onset and evolution of an illness. It must also give an insight into the patient's personality, the ability of the patient to cope with the medical problem, and the effects of the problem on the patient. It serves as the basis for the relationship between patient and interviewer.

Whenever possible, the interview should take place in privacy. The patient should be put at ease and assured that there will be time enough to discuss fully any matter of concern. When confronted with a confused patient or a patient who minimizes, denies, or conceals symptoms, it is essential to interview a reliable relative or friend.

1. The first step in history taking is to invite the patient to express the reason for seeking medical advice. In order to obtain the patient's chief complaint, a question of a general nature, such as, "What can I do for you?" or "Please tell me about your trouble," is frequently necessary. Avoid asking the patient, "What is wrong with you?" as the answer might be, "That's why I came to you!"

The patient should then be asked to give, in the patient's own terms, a full account of his or her illness. All facts believed associated with the complaint should be brought out, and the patient should be encouraged to give his or her feelings about the symptoms. Except in case of rambling, the patient should be allowed to discuss problems uninterrupted as they come to mind.

Do not disregard too rapidly details which seem irrelevant or even bizarre, or which do not fit with your initial hypothesis. *All* facts mentioned by the patient must be taken into account; they should be carefully analyzed before being eventually discarded.

When the patient seems to come to a stop, prompting with nonspecific questions, such as, "And then?" or "Are there any other problems?" is indicated.

A patient who has several complaints should be asked which one seems the most important.

2. After having afforded the patient the opportunity to describe his or her illness, the interviewer should then proceed methodically to analyze the complaint within the following framework: mode of onset and chronology; location and, if applicable, radiation of the symptom; character (or quality) of the symptom; intensity (or quantitative aspects) of the complaint; precipitating or aggravating factors; relieving factors; accompanying symptoms; iatrogenic factors; personal and social factors; personal and relevant family medical history pertaining to the complaint; evolution of the illness and its effects on the patient.

The exploration of these features need not be done in a rigid sequence. For instance, when dealing with a pain problem, the first step should be to locate exactly the site of discomfort. With other complaints, such as fatigue or vertigo, the interviewer should first try to define exactly what the patient means, i.e., the character (or quality) of the complaint should be assessed first. Flexibility in the order of the questions is also required to avoid inhibiting any beneficial association of thoughts by the patient.

Inquiry into each of these topics should begin with nondirective questions, such as, "Does the discomfort remain localized? Does it move?" Asking a patient with chest pain on exertion, "Does the pain disappear rapidly when you stop walking?" is bad technique. The very formulation of the question may influence the patient. In a desire to be cooperative, the patient may provide information that the interviewer appears to want. The significance of "rapidly" may be quite different to the patient than to the interviewer. Finally, this type of questions is too complex. It actually contains two separate questions: (1) "Does the pain disappear when you stop walking?" and (2) "Does the pain disappear rapidly?" Questions must explore one item at a time. The correct sequence would be: "When you stop walking, does it affect your discomfort?" and, if so, "In how much time does the pain disappear?"

Some patients will give a clear, lucid description of their illness, and satisfactorily answer the interviewer's questions. However, in the majority of patients, verbosity, limited vocabulary, and/or forgetfulness will eventually force the interviewer to guide the patient by asking specific, directive questions to help clarify the subject. For example, with a patient complaining of lower back pain, the interviewer should first ask, in a neutral manner, "Does the pain move anywhere?" If the response is not explicit, the interviewer should specify, "Does the pain radiate to the buttock? The calf?"

Nondirective as well as directive questions must be concise and easily understandable by the patient. Avoid medical terms and technical expressions. Use the patient's own words ("trouble," "discomfort," etc.). This way you will not distort the patient's thoughts and substitute your own interpretation. Sometimes, it is useful deliberately to repeat the question (perhaps phrased differently) later in the interview if the original response appears doubtful.

The different aspects of the full analysis of a complaint will now be briefly discussed.

Mode of Onset and Chronology

The exact manner in which the illness began must be defined: What was the patient doing at the time of onset? Where was the patient? What were the precise circumstances of the onset? Many patients believe that their illness began later than it actually did. If the patient has difficulty in recalling precisely the date of onset of the illness, the interviewer can help by referring to chronological landmarks, such as seasons or holidays: "How were you feeling during the summer vacation? the Christmas holidays?" Another useful reference point is the patient's last thorough medical examination for employment or insurance. Time relationship must be established by date. If the complaint is intermittent, ask the patient to specify the periodicity and frequency of the symptom, and to describe fully a typical episode.

Location and Radiation of Symptom

The patient should be invited to point (with a finger if possible) to the site of the discomfort and to its eventual radiation. He or she should also locate the depth at which the abnormal sensation seems to arise.

Character (or Quality) of Symptom

Generally, a patient will have difficulty describing this aspect of the complaint and will often resort to comparisons. For example, a patient with tension headache might say, "I feel as if my head were in a vise." The interviewer may aid the patient by presenting various descriptive terms or phrases. If the symptom is a pain, the question might be: "What sort of pain is it? dull? burning? constrictive?" The interviewer should be careful not to emphasize one descriptive term or one comparison more than another.

Intensity (or Quantity) of Symptom

Any complaint that lends itself to quantification should be defined in some measurable way. Diarrhea must be expressed in the number of stools per day, dyspnea or intermittent claudication in terms of level blocks walked before it is felt.

Precipitating, Aggravating, and Relieving Factors

Some patients will spontaneously tell the interviewer that their complaint becomes better or worse under certain circumstances. For instance, a patient may indicate that a pain in the calves appears on walking and disappears on stopping. However, the interviewer generally must ask specific questions. For example, the interviewer, knowing that the pain of a peptic ulcer appears within hours after a meal and subsides after eating, will specifically ask about these circumstances. Again, the questions should be worded to avoid influencing the answers. Thus it is better to ask, "What effect does eating have on your pain?" rather than, "Does eating relieve your pain?"

Accompanying Symptoms

Most often, the patient's complaint is only part of a constellation of symptoms grouped into clinical syndromes. Some patients frequently fail to realize that other symptoms they are presenting are related to the chief complaint, and they may even fail to mention the other symptoms, having become accustomed to them. For instance, a man complaining about edema in the lower extremities may not volunteer that he has been short of breath when walking and has been sleeping with two pillows for months. The interviewer must anticipate the missing symptoms in the patient's account of the illness and must inquire, in a directive manner, about associated phenomena that the patient may have failed to mention.

Iatrogenic Factors

In this era of universal polypharmacopeia, the interviewer should never omit to have patients give a full account of all drugs they are currently taking. Many patients taking sleeping pills, tranquilizers, analgesics, laxatives, oral contraceptives, may become so accustomed to these medications that they do not consider them as drugs. It is not enough to ask the patient, "Do you take any medications?" Questions should be specific: "Do you take aspirin? sleeping pills? laxatives?" It is wise to ask the patient whether the drugs were prescribed by a physician or bought over the counter. Knowing that a patient uses drugs indiscriminately enables the physician to anticipate poor compliance with his or her own prescriptions.

Personal and Social Profile

The patient's life-style, environment, job, hobbies, domicile, travels are all possible etiologic factors. It is important to inquire about the patient's sexual practices or concerns, to know that the patient with cough and sputum of recent onset has a parrot at home, or to learn that the present fever and recurrent chills appeared after a travel in a malaria-infested area. Direct questioning is imperative here.

Personal Antecedents and Family Medical History Pertaining to the Complaint

The patient's personal antecedents and the family medical history may provide useful information on the present illness. For instance, it is important to learn that a jaundiced patient with acute pain in the right hypochondrium has a history of anemia and that relatives have undergone splenectomy to cure an anemia. What might have initially been interpreted as gallbladder colic now seems likely to be cholelithiasis complicating hereditary spherocytosis. Do not accept at face value the patient's version of past diagnoses by other physicians. Patient's terms such as "pneumonia," "heart attack," "pleurisy," must be critically analyzed. For instance, the details of a past "gallstone attack" should be elicited: "Where was the pain located? Did the color of the skin and/or urine change? Was there fever, chills?" etc.

Evolution of the Illness and Its Effects on the Patient

The interviewer should ask the patient a series of questions aimed at exploring the evolution of the illness and its overall effects on the patient's normal activities. A useful question always to be asked is "Why did you select this particular time to seek medical advice?" It occasionally brings out an important recent change in symptoms that the patient has omitted. Never forget to inquire about the patient's opinion regarding the illness: this question may reveal the patient's fear, apprehensions, or fantasies.

   3. After full characterization of the symptom, the following areas are explored: complete personal and family medical history; review of systems; and finally the personal and social profile.

Personal Past Medical History

Information about previous illnesses, operations, and accidents should be obtained, preferably in chronologic order, with the dates and locations of occurrence, the names of the physicians involved, and the treatments applied. Specific questions will need to be asked of the patient. Again do not forget that the diagnoses reported by the patient may not be correct because of misinterpretation or misdiagnosis. On the other hand, diagnoses made by previous physicians should not be discarded lightly.

Family Medical History

The health of family members should be ascertained. Diseases with hereditary or environmental factors should be mentioned specifically. Knowledge of the ethnic origin of the parents and of any consanguinity may be important.

Review of Systems

In this part of the history taking, the interviewer specifically checks each system, from head to extremities, to make certain that neither physician nor patient has overlooked any symptom or sign of significance. Direct questions have to be asked. Whenever a positive answer is obtained, the interviewer should clarify the newly elicited symptom by shifting back to nondirective questions and encouraging a description of the symptoms in the patient's own terms. If ambiguity still persists, leading questions should be asked. Chronology of events must be delineated. When a patient responds positively to nearly every question, a multisystem disease or a psychologic illness should be suspected.

Personal and Social Profile

The patient's ethnic, familial, educational, and social background, employments, habits, and moods should be explored. These features may play an important role in the health problem, and may help evaluate the personality of the patient. For example, multiple jobs in a short period of time are suggestive of psychological difficulties; alcoholics are liable to certain diseases such as cirrhosis, acute pancreatitis, neurologic disorders, while homosexual men are at risk for human immunodeficiency virus infection and other infectious diseases.

Some patients are reluctant to discuss their personal problems. Questions about these matters should initially be general and not probe too deeply so that the patient is not put on the defensive. When highly private problems are being discussed, it is better for the interviewer to lay aside his or her pen, as note taking may have an inhibitory effect on the patient.

At the end of the interrogation, the interviewer should always inquire whether the patient has questions to ask or anything to add: previous hidden anxieties may be revealed.

The above suggested sequence need not be rigidly adhered to; each patient demands an individual procedure. Particularly, patients who so wish should be allowed to speak freely about emotional problems at any time during the interview. However, it is psychologically wise to close the interview with the personal and social profile. In this way, inquiry about more intimate matters is postponed until after the medical aspects have been explored and sufficient time has elapsed to create a satisfactory patient-interviewer relationship.

PART ONE

Problem-Centered History Taking

Cardiorespiratory System

2
Chest Pain

INTRODUCTION

Chest pain may have its origin in the various tissues of the chest wall, the intrathoracic structures, the neck, or areas below the diaphragm.

Cardiac Pain

The myocardium gives rise to pain when the oxygen supply to the heart is deficient in relation to the oxygen needs; this occurs when coronary blood flow is inadequate (e.g., coronary atherosclerosis). Pain from myocardial disease is felt to arise within the first to fourth or fifth thoracic segments. These spinal segments also receive sensory fibers from other structures: the esophagus, mediastinal contents, osseous and muscular structures; diseases of these structures may cause pain that is difficult to distinguish from cardiac pain. The pain of myocardial ischemia may be felt along the inner aspect of the left arm, owing to the common innervation of the heart and the affected area of the skin by the eighth cervical and first thoracic segments. However, almost any disorder involving the deep afferent fibers of the left upper thoracic region may produce pain in the chest, the left arm, or both areas. Pain associated with *pericarditis* is believed to be due to inflammation of the adjacent parietal pleura; the visceral surface of the pericardium is ordinarily insensible to pain.

Pleuritic Pain

The parietal pleura is supplied by pain nerve endings whose impulses are transmitted by the intercostal and phrenic nerves. The parenchyma of lung and its visceral pleura are insensitive to pain.

Pain Arising in the Chest Wall

The pain-sensory innervation of the integuments and the muscles of the chest wall is conveyed to the dorsal roots through the cutaneous and the intercostal nerves.

9

Generally pain arising from the thoracic integuments and other superficial tissues is sharply localized.

The coexistence of two different types of chest pain in the same patient is a frequent cause of a confusing history.

ETIOLOGY

Cardiac

Myocardial ischemia: coronary atherosclerosis: angina pectoris, myocardial infarction,* aortic stenosis and/or regurgitation, marked right ventricular hypertension
Mitral valve prolapse
Pericarditis: viral; tuberculosis; uremia; trauma; neoplasm; collagen-vascular disease; postinfarction (Dressler's syndrome); postcardiac-injury syndrome
Cardiomyopathies

Noncardiac Intrathoracic

Aortic dissection*
Pulmonary thromboembolism*
Pleural pain: fibrinous pleurisy, pneumonia, pneumonic processes; pneumothorax;* tumors involving the pleural space
Mediastinal emphysema; mediastinal tumors; mediastinitis

Chest Wall

Musculoskeletal disorders: muscle spasm (precordial catch syndrome); muscle strain; costochondritis (Tietze's syndrome); rib fracture; subacromial bursitis; arthritis of the shoulder and spine; ruptured cervical disk
Neurologic disorders: herpes zoster; thoracic outlet syndrome; nerve root compression
Mammary glands

Gastrointestinal

Esophageal disorder: esophageal spasm; reflux esophagitis; esophageal rupture;* Mallory-Weiss syndrome; tumors; ulcerations; diverticuli
Subdiaphragmatic structures: peptic ulcer; pancreatitis, gallbladder (cholecystitis, biliary colic); splenic flexure syndrome

Psychogenic

Anxiety; depression; malingering

Iatrogenic Causes of Chest Pain

Exacerbation of angina: adrenergic agents; alpha blockers; ergotamine; hydralazine; methysergide; oxytocin; propranolol withdrawal; vasopressin; excessive thyroid therapy; oral contraceptives
Pericarditis: emetine, hydralazine, methysergide, procainamide

*Urgent condition

HISTORY TAKING*

Possible meaning of a positive response

1 Location and Radiation of the Pain

1.1 Where do you have pain? discomfort?

Pain arising in the skin or superficial structures is usually accurately localized by the patient: chest-wall pain; Tietze's syndrome (if costochondral area). The patient with angina pectoris may *clench his fist* and hold it *over the sternum*, illustrating the constrictive nature of the discomfort

1.1a *Can you point with a fingertip to the pain?*

Pain in a sharply delineated area of the chest: excludes anginal pain

1.1b Is the pain diffuse? difficult to localize?

Pain arising in deeper structures

1.2 Is the pain localized
• *in the middle of your chest?*

Substernal: coronary artery disease; pericarditis, aortic, mediastinal; esophageal origin; **pulmonary embolism**

• under the left nipple? in the left hemithorax?

Precordial: usually a noncardiac condition: anxiety state, osteoarthritis, splenic flexure syndrome; gaseous distention of the stomach

• in the anterior part of the chest?

Myocardial infarction; dissecting aneurysm of aorta (proximal dissection, above the aortic valve)

• in the breast?

Inflammatory breast disease; mastodynia; tumor

• between the shoulder blades?

Myocardial infarction; esophageal dysfunction; dissecting aortic aneurysm (distal dissection, beyond the left subclavian artery)

• in an upper costochondral junction?

Anterior chest wall (Tietze's) syndrome

1.3 Is the pain
• superficial?

Chest-wall conditions; herpes zoster; pain of pleural origin; mitral valve prolapse

• deep?

Visceral pain; myocardial ischemia

*In this section, items in *italics* are characteristic clinical features, and items in **boldface** are potentially life-threatening or urgent conditions.

1.4   Does the pain radiate to the
      • ulnar aspect of the left arm? left
        shoulder?

Coronary artery disease; pericarditis (almost any condition capable of causing chest discomfort may induce radiation to the left arm); disorders of the cervical spine

      • right arm? right shoulder?

Occasionally observed in angina pectoris; disorders of the cervical spine

      • right lower chest?

Probably noncardiac pain: functional; osteoarthritis; gaseous distention of the stomach; splenic flexure syndrome

      • both arms?

Occasionally observed in myocardial infarction; dissecting aortic aneurysm

      • neck? jaw? teeth?

Angina; myocardial infarction; pericarditis

      • back? interscapular region?

Coronary artery disease; dissecting aortic aneurysm (rupture distal to the left subclavian artery); concomitant spinal arthritis

      • abdomen?

(Rare in angina.) Dissecting aortic aneurysm; concomitant spinal arthritis; concomitant upper abdominal disorder: esophageal dysfunction, gallbladder disease, pancreatitis, peptic ulcer (the presence of one condition may affect the radiation of the pain produced by another disorder)

2   Mode of Onset and Evolution

2.1   (Acute episode): How long have you had pain in your chest?

To be kept in mind when interpreting blood enzyme changes. Anginal pain is of brief duration, usually lasting from 2 to 10 minutes. Pain persisting for 20 minutes or longer: myocardial infarction, dissecting aneurysm, pulmonary embolism, acute pericarditis, herpes zoster, gallbladder colic, acute pancreatitis

2.1a Did the pain
      • set in abruptly?
      • reach its peak of intensity almost
        instantly?

Tissue disruption: aortic dissection; pneumothorax; mediastinal emphysema; cervical disk syndrome; rupture of the esophagus

2.2   Do you have recurrent episodes of chest pain?

Angina pectoris; cervical radiculitis; anterior chest-wall condition; GI disorders; anxiety

2.2a How long have you had attacks of chest pain?

2.2b What is the duration of the episodes?
- only a few seconds?

"Precordial catch": may be associated with poor posture. Anginal pain may be excluded; musculoskeletal pain; functional pain

- 2 to 3 minutes?

Hyperventilation

- 2 to 10 minutes?

Anginal pain

- up to a half hour or longer?

Musculoskeletal disease; mitral valve prolapse; esophageal reflux; esophageal spasm; psychogenic pain; gallbladder colic

- variable duration?

Musculoskeletal condition; anxiety states

2.2c What is the frequency of the episodes per day? per week?

If angina pectoris is present: reflects the intensity of the process

2.2d Are the frequency, the intensity, the duration, of the attacks
- increasing?

Recent coronary thrombosis; unstable angina; may presage an impending myocardial infarction

- decreasing?

May be due to limited activity to avoid anginal attacks

- *of the same character?*

Uniformity of the attacks: angina pectoris

3 Intensity of the Chest Pain

There is little correlation between the severity of chest pain and the gravity of its cause

3.1 Is the pain
- mild? moderately severe?

Angina pectoris induced by exertion is usually mild at the onset and becomes progressively more severe until the patient is forced to rest; pericarditis

- severe? unbearable?

Myocardial infarction; massive pulmonary embolism; dissecting aortic aneurysm

4 Character of the Pain

4.1 Is the pain
- choking? *squeezing? constricting?* bursting? burning? pressing? boring? gripping?

Angina pectoris; esophageal dysfunction

• *like a weight on your chest? a band across the chest? in the center of the chest?*	Coronary artery disease: angina pectoris
• crushing? severe?	True pain in: myocardial infarction; unstable angina; some cases of pericarditis; aortic dissection
• dull? aching? long lasting?	Against ischemic origin: musculoskeletal pain; lesion of bone; psychogenic chest pain
• sticking? jabbing?	Musculoskeletal pain (excludes anginal pain)
• throbbing?	Chest-wall pain; lesion of bone
• sharp? knifelike? fleeting?	Not typical of angina; lesion of the pleura, muscles, the spinal cord, and nerve roots; pericarditis; anxiety states
• like an indigestion?	Gastrointestinal pain; angina pectoris

5   Precipitating or Aggravating Factors

5.1   (Acute episode): Did the pain appear

• at rest?	Myocardial infarction; pneumothorax; pleural disorder
• *on exertion?*	Angina; pneumothorax; myocardial infarction (may appear without relation to effort)
• after unusual activity? unaccustomed exercise? trauma?	Chest-wall pain: muscle or ligament strain
• after protracted vomiting?	Mallory-Weiss syndrome: tear in the lower portion of the esophagus

5.2   (Recurrent chest pain):
Does the pain appear

• at rest?	Anxiety states; radicular pain; unstable angina; Prinzmetal's (variant) angina: coronary artery spasm
• while bending over?	Radicular pain; disk pain; osteoarthritis with involvement of the nerve roots of the cervical and upper thoracic spine; esophageal pain
• when moving your neck?	Herniated cervical intervertebral disk
• while eating?	Spasm of the esophagus
• after a large heavy meal?	Gastrointestinal pain; angina pectoris
• when under emotional strain? excitement? anger? fright?	Angina pectoris; psychogenic pain
• when exhausted?	Psychogenic pain
• at night? when lying down?	Angina decubitus; esophageal pain

• *on exertion? (moving the body as a whole)* • *on walking?: on cold days? against the wind? uphill? after meals?* • *during sexual intercourse?*	Angina pectoris; occasionally: right ventricular hypertension
• in the morning, but not later in the day?	In some patients, the anginal threshold is lower in the morning than at any other time of day
5.2a If the pain is induced by walking: Does it force you to stop? to reduce speed?	Angina pectoris
5.3 Is the pain induced or made worse by	
• swallowing?	Esophageal spasm; esophagitis; acute pericarditis
• lying flat? recumbency?	Reflux esophagitis; acute pericarditis; expanding thoracic aortic aneurysm eroding vertebral bodies
• nitroglycerin?	May occur in hypertrophic cardiomyopathy (reduction of left ventricular cavity size)
• *inspiration?*	Pleural, pericardial, mediastinal disorders; muscle or ligament strain
• coughing?	Pleural disorder; pericardial or mediastinal disorder; radicular pain; herniated cervical disk; tracheobronchitis; muscle strain
• sneezing? straining at stool?	Radicular pain
• movements of the neck? trunk? chest? arm? head? local exercise?	Lesion of the cervicodorsal spine; muscle strain; subacromial bursitis; arthritis of the shoulder and spine
• exhaustion?	Functional pain

6 Relieving Factors

6.1 Is the pain relieved by	
• *remaining immobile?*	Angina pectoris (the pain of myocardial infarction is not relieved by rest)
• exertion?	Psychogenic chest pain
• belching? passing gas?	Gaseous distention of the stomach or splenic flexure; angina pectoris
• sitting up? standing erect?	Reflux esophagitis; acute pericarditis; angina decubitus
• *leaning forward?*	Pericardial pain: acute pericarditis
• holding the breath in deep expiration?	Pleural lesion
• food? antacids?	Reflux esophagitis; peptic ulcer

• *nitroglycerin?*

Angina pectoris (nitroglycerin deteriorates with age: failure to relieve the pain may be due to an old preparation). The pain of myocardial infarction and mitral valve prolapse is poorly responsive to nitroglycerin. The pain of esophagitis or esophageal spasm may be relieved by nitroglycerin

6.1a Does the pain disappear more rapidly and more completely with nitroglycerin than with rest alone?

Angina pectoris

6.1b How quickly is the pain relieved by
• nitroglycerin? rest?
  • within a few seconds?
  • within 5 minutes or less?
  • 10 minutes or more?

Unlikely in angina
Angina pectoris
Unstable angina; acute myocardial infarction; noncardiac pain. Evidence against the diagnosis of chronic stable angina pectoris

7 Accompanying Symptoms of the Painful Episode

7.1 Is (was) the chest pain accompanied by
• sweating? nausea? vomiting?
• belching?

Serious disorder: myocardial infarction
The need to belch during an anginal attack is common

• shortness of breath?

Congestive heart failure; pulmonary edema secondary to myocardial infarction; pneumothorax; pulmonary embolism; hypertrophic cardiomyopathy

• palpitations?

Arrhythmias accompanying a myocardial infarction; mitral valve prolapse; some angina occurs only with arrhythmias

• *a sensation of imminent death?*
• coughing?

Myocardial infarction
Pulmonary or pleural origin of pain: pneumonia; lung tumor

• bloody expectorations?

Hemoptysis in pulmonary infarction; lung tumor

• fever?

Pneumonia; pleurisy; viral pericarditis; low-grade fever frequently appears on the second or third day after myocardial infarction

• abdominal pain?

Thoracic pain referred from subdiaphragmatic structure

7.2 Do you have

- leg pain or swollen leg?   Deep-vein thrombosis with pulmonary embolism

- pain in your calves when walking?   Intermittent claudication: atherosclerosis of the vascular beds

- episodes of dizziness? transient loss of vision? paresis?   Transient ischemic attacks. Manifestations of extracardiac atherosclerosis lend weight to the diagnosis of myocardial ischemia

- *frequent sighing?* anxiety? depression?   Psychogenic pain

- difficulty swallowing? water brash?   Esophageal disease

8 Iatrogenic Factors   See Etiology

9 Personal and Social Profile

9.1 Do you smoke? How many cigarettes a day?   Smoking is a major, and preventable, risk factor for coronary artery disease

9.2 What is your occupation?   Exacerbation of coronary artery disease caused by exposure to
- carbon monoxide: in garage mechanics, toll collectors, foundry workers, firefighters
- nitrates: in explosive workers
- carbon disulfide: in dry cleaners, paint workers, rayon workers

9.3 What is your daily physical activity?   Sedentarity is a risk factor for coronary disease

9.3a Does the pain interfere with your activities?   Many patients with angina pectoris learn to modify their daily activity to avoid pain

9.4 Do you have emotional tensions? at home? at work?   Risk factors for coronary disease

9.5 According to you, what is your type of personality? highly competitive? impatient? in constant struggle with your environment?   Type A behavior: a risk factor for coronary artery disease (controversial)

9.6 What is your alcohol consumption?   Rib fracture is a frequent cause of chest pain in alcoholics (these patients frequently do not recall a history of trauma)

10   Personal Antecedents Pertaining to the Chest Pain

10.1   Have you ever had an ECG? a chest
         x-ray? past cardiac catheterization?
         When? With what results?

10.2   Have you recently had
         • an operation?   Deep-vein thrombosis with pulmonary
                                                embolism

         • an upper respiratory infection?   May precede acute viral pericarditis

10.3   Do you have any of the following
         conditions:
         • high blood pressure?   A major risk factor for coronary artery
                                                disease

         • a cardiac disease?   Aortic stenosis, hypertrophic cardio-
                                                myopathy, aortic regurgitation, mitral
                                                valve prolapse, mitral stenosis or septal
                                                defects associated with pulmonary
                                                hypertension: may be associated with
                                                anginal pain
         • emphysema? chronic bronchitis?   Proneness to pneumothorax
         • high serum cholesterol level?   Hypercholesterolemia is one of the
                                                three primary risk factors (with tobacco
                                                smoking and hypertension) for coro-
                                                nary artery disease

11   Family Medical History Pertaining to the Chest Pain

11.1   Does someone in your family have
         high cholesterol? diabetes? hyper-
         tension? (premature death?)

PHYSICAL SIGNS PERTAINING TO CHEST PAIN*

Possible significance

At the time of an acute episode of pain:

Tachycardia; rise in blood pressure;   Coronary ischemia with left ventricular
fourth heart sound; abnormal parasternal   dysfunction and localized noncontract-
heave   ing myocardium

Systolic murmur at apex   Angina pectoris with papillary muscle
                                            dysfunction secondary to localized
                                            ischemia

*In this section, items in *italics* are characteristic clinical features, and items in **boldface** are
potentially life-threatening or urgent conditions.

Anxious, restless patient; cool skin; sweating; fourth heart sound; thready pulse; reduced blood pressure; basilar crackles; friction rub; arrhythmias	Acute myocardial infarction
Precordial friction rub	Acute pericarditis
Pleural friction rub, crackles, rhonchi	Pleurally based lesion; pulmonary thromboembolism, pneumonia, tumor
Hypertension; unequal peripheral pulses; aortic insufficiency murmur; neurologic abnormalities	Dissecting aortic aneurysm
Tachycardia; tachypnea; accentuation of P_2; S_3 or S_4 gallop; crackles; friction rub; deep-vein thrombosis	Pulmonary thromboembolism
On affected side: **hyperresonance; diminished breath sounds**	Pneumothorax
Fever	Infectious cause of pain: bacterial or viral pneumonia; viral pericarditis
Localized swelling or tenderness to palpation	Local musculoskeletal disease; fractured rib. Pressure on the chondrosternal and costochondral junctions is an essential part of the examination of every patient with chest pain
• of upper costochondral cartilages	Tietze's syndrome
Crepitus in the neck; crushing noise synchronous with the heartbeat	Mediastinal emphysema

LABORATORY TESTS PERTAINING TO CHEST PAIN[†]

Test	Finding	Diagnostic Possibilities
Blood		
Creatine kinase (CK) and MB-CK	Elevated	Myocardial infarction; intramuscular injection; muscle disease; electrical cardioversion; cardiac catheterization

[†]See the appendix on Laboratory Reference Values for the associated normal laboratory values.

LABORATORY PROCEDURES PERTAINING TO CHEST PAIN

Procedure	To Detect
Resting ECG	Ischemic heart disease; pulmonary embolism; pericarditis. The resting ECG is frequently normal in patients with angina
Exercise stress testing	Plateau-type ST segment depression of more than 0.1 mV lasting more than 0.08 s: myocardial ischemia
Exercise thallium scan*	Coronary artery disease
Coronary angiography*	The most accurate method for diagnosing coronary artery disease
Echocardiography*	Mitral valve prolapse; valvular aortic stenosis; hypertrophic obstructive cardiomyopathy; pericardial effusion
Chest x-ray	Pericarditis; pneumothorax; pleural effusion; pneumomediastinum; pulmonary thromboembolism; widening of aortic shadow: dissecting aortic aneurysm
X-ray of cervical and thoracic spine, sternum, and ribs	Skeletal disease pain; cervical rib; thoracic outlet syndrome; traumatic injury
Lung scan*; pulmonary angiography*	Pulmonary thromboembolism
Barium swallow and esophageal manometry*	Esophageal origin of thoracic chest pain; reflux esophagitis

*When indicated

SELECTED BIBLIOGRAPHY

Brundage BH: A sensible approach to chest pain. *Postgrad Med* 69(3):120–143, 1981.
Donat WE: Chest pain: Cardiac and noncardiac causes. *Clin Chest Med* 8(2):241–252, 1987.
Goldman L: Acute chest pain: Emergency room evaluation. *Hosp Pract* 21(7):94A–94T, 1986.
Horwitz LD: Chest pain, in Horwitz LD, Groves BM (eds). *Signs and Symptoms in Cardiology*, pp. 1–27, Philadelphia: Lippincott, 1985.

3
Cough and Expectorations

INTRODUCTION

Cough   An explosive expiration which provides a means of clearing the tracheo-bronchial tree of mucus and foreign material.

Expectoration   Ejection, by coughing and spitting, of fluid or semi-fluid matter from the lungs and respiratory passages.

The afferent pathways of the cough reflex are in the trigeminal, glossopharyngeal, superior laryngeal, and vagus nerves. The efferent pathways lie in the recurrent laryngeal nerve, which causes closure of the glottis, and in the phrenic and spinal nerves, which cause contraction of the thoracic and abdominal musculature. The nerve endings in the airway passages are sensitive to contact with foreign material and inflammatory, mechanical, thermal, and chemical stimuli. The acinar units have no nerve supply; material from those areas has to move up into larger airways into the presence of nerve endings to initiate coughing. A cough may also occur as a result of stimulation of the parietal pleura and of afferent pathways originating in other viscera.

The normal adult produces about 100 mL of mucus from the respiratory tract in a day. It takes about 30 to 60 min for mucus and/or foreign material to be swept from the levels of the respiratory bronchioles up to the mouth. When excess mucus is formed, the normal process of removal may be ineffective and accumulation of mucus may occur, so that the mucus membrane is stimulated and the mucus coughed up as sputum.

ETIOLOGY

Respiratory

Acute upper respiratory tract infection: viral, bacterial
Acute and chronic bronchitis
Asthma
Bronchiectasis
Pneumonia; tuberculosis; fungal infections; parasitic lung disease
Neoplasm
Interstitial lung disease (sarcoidosis, fibrosis); cystic fibrosis
Foreign body
Irritants: cigarette smoke; chemical fumes

Cardiovascular

Left ventricular heart failure; pulmonary edema; pulmonary infarction; aortic aneurysm

Miscellaneous

Sinusitis; postnasal drip; mediastinal neoplastic or inflammatory process; gastroesophageal reflux; external ear canal and tympanic membrane; nervous habit

Iatrogenic Causes of Cough

Beta-blockers; angiotensin-converting enzyme inhibitors

HISTORY TAKING*

Possible meaning of a positive response

1   Duration and Mode of Onset

1.1   How long have you had a cough?
expectorations?
   • up to 3 weeks?

Acute process: viral laryngotracheobronchitis; bacterial bronchopneumonia; inhalation of irritative substances

   • more than 3 weeks?

Process becoming chronic: pulmonary tuberculosis; pulmonary neoplasm. In mycoplasmal infection, the cough may persist for 1 to 3 months

   • 2 years or more?

Chronic bronchitis; bronchiectasis; postnasal drip (a common cause of chronic cough); chronic cigarette cough (exclude underlying lesion); chronic persistent cough may be the sole symptom of bronchial asthma

1.2   Was the onset of cough acute?

If dry cough: inhalation of a foreign body; irritant substance; acute bronchitis, pneumonia (viral); pulmonary embolization

2   Character of Cough and/or Expectorations

Observation by the physician of the patient's sputum is mandatory

*In this section, items in *italics* are characteristic clinical features.

2.1 Do you have a chronic nonproductive cough?

Irritative stimulus: mechanical, chemical, or thermal; chronic bronchitis; asthma; environmental irritants; postnasal drip; tuberculosis (early stage); endobronchial tumor; extrinsic pressure on the trachea or on a bronchus; interstitial lung infiltration or fibrosis; early heart failure with pulmonary congestion (particularly in the recumbent position, at night); nervous habit; impaction of cerumen or hair in the ear canal, with irritation of the external auditory canal or tympanic membrane, which receives a nerve supply from the vagus (rare)

2.1a Is the chronic cough
- "hacking": short, dry, often repeated?

Cough originating in the upper respiratory tract; chronic postnasal drip

- dry, irritating, spasmodic? (and nocturnal)

Early symptom of left heart failure; cough due to pulmonary venous hypertension

- "barking", harsh, painful?

Acute laryngitis; epiglottal involvement

- loud, "brassy", high-pitched, dry?

Tracheal or major airway involvement

- deep, "loose", moist?

Cough originating in bronchi or lung parenchyma: acute bronchitis; pneumonia; bronchiectasis. A moist cough indicates that sputum is present. Most dry coughs, if sufficiently prolonged, eventually become productive

2.2 Does the cough occur in prolonged paroxysms?
- with "whoops"?

Characteristic of pertussis

- without expectorations?

In chronic bronchitis: exhausted patient abandons attempts to clear the bronchi of secretions; asthma. Female patients are inclined to swallow sputum and not to expectorate; the character of the cough, if it is loose or moist, may indicate that sputum is present

- culminating in the production of sputum?

Productive cough: implies an underlying inflammatory process, often infectious; chronic bronchitis

2.3   In case of productive cough, is the
      sputum
      • clear? white?   Mucoid sputum: viral infection; foreign
                                             substances (smoke, atmospheric pollu-
                                             tion); any form of long-standing bron-
                                             chial irritation; bronchoalveolar carci-
                                             noma (abundant frothy saliva-like
                                             sputum)
      • foamy and pink-tinged?   Pulmonary edema
      • sometimes black, with soot parti-   Chronic bronchitis; coal miners' spu-
        cles?   tum may contain coal dust
      • thick and yellowish, or greenish?   Purulent: infection in the tracheo-
                                             bronchial tree or lung; bronchiectasis;
                                             bacterial pneumonia; lung abscess;
                                             chronic or recurrent mucopurulent
                                             bronchitis
      • gelatinous and rusty? "prune-   Pneumococcal pneumonia
        juice"?
      • similar to currant jelly? tena-   *Klebsiella* pneumonia (in only 25 to 50
        cious?   percent of patients)
      • containing threads?   Casts of the bronchial tree (inspissated
                                             mucus); bronchitis; bronchial asthma
      • blood-streaked?   Tuberculosis; bronchiectasis; lung tu-
                                             mor; pulmonary infarction
      • bloody?   Pulmonary infarction; bronchogenic
                                             carcinoma; tuberculosis (See Chapter 8,
                                             "Hemoptysis")

2.3a Is your expectoration difficult to   Mucoid sputum is more viscous than
      eliminate?   purulent sputum and therefore often
                                             more difficult to cough up; asthma

2.4   Has your expectoration an offen-   Bronchiectasis; infection from anaero-
      sive odor? Does it taste or smell   bic organisms: aspiration, lung abscess,
      bad? ("rotten eggs")   necrotizing pneumonia

2.5   Do you cough and/or expectorate
      • *mostly early in the morning? upon* Pooling of secretions during the night in
        awakening?   the larynx and trachea: chronic bron-
                                             chitis; bronchiectasis; chronic sinusitis;
                                             postnasal drip
      • all day?   Active and/or persistent underlying
                                             process
      • at night?   Left-heart failure (dry cough); bron-
                                             chial asthma

2.6   In case of chronic cigarette cough: Initiate immediate diagnostic evalua-
      Has it changed in character or pat-   tion to detect bronchogenic malignancy
      tern?

3 Intensity of the Cough and Expectorations

3.1 Do you cough and/or expectorate
- daily? — Chronic bronchitis
- *for at least 3 months of 2 consecutive years?* — Characteristic of chronic bronchitis; bronchiectasis

3.2 Can you estimate the amount of your expectorations?
- 1 or 2 spits per day? — Reliable: very small amounts
- a teacupful per day? — Very large amounts
- *daily small quantities (usually mucoid)?* — Simple chronic bronchitis
- copious and purulent sputum? — Chronic mucopurulent bronchitis; bronchiectasis, lung abscess

4 Precipitating or Aggravating Factors

4.1 Does the cough occur
- *with, or shortly after, ingestion of food?* — Tracheoesophageal fistula; esophageal diverticulum

4.2 Is your cough and/or sputum provoked or worsened by
- *a change in position?* — Localized area of bronchiectasis; lung abscess
- recumbency at night? — Congestive left heart failure; bronchiectasis; postnasal drip (more mucus drips into the throat); asthma; reflux esophagitis (aspiration of gastroesophageal contents)
- sudden changes in temperature? — Chronic bronchitis
- smoke? fumes or dust? smog? — Bronchial irritants can produce cough, particularly in patients with chronic bronchitis, postviral bronchitis, asthma
- *exercise?* — Asthma: particularly in young adolescent patients; chronic bronchitis: sudden increase in the depth of ventilation

5 Relieving Factors

5.1 In case of nocturnal (and dry) cough, is it relieved
- *if you sit up? if you use more than one pillow?* — Pulmonary congestion: left ventricular failure

6 Accompanying Symptoms

6.1 Do you have
- fever? chills? pain in your muscles? — Acute infection; early symptoms of acute bronchitis or pneumonia
- a sore throat? a running nose? — Upper respiratory infection
- severe headache? — *Mycoplasma;* psittacosis; AIDS (cryptococcosis, nocardiosis)

- night sweats?

Pulmonary tuberculosis; lymphoma

- chest pain?

Chest muscle pain associated with infection of the upper respiratory tract, with dry paroxysmal cough. Strenuous coughing may cause rupture of an emphysematous bleb; it may produce rib fractures ("cough fractures" may occur in otherwise normal patients; suspect underlying disorder: osteoporosis, osteolytic metastases, multiple myeloma)

- *worsened by inspiration?*

Pleuritic pain: pneumonia; lung abscess; lung tumor with pleural involvement

- shortness of breath?

Chronic bronchitis; congestive heart failure; bronchial asthma

  - *having preceded the chronic cough?*

Chronic obstructive pulmonary disease, predominant emphysema

  - *having appeared after a long period of chronic cough?*

Chronic obstructive pulmonary disease, predominant bronchitis

- a loss of weight?

Bronchogenic carcinoma; tuberculosis; opportunistic infection in an AIDS-patient

- difficulty swallowing?

Recurrent aspiration: in elderly patients, in patients with esophageal disease

- diarrhea?

Legionella, Mycoplasma infection

- hoarseness?

Bronchogenic carcinoma involving the recurrent laryngeal nerve; laryngeal tumor; secondary laryngeal lesions in pulmonary excavated tuberculosis; viral laryngotracheobronchitis; pressure of a greatly enlarged left atrium on an enlarged pulmonary artery compressing the recurrent laryngeal nerve

- the sensation of having something drip down into your throat? frequent throat-clearing? hawking? mucus swallowing? a cough that is worse in the morning?

Postnasal drip

- wheezing?

Obstruction to air flow: acute bronchospasm: asthma; acute or chronic bronchitis

- loss of consciousness during a coughing fit?

"Cough syncope": increased intrathoracic pressure on venous return and cardiac output: in chronic bronchitis (in obese patients who smoke and drink heavily); also in neoplastic or vascular cerebral lesions

7 Iatrogenic Factors   See Etiology

8 Personal and Social Profile

8.1 Do you smoke?

Smoking, the most common cause of chronic coughing, may stimulate the cough reflex by bronchial irritation or it may induce chronic inflammatory changes with the presence of secretions. Heavy cigarette smokers are liable to chronic bronchitis and lung tumor

8.2 What is your alcohol consumption?

Alcoholism may facilitate the development of infections that produce coughing: pneumococcosis, tuberculosis, aspiration pneumonia, *H. influenzae*, *Klebsiella* infections; lung abscess

8.3 What is your occupation?

Dry cough due to formaldehyde, toluene diisocyanate, animal dander in: exposure to textiles, plastics, polyurethane kits, lacquer use, animal handler. Silicosis, tuberculosis in coal mine workers; exposure to beryllium, asbestos, rock dust, irritant substances (asbestosis and exposure to radioactive materials predispose to bronchogenic carcinoma).
Legionnaire's disease, histoplasmosis, blastomycosis: construction workers.
Psittacosis: pet shop owners, taxidermists

8.4 Do you have any pets? birds? pigeons?

Psittacosis

8.5 Have you ever been exposed to someone with tuberculosis?

8.6 What are your sexual preferences?

Persistent cough in a homosexual man suggests: *Pneumocystis carinii*, pulmonary *Mycobacterium avium-intracellulare*, cytomegalovirus pneumonia

8.7 Do you use intravenous drugs?

Septic pulmonary embolism; *Pneumocystis carinii* infection (AIDS)

8.8 Have you recently traveled to
  • the southwestern United States?
  • the central United States?
  • foreign countries?

Coccidioidomycosis
Histoplasmosis
Tuberculosis; Q fever

9   Personal Antecedents Pertaining to the Cough

9.1   Have you ever had a chest x-ray? a
      tuberculin skin test? a bronchos-
      copy? a bronchography? lung
      tests? When? With what results?

9.2   Do you have
      • frequent episodes of lung infec-   Chronic bronchitis; bronchiectasis; im-
        tion? recurrent pneumonias?   munodeficiency diseases; mitral ste-
                                                    nosis; foreign body; obstructing tumor

      • a heart condition?   Congestive heart failure with (noctur-
                                                    nal) cough

      • a recent choking episode?   Aspiration of foreign body (may not be
                                                    recalled)

      • allergy?   Bronchial asthma
      • chronic sinusitis? allergic rhi-   May cause postnasal drip with cough;
        nitis?   sinusitis is a common accompaniment
                                                    of diffuse bronchiectasis

10   Family Medical History Pertaining to the Cough

10.1 Does anyone in your family have a   In several members of a household:
      lung disease?   acute bronchitis of epidemic infectious
                                                   origin; tuberculosis; asthma; cystic fi-
                                                   brosis

PHYSICAL SIGNS PERTAINING TO THE COUGH*

	Possible significance
Inspiratory stridor; wheezing	Partial obstruction of the larynx or trachea
Inspiratory and expiratory rhonchi	Tracheal and major airway involvement
Coarse, inspiratory crackles	Involvement of terminal bronchioles; interstitial fibrosis and/or edema
Fine end-inspiratory crackles	Fluid accumulation in alveoli: pneumonitis; pulmonary edema
Pharyngitis; normal chest examination	Upper respiratory infection
Fever; localized dullness; increased breath sounds; crackles, wheezes	Bacterial and *Mycoplasma* infection
Prolonged expiration; hyperresonant lung fields; distant breath sounds; scattered rhonchi or wheezes	Chronic obstructive pulmonary disease

*In this section, items in *italics* are characteristic clinical features, and items in **boldface** are
potentially life-threatening or urgent conditions.

Localized wheezing; atelectasis; supraclavicular lymphadenopathy; clubbing	Bronchogenic carcinoma
Fever; weight loss; posttussive fine crackles	Tuberculosis
Bilateral basilar crackles; gallop rhythm; hepatomegaly; ankle edema	Congestive heart failure
Sinus tenderness	Chronic sinusitis accompanying bronchiectasis
Foul breath (halitosis)	Bronchiectasis; lung abscess

LABORATORY TESTS PERTAINING TO THE COUGH[†]

Test	Finding	Diagnostic Possibilities
Sputum		
Gram's stain	Polymorphonuclear leukocytes	Infectious process
Acid-fast stain	Positive	Tuberculosis
Wright's stain	Eosinophilia	Asthma
Culture	Positive	Bacterial, mycoplasmal, fungal infection
Cytology	Positive	Bronchogenic carcinoma
Blood		
RBCs	Anemia	Lung cancer; tuberculosis; lung abscess
WBCs	Leukocytosis	Infectious process
Cold agglutinins	Positive	Mycoplasmal pneumonia

[†]See the appendix on Laboratory Reference Values for the associated normal laboratory values.

LABORATORY PROCEDURES PERTAINING TO THE COUGH

Procedure	To Detect
Pulmonary function tests	Reversible airflow obstruction in asthma. Abnormalities of airflow and/or lung volumes

Procedure	To Detect
Chest x-ray	Pneumonic lesion; tuberculosis; tumor; infiltrative lung disease
	Bilateral hilar adenopathy: sarcoidosis, lymphoma
	A normal chest x-ray may occur in diseases of the lung parenchyma (sarcoidosis, scleroderma), pleura (acute pleuritis), airways (irritants, chronic bronchitis, asthma, partially obstructing endobronchial masses, acute tracheobronchitis, bronchiectasis, otorhinolaryngeal conditions)
X-ray of sinuses	Chronic sinusitis with thickened membranes

When indicated: Skin testing for tuberculosis, fungal serologic study, fiberoptic bronchoscopy with biopsy and/or brushing; bronchography; mediastinoscopy

SELECTED BIBLIOGRAPHY

Braman SS, Corrao WM: Cough: Differential diagnosis and treatment. *Clin Chest Med* 8(2):177–188, 1987.

Irwin RS, Corrao WM, Pratter MR: Chronic persistent cough in the adult: The spectrum and frequency of causes and successful outcome of specific therapy. *Am Rev Respir Dis* 123:413–417, 1981.

Stulbarg M: Evaluating and treating intractable cough. Medical Staff Conference, University of California, San Francisco. *West J Med* 143:223–228, 1985.

4
Cyanosis

INTRODUCTION

Cyanosis A bluish discoloration of the skin, the mucous membranes, and nail beds resulting from an increased amount of reduced hemoglobin or of abnormal hemoglobin pigments in the blood and in the tissues of those areas.

Peripheral cyanosis is a result of diminished peripheral blood flow and vasoconstriction. Blood flow is slow, each red cell remains in contact with the tissue for a longer period, more oxygen is extracted from normally saturated arterial blood, and more unsaturated hemoglobin is present in the venous blood. Peripheral cyanosis is usually observed in the peripheral tissues, central tissues such as the mucous membranes of the mouth or beneath the tongue being spared.

Central cyanosis is caused by arterial unsaturation. This results from impaired pulmonary function (alveolar hypoventilation, ventilation-perfusion abnormality, impaired oxygen diffusion), or from right-to-left shunts inside the heart (septal defect), between the great vessels (patent ductus arteriosus), or in the lungs. Central cyanosis may also be produced by circulating abnormal hemoglobin derivatives (methemoglobin, sulfhemoglobin).

Cyanosis becomes apparent at a mean capillary concentration of 5 g reduced hemoglobin, 1.5 g methemoglobin, or 0.5 g sulfhemoglobin per 100 mL. In patients with severe anemia and marked arterial desaturation, cyanosis may be absent because the absolute amount of reduced hemoglobin is small. Conversely, patients with marked polycythemia will be cyanotic at higher levels of arterial oxygen saturation than patients with normal hemoglobin values.

ETIOLOGY

Peripheral Cyanosis

Vasoconstriction: exposure to cold
Low cardiac output: congestive heart failure; shock
Peripheral vascular disease: arterial obstruction (embolus); arterial constriction (Raynaud's phenomenon); venous obstruction
Acrocyanosis; livedo reticularis

Central Cyanosis

Decreased arterial oxygen saturation
    Decreased atmospheric pressure: high altitude
    Impaired pulmonary function: alveolar hypoventilation; perfusion of nonventilated or underventilated lung; impaired diffusion of oxygen
    Anatomic right-to-left shunts: certain types of congenital heart disease (tetralogy of Fallot, patent ductus arteriosus); pulmonary arteriovenous fistulas; multiple small intrapulmonary shunts

Hemoglobin abnormalities (rare): methemoglobin (hereditary, acquired); sulfhemo-globin (acquired); low affinity hemoglobins

Iatrogenic Causes of Methemoglobin

Antipyretic drugs: acetanilid, phenacetin; benzocaine; lidocaine; chlorates; nitrites, nitrates; primaquine; quinones; certain sulfonamides: sulfathiazole, sulfapyridine (not sulfadiazine)

HISTORY TAKING*

Possible meaning of a positive response

1   Mode of Onset and Duration

1.1   When has the cyanosis appeared?
• present since birth?

Congenital heart lesion, right-to-left shunt (cyanosis in congenital heart disease appears in patients with normal hemoglobin when the volume of a right-to-left shunt exceeds 25 percent of the left ventricular output); hereditary methemoglobinemia (rare)

• between ages 5 and 20 years?

Eisenmenger's syndrome: large communication at the atrial, ventricular, or aortopulmonary level with marked increase in pulmonary vascular resistance and right-to-left shunt

1.2   If the cyanosis has recently appeared, has the onset of the cyanosis been
• acute? (within hours)

Extensive pneumonia; acute pulmonary edema; upper-airway obstruction by a foreign body (café coronary); **massive pulmonary embolus; pneumothorax; cardiovascular collapse** (following myocardial infarction); **acquired methemoglobinemia**

• gradual? (weeks to months)

Severe (chronic obstructive) pulmonary disease (emphysema)

2   Location of Cyanosis

2.1   Is the cyanosis localized?

Peripheral cyanosis: decreased rate of blood flow

---

*In this section, items in *italics* are characteristic clinical features, and items in **boldface** are potentially life-threatening or urgent conditions.

- to "cold areas": nose, ears, cheeks, fingers (nail beds), ear lobes?

Peripheral cyanosis (e.g., secondary to heart failure)

- to the lower limbs?

Peripheral vascular disease; cyanotic feet and toes with pink hands and fingers ("differential cyanosis") in patients with patent ductus arteriosus, pulmonary hypertension, and right-to-left shunt; livedo reticularis: bluish mottling of the skin on the lower legs occurring predominantly in young females, not to be confused with cyanosis: may occur in systemic lupus erythematosus, polyarteritis nodosa, cryoglobulinemia, cholesterol embolization, Cushing's syndrome, or amantadine hydrochloride administration

- to the head, neck, and upper limbs?

Superior vena cava obstruction (bronchogenic carcinoma)

- to the hands?

Raynaud's phenomenon (episodic); acrocyanosis: constant, painless cyanosis, much more common in women

2.2 Is the cyanosis generalized?

Central cyanosis; peripheral cyanosis: shock

3 Precipitating or Aggravating Factors

3.1 Does the cyanosis occur or worsen
- during exertion?

Central cyanosis due to arterial oxygen unsaturation: increased extraction of oxygen from the blood by the exercising muscles; congenital heart disease with anatomic right-to-left shunt; interstitial lung infiltration and fibrosis with diffusion abnormalities

- after ingestion of certain drugs?

Hereditary methemoglobinemia, heterozygous; acquired methemoglobinemia

3.1a Is the cyanosis present at rest? constant?

Central cyanosis due to arterial unsaturation; cardiac failure, low-output varieties; chronic pulmonary lesion: perfusion of nonventilated areas of the lung; congenital heart lesion, right-to-left shunt; hemoglobin abnormalities (rare)

3.2 In case of cyanosis located in the upper limbs: Does it occur
- *in cold weather? when immersing the hands in cold water?*

Raynaud's disease or phenomenon: cyanosis may appear alone or follow initial pallor; acrocyanosis

4   Accompanying Symptoms

4.1   Do you have
• headaches?   In methemoglobinemia: indicates concentrations of 20 to 50 percent methemoglobin

• shortness of breath?   Chronic pulmonary disease; congestive heart failure with peripheral cyanosis; may be secondary to a congenital heart disease

   • *relieved by squatting?*   Right-to-left shunts: tetralogy of Fallot
• a chronic cough? expectorations?   Central cyanosis due to impaired lung function, chronic obstructive pulmonary disease, chronic bronchitis

• intestinal, nose bleeding? bloody expectorations?   Hereditary hemorrhagic telangiectasia associated with pulmonary arteriovenous fistula

• no complaints?   Cyanotic patients with hereditary methemoglobinemia or sulfhemoglobinemia are "more blue than sick"; acrocyanosis

5   Iatrogenic Factors   See Etiology

6   Personal and Social Profile

6.1   What is (was) your present (former) occupation?   Methemoglobinemia in arc welders (may inhale nitrous gases); exposure to aniline dyes, chlorates, chromates, nitrites, hydrogen peroxide (methemoglobinemia secondary to industrial exposure to chemicals is declining); occupational causes of chronic respiratory disease: silicosis, asbestosis, berylliosis; bagassosis

7   Personal Antecedents Pertaining to the Cyanosis

7.1   Do you have
• a cardiac condition?   Reduced cardiac output with peripheral cyanosis; congenital heart disease

• chronic bronchitis? emphysema? asthma?   Central cyanosis due to impaired pulmonary function: alveolar hypoventilation, perfusion of unventilated areas of the lung, impaired oxygen diffusion

• a blood disease?   Polycythemia vera or polycythemia secondary to chronic pulmonary disease or congenital heart disease: contributes to, or may produce, cyanosis

8   Family Medical History Pertaining to the Cyanosis

8.1 Do your parents, your children, also have a bluish tint?	Hereditary methemoglobinemia associated with abnormal hemoglobin M (autosomal dominant trait, rare)
8.1a If not, do your siblings?	Cytochrome b_5 reductase deficiency (autosomal recessive, rare)

PHYSICAL SIGNS PERTAINING TO CYANOSIS

	Possible significance
Bluish color of the skin and mucous membranes ("warm areas": tongue, inner surfaces of the lips)	Central cyanosis
Bluish color of the skin sparing mucous membranes	Peripheral cyanosis resulting from vasoconstriction and diminished peripheral blood flow: shock, congestive heart failure; cold exposure; peripheral vascular disease
"Red cyanosis"	Polycythemia vera: to be distinguished from true cyanosis
Abnormal percussion; crackles, wheezes	Severe pulmonary disease with impaired pulmonary function and central cyanosis
Heart murmur	Cyanotic congenital heart disease in adults (relatively frequent causes): tetralogy of Fallot, pulmonary atresia with ventricular septal defect, pulmonary stenosis with atrial right-to-left shunt, Eisenmenger's reaction (pulmonary hypertension) to ventricular septal, atrial septal, or aortopulmonary defect
Cardiomegaly; distended jugular veins; hepatomegaly; edema	Severe congestive heart failure with low cardiac output, cutaneous vasoconstriction, and peripheral cyanosis
Telangiectases on skin and mucosae	Hereditary hemorrhagic telangiectasia with pulmonary arteriovenous fistulas
Cyanosis of an extremity with	
• coldness; absent pulses	Arterial obstruction with diminution in blood flow not sufficient to cause blanching of the skin
• edema; varicose veins; ulcers	Venous obstruction

Cyanosis and swelling of head, neck, upper extremities; superficial venous collateral vessels

Clubbing

Superior vena cava syndrome: bronchogenic carcinoma; primary mediastinal tumor; aortic aneurysm

Central cyanosis (long-standing process); certain types of congenital cardiac diseases; chronic pulmonary disease; lung abscess; pulmonary arteriovenous shunts (clubbing is absent in peripheral cyanosis; abnormal hemoglobin pigments; acutely developing central cyanosis)

LABORATORY TESTS PERTAINING TO CYANOSIS[†]

Test	Finding	Diagnostic Possibilities
Blood		
RBCs	Polycythemia	Secondary to arterial unsaturation in central cyanosis
Arterial oxygen tension	Normal	Peripheral cyanosis
	Decreased	Central cyanosis
Arterial CO_2 tension	Elevated	Central cyanosis due to chronic alveolar hypoventilation
Spectroscopic analysis	Abnormal types of hemoglobin	Methemoglobinemia; sulfhemoglobinemia
Pulmonary function tests		
FEV_1/FVC	Reduced	Chronic obstructive pulmonary disease (COPD)
FEV_1/FVC	Normal or high	Restrictive pulmonary disease

[†]See the appendix on Laboratory Reference Values for the associated normal laboratory values.

LABORATORY PROCEDURES PERTAINING TO CYANOSIS

Procedure	To Detect
Chest x-ray	Congenital heart diseases; pulmonary diseases; pulmonary arteriovenous fistula
ECG	Congenital heart disease; right ventricular strain pattern in chronic obstructive pulmonary disease (COPD)
Cardiac catheterization; pulmonary angiography	Congenital heart disease; pulmonary arteriovenous fistula

SELECTED BIBLIOGRAPHY

Braunwald E: Cyanosis, Hypoxia, and Polycythemia, in Wilson J, Braunwald E, Isselbacher KJ et al (eds). *Harrison's Principles of Internal Medicine*, 12th ed., pp. 224–228, New York: McGraw-Hill, 1991.

Ditchey RV: Cyanosis, in Horwitz LD, Groves BM (eds). *Signs and Symptoms in Cardiology*, pp. 116–131, Philadelphia: Lippincott, 1985.

Jaffé ER: Methemoglobinemia in the differential diagnosis of cyanosis. *Hosp Pract* 20(12):92–110, 1985.

5
Dyspnea

INTRODUCTION

Dyspnea   The patient's subjective awareness of respiratory discomfort.

Dyspnea can be induced in healthy subjects by strenuous exertion and should be regarded as abnormal only when it occurs at rest or at a level of physical activity that could not normally be expected to cause respiratory discomfort.

As indicated by the above definition, dyspnea, i.e., difficult or uncomfortable breathing, is a subjective state. In metabolic acidemia, breathing may appear labored but dyspnea does not occur.

Dyspnea occurs whenever the work of breathing is excessive. It may be due to an increase in airway resistance, in the stiffness of the lung, in exercise ventilation, or, most commonly, to a combination of these factors. It can be viewed as an imbalance between the ventilating stimulus and the capacity to respond to the stimulus. It has been suggested that proprioceptive mechanisms in the respiratory muscles and thoracic cage create an awareness of disproportion between muscular effort and the level of ventilation produced.

Shortness of breath during exercise or at rest is a common manifestation of many forms of pulmonary and cardiovascular disease. In the patient with obstructive pulmonary disease (e.g., emphysema, asthma), the dyspnea is primarily related to the reduced capacity to respond to the ventilatory stimulus. In conditions where the lungs or thorax are stiffer than normal, dyspnea is a prominent symptom, because the inspiratory muscles have to develop greater tension to produce the same tidal volume. Dyspnea in pure left ventricular failure is primarily due to the increased stimulus from the congestion, which also causes some increase in stiffening of the lungs. Patients may use the term "shortness of breath" when the discomfort is actually an abnormal awareness of breathing resulting from anxiety states.

ETIOLOGY

Disorders of the Lungs

Obstructive Diseases of Airways

Upper Airway Obstruction

Acute: acute laryngopharyngitis; epiglottic and laryngeal edema; diphtheria; foreign-body aspiration; retained secretions; retropharyngeal abscess; laryngospasm (hypocalcemia)

Chronic: tumor of larynx or trachea; mediastinal tumor or nodes; aortic aneurysm; scarring of trachea (from previous tracheostomy, prolonged endotracheal intubation, or trauma)

Lower Airway Obstruction

Acute (or recurrent): asthma; inhalation of toxic vapors
Chronic: chronic bronchitis; emphysema; bronchiectasis; late complications of pulmonary fibrosis

Restrictive Lung Diseases

Interstitial Lung Diseases

Of known cause: inhaled gases, fumes, vapors, inorganic dusts (pneumoconiosis), organic dusts (hypersensitivity pneumonitis); drug-induced reactions; radiation; viral pneumonitis; uremia; lymphangitic carcinomatosis; shock
Of unknown origin: idiopathic pulmonary fibrosis; sarcoidosis; collagen-vascular disorders: rheumatoid arthritis; systemic lupus erythematosus (SLE); progressive systemic sclerosis; histiocytosis X; chronic eosinophilic pneumonia; pulmonary vasculitides; inherited disorders

Replacement of Pulmonary Parenchyma by Nonventilating Tissue

Atelectasis; bullae
Pneumonectomy
Compression of lung by space-occupying intrathoracic lesions: large tumors

Disorders of the Pleura

Pleural effusion; pleural fibrosis; pneumothorax*

Disorders of the Chest Wall

Thoracic cage limitations: kyphoscoliosis; pectus excavatum; spondylitis; obesity; trauma;* surgery
Paralysis of respiratory muscles

Diseases of the Heart and Circulation

Congestive heart failure, left and right; pulmonary edema;* pulmonary thromboembolism;* mitral stenosis; aortic stenosis; congenital heart disease
Pericardial effusion
Pulmonary hypertension

Miscellaneous

Psychogenic dyspnea (anxiety, hyperventilation*); anemia; obesity

Iatrogenic Causes of Dyspnea (Partial List)

Drug-Induced Interstitial Lung Disease

Amiodarone, beta-blockers, bleomycin, busulfan, chlorambucil, nitrosoureas, melphalan, procarbazine, azathioprine, nitrofurantoin, cyclophosphamide, methotrexate, methysergide, penicillins, sulfonamides, gold salts

*Causes of acute dyspnea

Drug-Induced Pulmonary Edema

Heroin, methadone, hydrochlorothiazide, propoxyphene, contrast media

Drug-Induced Bronchospasm (Asthma)

Nonsteroidal anti-inflammatory drugs (e.g., acetylsalicylic acid), beta-blockers, cholinergic drugs, penicillins, cephalosporins, pentazocine, tartrazine (drugs with yellow dye)

Drug-Induced Respiratory Muscle Paralysis

Aminoglycosides; polymyxins

HISTORY TAKING*

Possible meaning of a positive response

1   Mode of Onset

1.1   How long have you had shortness of breath?

Early age of onset: alpha-1-antitrypsin deficiency; cystic fibrosis; asthma.
In older patients: chronic obstructive pulmonary disease (COPD); left-heart failure

1.2   Did the dyspnea appear
• suddenly?

Pneumothorax; pulmonary embolism; pulmonary edema; bronchial asthma; pneumonia; angioneurotic edema of the glottis; upper airway obstruction: aspiration of food or foreign body; inhalation of noxious gases or fumes; farmer's lung; anxiety; hyperventilation

• progressively?
• over weeks or months?

Chronic dyspnea: congestive heart failure; severe anemia; obesity; pregnancy; pleural effusion; tuberculosis; pericardial effusion; subacute occlusion of a major airway (tumor)

• over months or years?

Chronic bronchitis and emphysema in older patients; interstitial lung disorder

1.2a   If the onset was acute, what were you doing before and at the onset of dyspnea?

Pulmonary embolism, spontaneous pneumothorax, or anxiety hyperventilation can occur at rest or sedentary activity; 20 percent of pneumothorax occur with strenuous physical activity

• eating?

Foreign-body aspiration

*In this section, items in *italics* are characteristic clinical features, and items in **boldface** are potentially life-threatening or urgent conditions.

2   Character of Dyspnea

2.1 Do you have any difficulty moving
     air
     • during inspiration?   Upper-airway obstruction
     • during expiration?   Lower-airway obstruction
     • in and out of the lungs?   Not specific: obstructive pulmonary dis-
                                          ease

2.2 *Do you feel that you do not breathe in*   Psychogenic dyspnea: anxiety neurosis
     a sufficient quantity of air?

2.3 Is the dyspnea
     • constant?   COPD: chronic bronchitis; bronchiec-
                                          tasis; chronic static course of pneumo-
                                          coniosis

     • variable?   Due to changes in bronchial secretions
                                          or the degree of bronchospasm: asthma;
                                          asthmatiform bronchitis

     • continuous,   with   paroxysmal   Asthma; any chronic pulmonary dis-
       episodes?   ease which is made worse by superim-
                                          posed infection

     • acute intermittent? paroxysmal,   Bronchial asthma; psychogenic dysp-
       with asymptomatic intervals?   nea; recurrent pulmonary emboli
     • paroxysmal nocturnal? awaken-   Paroxysmal nocturnal dyspnea: intersti-
       ing you from sleep?   tial pulmonary edema secondary to left
                                          ventricular failure; also in COPD, usual-
                                          ly with sputum production (increased
                                          accumulation of bronchial secretions in
                                          the   supine   position);   asthma   often
                                          occurs at night; anxious patients with
                                          nightmares and hyperventilation

2.3a In case of acute intermittent dysp-
     nea: What is the
     • frequency of the episodes?
     • duration of the episodes?

3   Intensity of Dyspnea

3.1 Are you short of breath on exer-   Quantitation of dyspnea is usually
     tion?   based upon the amount of physical ex-
                                          ertion required to produce the difficult
                                          breathing. Physical disabilities due to
                                          severe osteoarthritis of the hips or knees
                                          or to peripheral vascular insufficiency
                                          may preclude exertional dyspnea

3.2 Are you short of breath
     • on climbing stairs? walking up FEV_1 between 1.2 and 1.5 L
       hills? but not on level walking at
       your own pace?

- when walking with people your own age on level ground?
- on minimal exertion? on dressing? bathing? Do you have to pause on climbing one flight or walking a city block?
- at rest? Are you dependent on help for most needs?

FEV_1 near 1 L

FEV_1 near 700 mL

FEV_1: 500 mL or less

4   Precipitating or Aggravating Factors

4.1   Does the dyspnea occur or intensify
- *on exertion?*

Strong evidence for organic disease: early congestive heart failure; COPD (emphysema); early interstitial lung disease; pulmonary hypertension; post-exercise asthma (bronchospasm due to airway thermal changes); severe anemia; obesity; pregnancy; constrictive pericarditis. Dyspnea on exertion may represent transient myocardial ischemia with left ventricular failure

- at rest?

Pneumothorax; bronchial asthma; pulmonary edema; massive pulmonary embolism; pneumonia; pleural effusion; obstruction of airways; psychogenic dyspnea

- at rest, after many years of exertional dyspnea?

COPD with predominant emphysema; advanced form of interstitial lung disease; severe heart failure (cardiac dyspnea)

- *only at rest and not on exertion?*
- in the upright position?

Almost invariably psychogenic dyspnea
Platypnea: in severe COPD (relieved by recumbency)

- *when lying flat?*

Orthopnea: suggests the presence of organic disease: left-heart failure (redistribution of blood volume with little gravitational influence, increased intrathoracic blood volume at the expense of the air volume, and reduced lung's air-containing capacity). May also occur in asthma, COPD, and bilateral diaphragmatic paralysis. Rare in interstitial lung disease

- when lying flat in the left or right lateral position?

Trepopnea: suggests heart disease (positional alterations in ventilation-perfusion relations)

4.2   Is the dyspnea precipitated or aggravated by

- atmospheric conditions? exposure to cold? smog? dusts? smoking?
- allergens? with seasonal exacerbations?
- respiratory infection?

- cough? emotions? laughing?

All varieties of COPD; asthma

Allergic asthma

Increases the cough, sputum and dyspnea in chronic bronchitis; asthma
Causing sudden variations in the level of pulmonary ventilation

5   Relieving Factors

5.1   Is the dyspnea relieved by
- bronchodilators? corticosteroids?
- digitalis? diuretics?
- exertion? taking a few deep breaths? sedatives?
- rest?

- leaning forward while seated?

Asthma
Left-heart failure
Functional origin of dyspnea

Occasionally dyspnea is an anginal equivalent, secondary to myocardial ischemia
Severe COPD (this position increases the efficiency of diaphragmatic movement and facilitates the use of the accessory muscles of respiration)

5.2   In case of nocturnal dyspnea: Is it relieved by
- *supporting head and thorax by two or more pillows? sitting up in bed?*
- *standing up?* going to a window for air?
- cough and expectoration of sputum?

Paroxysmal nocturnal dyspnea in left ventricular failure. The nocturnal attack of asthma is not relieved by sitting or standing up
Chronic bronchitis; nocturnal attack of asthma

5.3   In case of exertional dyspnea: Does cessation of exercise relieve the dyspnea?
- rapidly? (a few minutes)
- gradually? slowly?

Pulmonary cause of dyspnea
Cardiac cause of dyspnea

6   Accompanying Symptoms

6.1   Is the dyspnea accompanied by
- wheezing?

- fever?

- nonproductive cough?

Bronchial obstruction; acute pulmonary embolism
Pneumonia; diffuse bronchiolitis; tuberculosis
Interstitial lung disease; left-heart failure (reflexes from the congested lungs and bronchi)

- cough and/or expectorations?

  Acute infection. With chronic dyspnea: chronic bronchitis; bronchiectasis; tuberculosis

  - occurring over many years before the appearance of exertional dyspnea?

    Chronic bronchitis ("blue bloater")

  - following a long history of progressive dyspnea?

    Chronic bronchitis, emphysema type ("pink puffer")
- frothy, blood-tinged sputum?

  Pulmonary edema; adult respiratory distress syndrome
- frankly bloody sputum?

  Hemoptysis in cancer; pulmonary infarction; acute bronchitis; bronchiectasis; tuberculosis
- chest pain?

  Could be myocardial infarction with congestive heart failure; pulmonary embolism; substernal discomfort when pulmonary hypertension develops; dyspnea as an anginal equivalent secondary to myocardial ischemia

  - *increased when you take a deep breath?*

    Pleuritic or pericardial involvement: pneumonia; pneumothorax; pulmonary infarction; lung tumor; pericarditis

  - sharp? fleeting? in various loci?

    Anxiety neurosis with psychogenic dyspnea
- palpitations?

  Cardiac arrhythmia with resultant congestive heart failure
- hoarseness?

  Upper-airway obstruction; recurrent laryngeal nerve involvement in lung cancer
- sighing? anxiety? yawning? tingling and/or numbness of the extremities or around the mouth? light-headedness?

  Psychogenic dyspnea: anxiety; hyperventilation, respiratory alkalosis; mitral valve prolapse
- weight gain?

  Possible water retention in congestive heart failure
- swollen legs?

  Congestive heart failure; deep-vein thrombosis
- difficulty swallowing?

  Dysphagia: esophageal disease (e.g., scleroderma) with aspiration of foreign material
- pain in your joints?

  Sarcoidosis; collagen-vascular diseases; rheumatoid arthritis with interstitial lung disease; Caplan's syndrome: coal miners with rheumatoid arthritis and progressive massive pneumoconiosis
- diarrhea?

  Carcinoid syndrome; parasitic disease of the lung; cystic fibrosis

7   **Iatrogenic Factors   See Etiology**

7.1 In a patient with asthma:
  • Do attacks of asthma follow the ingestion of aspirin? other nonsteroidal anti-inflammatory drugs?

About 10 percent of patients with nonallergic asthma have bronchospasm, nasal polyps, and sensitivity to aspirin

8 Personal and Social Profile

8.1 Do you smoke? How many cigarettes a day?

The inhalation of tobacco smoke is a powerful factor in causation and progression of COPD, and is the leading cause of lung cancer

8.2 What is (was) your current (past) occupation?

Asthma due to formaldehyde, toluene diisocyanate, animal dander in: textiles, plastics, lacquer use, polyurethane kits, animal handler.
Pulmonary fibrosis due to asbestos, silica, beryllium, coal, aluminum in: mining, insulation, sandblasting, quarrying, metal alloy work.
Pulmonary edema, pneumonitis due to nitrogen oxides, phosgene, halogen gases, cadmium in: fuming, welding, chemical operations.
Chronic bronchitis, emphysema due to cotton dust, cadmium, coal dust, organic solvents in: textile industry, battery production, soldering, mining, solvent use.
Lung cancer due to asbestos, arsenic, nickel, uranium, coke-oven emissions in: insulation, pipefitting, smelting, coke ovens, shipyard workers, nickel refining, uranium mining

8.2a Are you short of breath at your workplace? symptom-free after work? on weekends?

Occupational precipitents of dyspnea

8.3 Do you have any pets? birds? pigeons?

Psittacosis; allergy to cat or dog dander

8.4 Have you ever lived in
  • the southwestern United States?
  • the central United States?

Coccidioidomycosis
Histoplasmosis

8.5 Have you ever been exposed to someone with active tuberculosis?

8.6 Do you use intravenous drugs?

Pulmonary vasculitis

8.7 What is your sexual orientation?

Dyspnea in a homosexual man: *Pneumocystis* pneumonia, pulmonary *Mycobacterium avium-intracellulare*, cytomegalovirus pneumonia

9 Personal Antecedents Pertaining to Dyspnea

9.1 Have you ever had a chest x-ray? breathing tests? allergic skin tests? When? With what results?

9.2 Do you have any of the following conditions: emphysema? chronic bronchitis? asthma? allergy? tuberculosis? a past chest operation?

• a heart disease? hypertension? an antecedent myocardial infarction?   Congestive heart failure

• repeated colds or bronchitis?   COPD; bronchiectasis; cystic fibrosis; immunologic deficiencies

• a recent operation? a recent pregnancy? prolonged recumbency? phlebitis?   Pulmonary embolism

• past radiation therapy to the chest?   Pneumonitis and/or fibrosis in exposed area

10 Family Medical History Pertaining to Dyspnea

10.1 Is there someone in your family with a pulmonary condition?   COPD tends to cluster in families; tuberculosis; alpha-1-antitrypsin deficiency; cystic disease of the lung; asthma; cystic fibrosis

PHYSICAL SIGNS PERTAINING TO DYSPNEA*

Possible significance

Stridor; retraction of the supraclavicular fossae and intercostal spaces with inspiration   Acute upper-airway obstruction

Cardiomegaly; basilar crackles; distended jugular veins; hepatomegaly; pitting edema   Cardiac origin of dyspnea: congestive heart failure

Numerous bilateral crackles; gallop rhythm; cardiomegaly   Acute left ventricular failure: pulmonary edema

Fever; tachypnea; localized dullness; increased tactile and vocal fremitus; bronchial breath sounds, crackles, wheezes   Pulmonary signs of consolidation: bacterial pneumonia; lung abscess

*In this section, items in *italics* are characteristic clinical features, and items in **boldface** are potentially life-threatening or urgent conditions.

Prolonged expiration; generalized wheezing and rhonchi	Obstruction of intrathoracic airways; asthma; chronic bronchitis. Sudden acute dyspnea with generalized wheezing may be due to acute pulmonary embolism or pulmonary edema
Unilateral wheezing	Bronchial obstruction: tumor; foreign body; mucous plug
Dry ("Velcro") crackles at both bases	Interstitial lung disease
Underweight patient; overinflated chest; prominent accessory muscles; hyperresonance; prolonged expiration; distant breath sounds, end-expiratory wheezes, pink mucous membranes	COPD, emphysema, type A ("pink puffer")
Plethoric patient; cyanosis at rest; prolonged expiration; well-heard breath sounds, rhonchi, right ventricular failure	COPD, chronic bronchitis, type B ("blue bloater")
Dullness to percussion; decreased fremitus; decreased to absent breath sounds; pleural friction rub in some cases	Pleural effusion
On affected side: decreased chest movement; hyperresonance; decreased fremitus and breath sounds; tracheal deviation to the opposite side	Pneumothorax
Deep-vein thrombosis; tachypnea; accentuation of the pulmonary second sound; gallop rhythm; crackles, pleural friction rub	Pulmonary embolism and infarction (nonspecific signs)
On affected side: diminished chest movement; deviation of mediastinum toward the affected side; dullness to percussion; absent breath sounds	Atelectasis
Deformed chest; severe kyphoscoliosis; spondylitis; pectus excavatum	Thoracic cage abnormalities with hypoventilation
Neurologic or muscular disorder	Neuromuscular disease with weakness of respiratory muscles
Clubbing	Bronchial carcinoma; suppurative disease (pulmonary abscess; bronchiectasis); idiopathic pulmonary fibrosis; congenital heart disease; asbestosis (clubbing is not associated with COPD)
Nicotine stains on the fingertips	Prolonged excessive cigarette smoking

LABORATORY TESTS PERTAINING TO DYSPNEA[†]

Test	Finding	Diagnostic Possibilities
Blood		
Hematocrit	Increased (>55 percent)	Polycythemia secondary to chronic hypoxemia, e.g., COPD, bronchitic type
WBCs	Hyperleukocytosis	COPD with superimposed infection; bacterial pneumonia
	Eosinophilia	Asthma
Arterial oxygen tension	Decreased (<75 mmHg)	Hypoxemia may be present in all pulmonary causes of chronic dyspnea
Arterial carbon dioxide tension	Increased (>50 mmHg)	Hypercapnea: in COPD, predominant bronchitis
	Low to normal	Due to tachypnea in: COPD, predominant emphysema; interstitial lung disease
Alpha-1-globulin	Decreased	Alpha-1-antitrypsin deficiency
Pleural Fluid (PF)		
PF protein/serum protein	>0.5	One or more of these three characteristics present: exudate: malignancy, tuberculosis, parapneumonic effusion, pulmonary infarction. None present: transudate: congestive heart failure, cirrhosis, nephrotic syndrome
Lactic dehydrogenase (LDH)	>200 U	
PF LDH/serum LDH	>0.6	
Pulmonary Function Tests		
Forced vital capacity (FVC)	Decreased	COPD; restrictive lung disease
Forced expiratory volume in 1 s (FEV$_1$)	Decreased	COPD
	Normal	Restrictive lung disease
FEV$_1$/FVC	Decreased	COPD
	Normal or increased	Restrictive lung disease

[†]See the appendix on Laboratory Reference Values for the associated normal laboratory values.

Test	Finding	Diagnostic Possibilities
Carbon dioxide diffusion capacity (DLCO)	Normal (=25 mL CO/min/mmHg)	Asthma; chronic bronchitis
	Decreased	Emphysema; restrictive lung disease
Residual volume	Increased	Obstructive pattern
	Decreased	Restrictive pattern
Total lung capacity	Normal or increased	Obstructive pattern
	Decreased	Restrictive lung disease

LABORATORY PROCEDURES PERTAINING TO DYSPNEA

Procedure	To Detect
Chest x-ray	Hyperinflation of the lungs, cor pulmonale: COPD
	Interstitial infiltrate: infiltrative lung disease
	Lobar consolidation: bacterial pneumonia
	Interstitial edema, pulmonary vascular redistribution, cardiomegaly: left ventricular failure
	Pneumothorax; pleural effusion; acute pulmonary embolism
ECG	Right axis deviation, P pulmonale, right ventricular strain pattern: chronic pulmonary disease; acute dyspnea in pulmonary embolism
Lung scan, ventilation/perfusion scan, pulmonary angiogram*	Pulmonary embolism; parenchymal lung disease
Fiberoptic bronchoscopy*	Tumors, granulomatous lesions
Lung biopsy*	Type of diffuse infiltrative disease of the lungs

Procedure	To Detect
Radionuclide ventriculography at rest and during exercise*	Left ventricle ejection fraction: depressed in left ventricular failure
	Right ventricular fraction low (at rest), may decline further during exercise in severe lung disease
	Both ejection fractions are normal in anxiety or malingering

*When indicated

SELECTED BIBLIOGRAPHY

Angelillo VA: Evaluation of dyspnea. *Postgrad Med* 73(2):336–345, 1983.

Flenley DC: Chronic obstructive pulmonary disease. *DM* 34(9):537–599, 1988.

Krumpe PE, Lum CC, Cross CE: Approach to the patient with diffuse lung disease. *Med Clin North Am* 72(5):1225–1246, 1988.

Mahler DA: Dyspnea: Diagnosis and management. *Clin Chest Med* 8(2):215–230, 1987.

6
Edema

INTRODUCTION

Edema Swelling produced by an increase in the extravascular component of the extracellular fluid volume.

The movements of fluid between the plasma volume and the interstitial space are governed by (1) the gradient in hydrostatic pressure between the intravascular and interstitial spaces, and (2) the colloid oncotic pressure gradient resulting from the difference in protein concentration between plasma and interstitial fluid. At the arterial end of the microcirculation, hydrostatic pressure favors movement of fluid into the interstitial spaces against the osmotic pressures exerted by the plasma proteins. At the venous end of the capillary bed, fluid returns to the vascular compartment because the hydrostatic pressure falls below plasma oncotic pressure. In addition, fluid is returned from the interstitial space into the vascular system by way of the lymphatic vessels.

Localized Edema

Movement of plasma fluid into the interstitium may be caused by a localized increase in capillary permeability (due to chemical, bacterial, thermal, or mechanical agents) or by any localized increase in the capillary pressure (due to local obstruction in venous and lymphatic drainage).

Generalized Edema

In congestive heart failure, the increased venous pressure produces an elevated capillary hydrostatic pressure, promoting the formation of edema. The decreased cardiac output is associated with a decreased effective arterial blood volume and a decreased renal blood flow. Renin is released, angiotensin is produced, stimulating aldosterone release with resultant sodium retention.

In cirrhosis, effective blood volume is diminished, probably as a consequence of splanchnic venous pooling, hypoalbuminemia, and diminished peripheral resistance. The increased portal venous pressure favors increased formation of intraperitoneal fluid (ascites). Hypoproteinemia causes a shift of plasma water into interstitial spaces, leading to generalized edema.

Hypoproteinemia resulting from protein loss (as in the nephrotic syndrome or in protein-losing enteropathy), or from nutritional deficiency, is associated with reduced oncotic pressure and increased fluid movement into the interstitium. This decreases plasma volume, and the kidney responds with salt and water retention.

Decreased glomerular filtration rate is usually not a major factor limiting sodium excretion until late in the disease. However, some causes of renal failure involve the renal vasculature and the glomeruli and impair sodium excretion early in their course.

ETIOLOGY

Generalized Edema

Congestive heart failure; constrictive pericarditis
Nephrotic syndrome; acute nephritic syndrome
Cirrhosis of the liver
Hypoalbuminemia: malabsorption; protein-losing gastroenteropathies; malnutrition
Endocrine: myxedema; secondary hyperaldosteronism; Cushing's syndrome
Allergy; serum sickness
Toxemia of pregnancy
Idiopathic cyclic edema

Regional Causes of Edema of Extremities

Acute cellulitis
Angioedema
Deep-vein thrombosis
Lymphatic obstruction: malignancy, resection of lymph nodes, irradiation
Lower extremities:
   Chronic venous insufficiency (postphlebitic syndrome)
   Gravitational: prolonged sitting or standing, pregnancy
   Pretibial myxedema
   Primary lymphedema; lipedema
Upper extremities: superior vena cava syndrome; thoracic outlet syndromes

Iatrogenic Causes of Dependent Edema

Diazoxide; propranolol; minoxidil; calcium-channel blocking agents; mannitol; phenylbutazone; indomethacine; corticosteroids; estrogens; testosterone; amantadine; monoamine oxidase inhibitors

HISTORY TAKING*

Possible meaning of a positive response

1   Location of edema

1.1   Is the edema localized?
   • around the eyes? the face?   Nephrotic syndrome, acute glomerulonephritis; hypoproteinemia; myxedema; constrictive pericarditis; tricuspid stenosis; allergic reactions; angioedema; trichinosis.

   • *the face, the neck, the upper arms?*   Superior vena cava syndrome (lung cancer)

*In this section, items in *italics* are characteristic clinical features, and items in **boldface** are potentially life-threatening or urgent conditions.

• in an (upper or lower) extremity?	Venous thrombosis; lymphatic blockage (secondary lymphedema); cellulitis (may be uni- or bilateral); lesions in the central nervous system affecting the vasomotor fibers on one side of the body (paralysis also reduces lymphatic and venous drainage on the affected side)
• in both arms?	Venous and/or lymphatic obstruction
• in the abdomen and legs?	Ascites: liver cirrhosis, congestive heart failure
• both legs?	Any cause of generalized edema; hypothyroidism; primary lymphedema

1.2 Is the edema
  • generalized?

Anasarca: nephrotic syndrome; severe congestive heart failure; hepatic cirrhosis; nutritional disorder; hypoproteinemia

2 Mode of Onset and Duration

2.1 When did you notice
  • a ring on a finger fitting more snugly than in the past?
  • difficulty in putting on shoes? particularly in the evening?

} Early symptoms of generalized edema

2.1a Has your abdominal girth increased?

Suggests the presence of ascites

2.2 For how long has (have) your leg(s) been swollen?
  • congenital?

Primary lymphedema is manifest at birth or becomes apparent before age 40 (more common in women)

  • noticed in childhood?
Lipedema (bilateral; in girls)
  • for years?
Repeated attacks of deep-vein thrombosis causing chronic edema; chronic lymphatic obstruction

2.3 In case of facial edema: Has the edema appeared
  • rapidly?
Angioedema; serum sickness; allergy
  • gradually?
Nephrotic syndrome

2.4 In case of edema of lower limb(s): Did the swelling occur
  • suddenly?
Venous thrombosis; acute cellulitis; cyclic edema
  • gradually?
Lymphedema; venous thrombosis; any cause of generalized edema

2.5   In case of ascites and edema of the
      legs: Has the ascites
      • *appeared first?*   Cirrhosis; constrictive pericarditis
      • *followed the edema of the legs?*   Cardiac or renal disease

3   Character of Edema

3.1   In case of edema of both legs: Is the
      edema
      • present or most pronounced in   Congestive heart failure; edema due to
        the evening?   gravitation or dependency
      • present all day?   Advanced stage of heart failure; hypo-
                                                proteinemia; venous or lymphatic fi-
                                                brosed edema

3.2   In case of generalized or localized   Angioedema; idiopathic cyclic edema
      edema: Is the edema intermittent?   (can be permanent)

4   Precipitating or Aggravating Factors

4.1   In case of generalized intermittent
      edema: Does the edema occur
      • after eating certain foods? expo-   Angioedema
        sure to animals? molds? cold?
      • *during the premenstrual period?*   Idiopathic cyclic edema

4.2   In case of edema of the face: Is the   Hypoproteinemia (because of the re-
      edema most pronounced in the   cumbent posture assumed during the
      morning?   night)

4.3   In case of edema in the lower ex-
      tremities: Does the edema appear
      or worsen
      • on prolonged standing?   Chronic venous insufficiency; idiopath-
                                                ic cyclic edema; congestive heart failure
      • in the evening? at the end of the   Congestive heart failure; chronic ve-
        day?   nous insufficiency; edema due to
                                                gravitation or dependency
      • in hot weather?   Chronic venous insufficiency; idiopath-
                                                ic cyclic edema
      • before or during the menstrual   Cyclic edema
        periods?

5   Relieving Factors

5.1   In case of edema in the lower ex-
      tremities: Does the edema
      • subside overnight?   ⎫ Gravitational edema; chronic venous
      • decrease by elevation of your   ⎬ insufficiency; right heart failure
        legs?   ⎭

6   Accompanying Symptoms

6.1	Has your weight increased?	Visible edema of both legs is preceded by a weight gain of at least 7 to 10 lb (5 kg) over weeks to months. Excess fluid retention may occur without a gain in weight because of concomitant malnutrition or excessive kidney or bowel loss of protein
6.2	*Does your evening weight exceed your morning weight by more than 2 lb (1 kg)?*	Increased fluid retention; idiopathic cyclic edema (large diurnal weight changes suggest an increase in capillary permeability which appears to fluctuate in severity)
6.3	Do you have shortness of breath?	Congestive heart failure; **pulmonary edema;** large bilateral pleural effusions; elevation of diaphragm due to ascites; **angioedema with laryngeal edema** (and stridor); **pulmonary embolism** secondary to deep-vein thrombosis. (Ascites and edema of the legs without orthopnea suggest tricuspid stenosis, constrictive pericarditis, or cirrhosis of the liver)
6.3a	Has shortness of breath preceded the edema of the legs?	Edema due to left ventricular dysfunction; mitral stenosis; chronic pulmonary disease with cor pulmonale

6.4 Do you have
- a decrease in the volume of your urine? → Acute glomerulonephritis; congestive heart failure; cirrhosis
- a smoky color of your urine? → Acute glomerulonephritis
- loss of appetite? nausea? vomiting? → May be due to venous congestion and edema of the bowel
- chronic diarrhea? → Malabsorption; protein-losing gastroenteropathy with hypoproteinemia
- abdominal pain? → Angioedema with gastrointestinal manifestations

6.5 In case of edema of lower extremities: Do you have
- pain in your leg(s)? → Local cause of edema: acute cellulitis; lymphangitis; acute thrombophlebitis; ulcer (cardiac edema usually does not cause pain because the tissues stretch gradually)
- fever? → Acute lymphangitis; venous thrombosis
- psychological, social difficulties? → Often present in women with idiopathic edema

7   **Iatrogenic Causes   See Etiology**

8   Personal and Social Profile

8.1   What is your intake of beer? alcohol? wine?

In an alcoholic patient: edema due to cirrhosis; alcoholic cardiomyopathy with heart failure; nutritional edema

8.2   Do you eat a particular kind of diet?

Possible nutritional deficiency with hypoalbuminemia and edema; the edema may be intensified by beriberi heart disease

8.3   What is your occupation?

An occupation involving relative immobility (sitting or standing) for long periods can be an aggravating factor

9   Personal Antecedents Pertaining to the Edema

9.1   Have you ever had liver, renal function tests? a chest x-ray? an ECG? When? With what results?

9.2   In case of edema of an extremity: Have you ever had phlebitis? surgery to the extremity? irradiation of involved area or near the edematous area?

9.3   Do you have any of the following conditions: a cardiac condition? a high blood pressure? a kidney disease? a liver disease? allergy? varicose veins?

10   Family Medical History Pertaining to the Edema

10.1 In case of edema of lower extremities: Does someone in your family have
      • varicose veins?
      • "edema" of the legs?

A positive family history is common
Lipedema; Milroy's disease: familial form of congenital lymphedema

PHYSICAL SIGNS PERTAINING TO EDEMA*

Possible significance

Generalized Edema

Cardiomegaly; gallop; basilar crackles; distended jugular veins; hepatomegaly

Congestive heart failure

Jaundice; hepatomegaly; spider angiomas; palmar erythema; gynecomastia

Edema of hepatic origin; cirrhosis

*In this section, items in *italics* are characteristic clinical features, and items in **boldface** are potentially life-threatening or urgent conditions.

Severe malnutrition	Edema of nutritional origin
Paradoxical pulse	**Pericardial tamponade;** occasionally in constrictive pericarditis; severe pulmonary disease with airway obstruction
Friction rub; distant heart sounds; pulsus paradoxus; distended jugular veins; hepatosplenomegaly; ascites; edema	Pericardial effusion; pericardial constriction (murmurs are usually absent)
Hypertension	Acute phase of glomerulonephritis

Localized Edema

Edema and cyanosis of head, neck, upper extremities; dilated venous collaterals over upper portion of chest and abdomen	Superior vena cava obstruction: bronchogenic carcinoma; mediastinal lymphoma; aneurysm of the aorta
Edema of one leg; edema of one or both arms	Venous and/or lymphatic obstruction
Symmetrical edema in the lower extremities	Systemic cause: cardiac, hypoproteinemia; lipedema
Asymmetrical edema in the lower extremities	Additional vascular or lymphatic factor; unilateral pelvic obstruction
Ulceration, pigmentation of the thickened, hard, red skin on the legs	Repeated episodes of prolonged edema; past attacks of deep-vein thrombosis with postphlebitic syndrome; chronic venous insufficiency
Localized edema with red, warm, tender area; fever	Inflammation or hypersensitivity; acute venous thrombosis; cellulitis; lymphangitis
Swollen leg with local cyanosis	Venous obstruction

LABORATORY TESTS PERTAINING TO EDEMA[†]

Test	Finding	Diagnostic Possibilities
Urine		
Proteinuria	Slight to moderate	Congestive heart failure; renal disease
	Heavy (>3.5 g/ 24 h)	Nephrotic syndrome
	Absent	Liver disease; protein-losing enteropathy; malnutrition (eliminates renal disease)

[†]See the appendix on Laboratory Reference Values for the associated normal laboratory values.

Test	Finding	Diagnostic Possibilities
Sediment	RBCs, RBC casts, proteinuria	Acute glomerulonephritis

Blood

Test	Finding	Diagnostic Possibilities
BUN, creatinine	Elevated	Acute glomerulonephritis; congestive heart failure with renal hypoperfusion
Liver function tests	Abnormal	Cirrhosis of liver
Serum proteins	Hypoalbuminemia (<2.5 g/100 mL)	Nephrotic syndrome; cirrhosis; severe malnutrition; protein-losing enteropathy
Cholesterol, low density lipoproteins	Elevated	Nephrotic syndrome
Thyroid function tests	Abnormal	Myxedema

LABORATORY PROCEDURES PERTAINING TO EDEMA

Procedure	To Detect
Chest x-ray	Cardiomegaly, pulmonary edema: congestive heart failure; pericardial effusion
Echocardiography;* radionuclide angiography*	Heart failure; pericardial effusion

*When indicated

SELECTED BIBLIOGRAPHY

Braunwald E: Edema, in Wilson J, Braunwald E, Isselbacher KJ et al (eds). *Harrison's Principles of Internal Medicine*, 12th ed., pp. 228–232, New York: McGraw-Hill, 1991.

Melby JC, Idiopathic edema: A clinical conundrum. *Hosp Pract* 20(12):68E-68T, 1985.

Naschitz JE: Yeshurun D: Local edema of the skin and subcutaneous tissue. *Hosp Pract* 24(6):53–60, 1989.

7
Heart Murmurs

INTRODUCTION

Murmur Any prolonged sound produced by the heart and blood vessels.

Normal blood flow is laminar and produces no audible murmur. Cardiac murmurs are attributed to vibrations arising in the heart or great vessels as a result of turbulent blood flow and/or the formation of eddies and bubbles. This occurs when the rate of blood flow is increased, when blood is propelled vigorously across a valvular or vascular constriction or into a dilated vessel, or when there is regurgitation, as in valvular insufficiency.

Systolic murmurs may be classified as (1) ejection murmurs (aortic and pulmonic stenosis), occurring predominantly in midsystole and related to a disproportion between blood flow and the size of the orifice which it traverses; and (2) regurgitant pansystolic murmurs (mitral and tricuspid insufficiency), involving two chambers which have widely different pressures throughout systole. Late systolic murmurs are attributed to papillary muscle dysfunction caused by infarction or ischemia of these muscles.

Early diastolic murmurs (aortic or pulmonic regurgitation) are due to a regurgitant flow of very high velocity. Middiastolic murmurs (mitral stenosis) usually arise from the atrioventricular valves and are due to disproportion between valve orifice size and flow rate.

Continuous murmurs depend on a continuous blood flow from a chamber or vessel of higher pressure to one of lower pressure, such pressure difference persisting in diastole as well as systole (patent ductus arteriosus).

ETIOLOGY

Systolic Murmurs

Pansystolic (regurgitant)

Mitral regurgitation (rheumatic, papillary muscle dysfunction, mitral valve prolapse)
Tricuspid regurgitation
Left-to-right shunt, ventricular level

Midsystolic (ejection)

Aortic

Obstructive: aortic stenosis; aortic sclerosis; hypertrophic obstructive cardiomyopathy; coarctation of aorta
Increased flow: aortic regurgitation; complete heart block; hyperkinetic states
Dilatation of ascending aorta; aneurysm of aorta

Pulmonary

Obstructive: pulmonic valve stenosis; infundibular stenosis; pulmonary arterial stenosis

Left-to-right shunt; atrial septal defect; ventricular septal defect

Dilatation of pulmonary artery

Diastolic Murmurs

Early diastolic

Aortic regurgitation: rheumatic, posttraumatic, postvalvulotomy, postendocarditis, aorta dissection, cystic medial necrosis, hypertension, syphilis, congenital bicuspid valve

Pulmonic regurgitation: rheumatic fever, carcinoid, endocarditis, pulmonary hypertension, Marfan's syndrome, congenital

Middiastolic

Mitral stenosis; tricuspid stenosis; acute rheumatic fever; increased flow across a nonstenotic atrioventricular valve (mitral regurgitation, ventricular septal defect, patent ductus arteriosus, tricuspid regurgitation, atrial septal defect)

Continuous Murmurs

Patent ductus arteriosus; coronary arteriovenous fistula; ruptured aneurysm of sinus of Valsalva; aortic septal defect; cervical venous hum; mammary souffle

HISTORY TAKING*

Possible meaning of a positive response

1   Mode Of Onset and Evolution

1.1   How long have you known that you have a heart murmur? When was the murmur first heard?

From birth and childhood: congenital heart disease; congenital aortic regurgitation; hypertrophic obstructive cardiomyopathy. In early adulthood: rheumatic cause of the heart murmur. In later years: degenerative changes in valvular structures

1.2   How was it detected?
   • during a routine examination?

The initial evidence of valvular heart disease is often a cardiac murmur on routine physical examination in an asymptomatic patient

   • because of health complaints?

*In this section, items in *italics* are characteristic clinical features.

1.3 How long have you known that you have a heart murmur without having any complaint?	Patients with mitral regurgitation, aortic stenosis, and aortic regurgitation remain relatively asymptomatic for 10 to 20 years; in rheumatic mitral stenosis, symptoms usually become apparent in young adulthood; mitral regurgitation is the best tolerated of all valvular diseases. The appearance of symptoms in a patient with aortic stenosis heralds a progressive downhill course

2 Accompanying Symptoms

2.1 Do you have shortness of breath?	Left heart failure with pulmonary congestion. Dyspnea is the earliest manifestation of mitral stenosis, mitral regurgitation, aortic stenosis; hypertrophic obstructive cardiomyopathy
• of sudden onset?	In a patient with mitral valve stenosis: development of atrial fibrillation, rupture of chordae tendineae, pulmonary embolism
• at rest?	Severe heart failure; congenital cyanotic heart disease
• on exertion?	Mitral stenosis: increased cardiac output and tachycardia of exercise with elevation of left atrial pressure, pulmonary venous hypertension, and increased lung stiffness. Aortic stenosis and regurgitation: elevation of the left ventricular end-diastolic, mean left atrial, and pulmonary capillary pressures
• at night?	Pulmonary edema: usually a late expression of valvular heart disease; indicates a decline in cardiac compensatory mechanisms and myocardial contractility
2.1a How long have you had shortness of breath on exertion?	Dyspnea beginning in early adulthood: mitral stenosis; in late adulthood (age 55 to 60): aortic stenosis or regurgitation
2.2 Do you have • chest discomfort? pain?	Reduction in myocardial perfusion may create chest discomfort. In severe mitral stenosis: may be due to pulmonary hypertension or myocardial ischemia; in aortic regurgitation: may be due to excessive cardiac pounding on the chest wall and/or myocardial ischemia; mitral valve prolapse. Severe pain of aortic dissection

• on exertion?

Aortic stenosis (angina pectoris occurs in one-third of patients); severe mitral stenosis (due to severe pulmonary hypertension?); hypertrophic obstructive cardiomyopathy; ischemic heart disease; aortic regurgitation with relative myocardial ischemia

• palpitations?

May be due to disturbances in rhythm. An early complaint in aortic regurgitation: awareness of the beating of a dilated left ventricle with a large volume change in systole; atrial fibrillation in mitral stenosis or regurgitation; mitral valve prolapse; aortic stenosis

• head pounding?

In aortic regurgitation: may be caused by sinus tachycardia with emotion or premature ventricular contractions

• swollen legs?

Congestive heart failure: late symptom in mitral regurgitation

• syncope?
  • *on exertion?*

Occurs in 10 to 20 percent of patients with aortic stenosis: due to decline in arterial pressure caused by vasodilatation in the exercising muscles unaccompanied by an increase in cardiac output or to transient arrhythmia due to the ischemia; primary pulmonary hypertension; hypertrophic obstructive cardiomyopathy; pulmonary stenosis

  • *with alterations in position?*

Atrial ball-valve thrombus in mitral stenosis obstructing the stenotic mitral valve; left atrial myxoma; orthostatic syncope may occur in aortic stenosis

• a dry cough?

Aortic aneurysm impinging on the trachea or bronchi; in mitral stenosis: cough due to left atrial enlargement and infringement on the mainstem bronchus

• bloody expectorations?

Hemoptysis: in mitral stenosis: may be due to rupture of pulmonary-bronchial venous connections, atrial fibrillation with pulmonary infarction, pulmonary edema, or bronchitis

• hoarseness?

Compression of recurrent laryngeal nerve by an aneurysm of the aorta; in mitral stenosis: compression of left recurrent laryngeal nerve between the enlarged hypertensive pulmonary artery, the aorta, and the ligamentum arteriosum (Ortner's syndrome)

- difficulty swallowing?

Dysphagia: compression of the esophagus by a dilated left atrium of mitral stenosis, an aneurysm of the aorta; coarctation of aorta, with the right subclavian artery passing behind the esophagus; aortic arch anomaly

- pain in the back? the joints? morning back stiffness?

Aortic regurgitation may be associated with ankylosing spondylitis and rheumatoid arthritis; bacterial endocarditis with arthralgia; acute rheumatic carditis

- *flushing of the upper chest and head? diarrhea? wheezing?*

Carcinoid heart disease with tricuspid regurgitation or pulmonic stenosis

- unusual sweating over the body?

Aortic regurgitation

- *fever?* sweating?

Subacute bacterial endocarditis superimposed on normal or abnormal valves; acute rheumatic carditis; atrial myxoma

- frequent episodes of bronchitis?

Pulmonary infections commonly complicate mitral stenosis

- headaches? weakness of the legs? pain in the calves when walking?

Coarctation of the aorta

2.3 Do you feel tired?

Early symptom in mitral regurgitation (low cardiac output); severe heart failure; subacute bacterial endocarditis; mitral valve prolapse; anemia with functional murmur

3 Personal and Social Profile

3.1 Has your heart problem affected your ability to work? your life at home? your social life?

Appraisal of physical activity is important to detect limitations in the patient and dictate the appropriate timing of noninvasive and invasive cardiac studies as well as the decision for surgical correction

3.2 Were you able some months ago to perform specific tasks which now cause symptoms?

Helps establish whether the patient's disability is stable or progressive

4 Personal Antecedents Pertaining to the Heart Murmur

4.1 Have you ever had a chest x-ray? an ECG? a cardiac catheterization? When? With what results?

4.2 Have you ever had
- rheumatic fever? "growing pains"? St Vitus' dance? (chorea)

Acute rheumatic fever producing chronic rheumatic heart disease; approximately 50 percent of patients with mitral stenosis recall a history of acute rheumatic fever

4.2a   How long after the episode of rheumatic fever was the murmur detected?

The murmur of mitral regurgitation is commonly heard during or soon after the acute rheumatic episode, in contrast to the relatively late development of the murmur of mitral stenosis

4.3   Have you ever had
- a trauma to the heart?
- a myocardial infarction?

Traumatic aortic regurgitation
Functional mitral regurgitation; papillary muscle dysfunction

4.4   Have you recently had
- dental extractions? urologic manipulations?

Subacute bacterial endocarditis (SBE) may be superimposed on rheumatic heart disease and mitral valve prolapse; SBE is rare in pure mitral stenosis but is not uncommon in combined mitral stenosis and regurgitation

4.5   Do you have a sexually transmitted disease?

Syphilitic aortic regurgitation

5   Family Medical History Pertaining to the Heart Murmur

5.1   Does someone in your family have a heart murmur? a cardiac disease? cyanosis?

Familial form of hypertrophic obstructive cardiomyopathy represents 50 percent of the disease. Heritable disorders of connective tissue: Marfan's syndrome; mitral valve prolapse; certain forms of cardiomyopathy and related murmurs occur in family members

5.2   Did your mother have a viral illness during her pregnancy?

Rubella in the first 2 months of pregnancy is associated with a number of congenital cardiac malformations: patent ductus arteriosus, atrial and ventricular septal defect, tetralogy of Fallot, supravalvular aortic stenosis syndrome; mitral valve prolapse

PHYSICAL SIGNS PERTAINING TO HEART MURMURS

Intensity of Heart Murmurs

Grade 1
very faint, just audible

Grade 3
moderately loud

Grade 2
faint, soft

Grade 4
loud

Grade 5

very loud

Murmur accentuated
  • during inspiration

  • with standing

  • with squatting

  • with sustained handgrip exercise

Crescendo middiastolic murmur at the apex, opening snap, loud first sound

Holosystolic murmur maximum at apex, radiating to axilla, soft first sound

Crescendo-decrescendo aortic ejection systolic murmur ending before the second heart sound, faint or absent second aortic sound; slow-rising peripheral arterial pulse

Decrescendo diastolic murmur at the base and along the left sternal border; elevated systolic pressure, depressed diastolic pressure; water-hammer pulse; capillary pulsations; to-and-fro murmur over compressed femoral arteries (Duroziez's sign)

Apical systolic click; mid- to late systolic murmur; slender body habitus

Systolic murmur, left second interspace; wide split of second sound unaffected by inspiration

Systolic murmur over the precordium, loudest along the left sternal border

Continuous murmur in interscapular region; hypertension; blood pressure lower in the legs than in the arms

Continuous machinery murmur; wide pulse pressure

Grade 6

audible with the stethoscope removed from contact with the chest

Possible significance

Murmur arising on the right side of the heart

Hypertrophic cardiomyopathy; mitral valve prolapse

Most murmurs except those of hypertrophic cardiomyopathy and mitral valve prolapse

Mitral regurgitation; aortic regurgitation; mitral stenosis (the murmurs of aortic stenosis and hypertrophic cardiomyopathy are diminished)

Mitral stenosis

Mitral regurgitation

Aortic stenosis

Aortic regurgitation

Mitral valve prolapse syndrome

Atrial septal defect

Ventricular septal defect

Coarctation of the aorta

Patent ductus arteriosus

A palpable delay between the apical impulse and the carotid upstroke	Significant aortic stenosis (aortic valve area < 1 cm² is highly likely)
Hypertension	Causing cardiomegaly with functional mitral regurgitation; ischemic heart disease; aortic dilatation in the elderly
Cyanosis	Congenital cyanotic heart disease; congestive heart failure with peripheral cyanosis
Systolic hepatic pulsations	Tricuspid regurgitation
Atrial fibrillation	A turning point in mitral stenosis: usually associated with accelerated rate of progress of symptoms
Fever	Subacute bacterial endocarditis; acute flare-up of the rheumatic process; atrial myxoma
Fever; petechiae; splinter hemorrhages; Osler's nodes (pulp of the fingers); splenomegaly; systemic emboli; anemia	Subacute bacterial endocarditis (systemic emboli may occur in left atrial myxoma)

LABORATORY PROCEDURES PERTAINING TO HEART MURMURS

Procedure	To Detect
Chest x-ray	Straightening of left-heart border, left atrial enlargement, prominence of the pulmonary arteries, Kerley B lines: mitral stenosis
	Left atrial and left ventricular enlargement, pulmonary congestion: mitral regurgitation
	Left ventricular hypertrophy, calcified aortic valve, dilated ascending aorta: aortic stenosis
	Left ventricular enlargement, dilated aortic root: aortic regurgitation
	Increased pulmonary vascularity with right ventricular enlargement: atrial septal defect
	Increased pulmonary vascularity with left atrial and left ventricular enlargement: ventricular septal defect

Procedure	To Detect
Chest x-ray *(continued)*	Decreased pulmonary vascularity: tetralogy of Fallot; primary pulmonary hypertension
ECG	Left atrial enlargement, right ventricular hypertrophy, right axis deviation: mitral stenosis
	Left ventricular hypertrophy: aortic stenosis; aortic regurgitation
	Left ventricular hypertrophy, left atrial enlargement: mitral regurgitation
Echocardiogram	Valvular anatomy and motion; orifice size; presence of infective endocarditis
Cardiac catheterization;* angiocardiography*	Nature and severity of a mechanical valvular defect; type of congenital heart disease

*When indicated

SELECTED BIBLIOGRAPHY

Lembo NJ, Dell'Italia LJ, Crawford MH, O'Rourke RA: Bedside diagnosis of systolic murmurs. *N Engl J Med* 318:1572–1578, 1988.
Paraskos JA: The innocent murmur. *Hosp Pract* 23(5A):20–29, 1988.
Perloff JK: Murmurs, in Horwitz LD, Groves BM (eds), *Signs and Symptoms in Cardiology,* pp. 227–260, Philadelphia: Lippincott, 1985.
Rothman A, Goldberger AL: Aids to cardiac auscultation. *Ann Intern Med* 99:346–353, 1983.

8
Hemoptysis

INTRODUCTION

Hemoptysis   Expectoration of sputum either streaked or grossly contaminated with blood.

Bleeding from the lungs and bronchi is influenced by the degree of aeration and the presence of mucus and pus. Hemoptysis in tuberculosis may be due to ulceration of the bronchial mucosa or slough of a caseous lesion; it is usually minor in degree, but massive hemorrhage occasionally occurs when a vessel is eroded. In severe pulmonary edema caused by acute left ventricular failure, the frothy fluid that pours from the bronchial tree is often blood-tinged, owing to the escape of red cells into the alveoli from the congested vessels of the lungs. In mitral stenosis, hemoptysis is caused by rupture of dilated endobronchial vessels which appear to form collateral channels between the pulmonary and bronchial venous systems; it tends to occur most frequently in patients who have elevated left atrial pressure without marked elevation of the pulmonary vascular resistance. Hemoptysis in pulmonary thromboembolism is present only when infarction, with necrosis and hemorrhage into the alveoli, has occurred. In lung carcinoma, hemoptysis of bright red blood or "rusty" sputum may be due to vascular invasion or to pneumonia developing behind the tumor. In bronchiectasis, bleeding from the lungs may result from necrosis of the mucosa or rupture of pulmonary-bronchial venous connections.

ETIOLOGY

Infections:* bronchitis, acute, chronic;* tuberculosis;* bronchiectasis;* lung abscess; pneumonia; necrotizing pneumonia; fungus infections; parasitic diseases
Neoplasms: bronchogenic carcinoma;* bronchial adenoma; miscellaneous rare tumors
Cardiac and vascular lesions: pulmonary thromboembolism; left ventricular failure; mitral stenosis; primary pulmonary hypertension; arteriovenous malformations; hereditary hemorrhagic telangiectasia; polyarteritis nodosa; Goodpasture's syndrome; Wegener's granulomatosis; idiopathic pulmonary hemosiderosis; intrabronchial leakage of an aortic aneurysm; Eisenmenger's syndrome
Miscellaneous: hemorrhagic diseases (purpura, leukemia, hemophilia); anticoagulant therapy; broncholith; foreign body; cystic fibrosis; trauma; lung contusion; amyloidosis

Iatrogenic Causes of Hemoptysis

Oral anticoagulants, heparin
Immunosuppressive drugs (with thrombocytopenic purpura)

*Common causes of hemoptysis in the adult

Contraceptive pills (deep-vein thrombosis with pulmonary infarction)
Medical and surgical procedures: bronchoscopy, transtracheal aspiration, Swan-Ganz
catheterization

HISTORY TAKING*

Possible meaning of a positive response

1 Character of Hemoptysis

1.1 Do you have bleeding from the nose? bleeding oral lesions?

Hemoptysis must be distinguished from epistaxis and other nonpulmonary bleeding

1.2 Was the blood coughed up preceded by
  • a tingling in the throat? a desire to cough?

The blood is coming from the respiratory tract, not from the gastrointestinal tract or nasopharynx with secondary aspiration of blood

  • nausea? vomiting? retching? abdominal discomfort?

Suggests hematemesis rather than hemoptysis

1.3 Is the sputum
  • streaked with blood?

Chronic bronchitis; bronchogenic carcinoma; bronchiectasis

  • intimately mixed with blood?

Bronchogenic carcinoma; lung abscess

  • "rusty"?

Pneumococcal pneumonia (due to degradation products of hemoglobin)

  • currant jelly? (dark blood intermixed with sputum)

Pulmonary infarction; *Klebsiella* pneumonia; necrotizing pneumonia

  • *pink frothy?*

Pulmonary edema; blood mixed with air from the lung (vomiting of blood excluded)

  • blood mixed with pus?

Pneumonia; bronchiectasis; lung abscess

  • frankly bloody? (without mucus or pus)

Pulmonary thromboembolism; mitral stenosis; bronchiectasis (now uncommon); tuberculosis (usually bright red); external trauma to the chest; bleeding tendency

  • at first red and becoming progressively darker for 24 to 48 h?

Prolongation of hemoptysis; common in pulmonary infarction

  • brown? magenta? mixed with food particles?

Vomiting of blood from the stomach rather than hemoptysis from the lung

1.4 After the initial bleeding, have you expectorated blood-tinged sputum for several days?

Usual in hemoptysis; unusual with hematemesis (bleeding from the deep respiratory tract usually recurs over a period of several hours or days)

*In this section, items in *italics* are characteristic clinical features, and items in **boldface** are potentially life-threatening or urgent conditions.

2   Duration of Bleeding

2.1   How long have you noticed the presence of blood in your sputum?

Recent onset in a patient over 45: bronchogenic carcinoma (hemoptysis is more frequent in non-small cell lung cancer, since small cell lung cancer is often submucosal without ulceration into the airway itself). Hemoptysis is rare in metastatic carcinoma to the lung

2.2   Do you have recurrent episodes of minor bleeding?

Chronic bronchitis; bronchiectasis; tuberculosis; mitral stenosis: may be due to rupture of pulmonary-bronchial venous connections, pulmonary edema, pulmonary infarction. Chronic recurrent hemoptysis in a young (otherwise normal) female: bronchial adenoma. Ascribing recurrent episodes of hemoptysis to a previously established diagnosis, such as chronic bronchitis or bronchiectasis, may result in missing a serious, potentially treatable lesion

3   Amount of Blood Coughed Up

3.1   Can you give an estimate of the amount of blood?

Most patients tend to exaggerate the amount of blood coughed up

3.2   Do you have
    • slight, persistent bleeding?

Of recent onset in a patient over 45: bronchogenic carcinoma

    • large amounts of blood coughed up? more than one-half cup?

Rupture of a pulmonary arteriovenous fistula; rupture of aortic aneurysm into the bronchopulmonary tree; inflammatory cause; pulmonary infarction; bleeding within a tuberculous cavity; upper lobe bronchiectasis; Goodpasture's syndrome. **Massive hemoptysis:** greater than 600 to 800 mL in 24 h (3 styrofoam coffee cups hold about 600 mL): high-risk patient

4   Precipitating Factors

4.1   Has hemoptysis occurred after
    • coughing?

Hemoptysis from the trachea, the bronchi, or the lung occurs typically after cough

    • exertion? excitement? sexual intercourse?

In mitral stenosis: sudden elevation in left atrial pressure

5   Accompanying Symptoms

5.1 Do you cough? expectorate?	The blood is usually mixed to some extent with sputum: chronic obstructive pulmonary disease (clear, gray sputum); pulmonary infection, lung abscess (purulent sputum)
• for days to weeks?	Bronchogenic carcinoma; acute bronchitis; pneumonia; tuberculosis. Occurrence of (usually scanty) hemoptysis during the course of a viral or bacterial pneumonia should raise the question of a more serious underlying process
• for months to years?	Chronic productive cough: bronchiectasis; chronic bronchitis
5.2 Do you have • chest pain? • burning? deep? • of sudden onset? *worse by inspiration?*	May localize the side of bleeding Pleural involvement: pulmonary thromboembolism, bronchogenic carcinoma, pneumonia; other pleurally based lesion: lung abscess; coccidioidomycosis cavity; vasculitis
• fever? (chills?)	Pulmonary infection: pneumonia; lung abscess; tuberculosis
• night sweats?	Tuberculosis
• shortness of breath?	Mitral stenosis; chronic bronchitis; pulmonary infarction; bronchogenic carcinoma
• palpitations?	Pulmonary infarction, pneumonia, with reflex tachycardia; atrial fibrillation with pulmonary thromboembolism
• hoarseness?	Bronchogenic carcinoma with recurrent laryngeal nerve compression; tuberculous laryngitis
• a loss of weight? a loss of appetite?	Bronchogenic carcinoma; tuberculosis; lung abscess
• a swollen, painful leg?	Deep-vein thrombosis with pulmonary thromboembolism
• bloody urine?	Goodpasture's syndrome; Wegener's granulomatosis
• purulent rhinorrhea? nasal or sinus pain?	(With renal disease): Wegener's granulomatosis; sinusitis may coexist with bronchiectasis

6   Iatrogenic Factors   See Etiology

7   Personal and Social Profile

7.1 Do you smoke?	The heavy smoker is liable to chronic obstructive pulmonary disease, bronchogenic carcinoma

7.2 Have you recently been exposed to a person with tuberculosis?

7.3 What is your occupation? — Pneumoconiosis in coal miners; possible exposure to toxic inhalants

7.4 Do you have any birds? pigeons? — Psittacosis

7.5 Do you use intravenous drugs? — Septic pulmonary emboli

7.6 Have you ever lived in
- the southwestern United States? California? Arizona? Texas? — Coccidioidomycosis (hemoptysis infrequent)
- the central United States? Mississippi, Missouri, Ohio River valleys? — Histoplasmosis
- the Far East? Vietnam? foreign countries? — Tuberculosis is more frequent in foreign countries

8 Personal Antecedents Pertaining to the Hemoptysis

8.1 Do you have
- frequent episodes of bronchitis? pneumonia? — Bronchiectasis; chronic bronchitis; mitral stenosis
- a prior history of tuberculosis? — Hemoptysis originating in a tuberculous cavity or a bronchiectatic segment
- a chronic sinusitis? — Frequently present in diffuse bronchiectasis
- a heart condition? — Congestive heart failure with deep-vein thrombosis and pulmonary infarction; left-heart failure with pulmonary edema; mitral stenosis; Eisenmenger's syndrome
- a renal disease? — Goodpasture's syndrome; Wegener's granulomatosis
- a bleeding tendency? — Telangiectasia of the lung (hemoptysis is rare in other bleeding tendencies)
- a recent operation? prolonged immobilization? — Deep-vein thrombosis with pulmonary thromboembolism
- a recent blunt trauma to the chest? — Lung contusion
- peptic ulcer? gastrointestinal bleeding? — Suggests hematemesis rather than hemoptysis

9 Family Medical History Pertaining to the Hemoptysis

9.1 Is there a history of blood sputum in your family? — Tuberculosis; hereditary hemorrhagic telangiectasia with pulmonary arteriovenous malformations

PHYSICAL SIGNS PERTAINING TO HEMOPTYSIS

	Possible significance
Examination of the nose, mouth, throat, larynx	The blood may be coming from the nasopharynx
Prolonged expiration; diffuse rhonchi and wheezes (with sputum production)	Significant bronchitis; bronchiectasis with airway obstruction
Increased tactile and vocal fremitus; bronchial breath sounds; crackles	Pulmonary signs of consolidation: bacterial pneumonia, lung abscess, lung tumor, pulmonary infarction
Localized wheeze	Bronchial obstruction: bronchogenic carcinoma, foreign body
Pleural friction rub	Pleurally based lesion: pulmonary embolism with infarction; pneumonia; lung abscess; vasculitis
Heart murmur	Mitral stenosis; congenital heart disease with pulmonary hypertension; Eisenmenger's syndrome
Deep-vein thrombosis; tachycardia	Pulmonary embolism with infarction
Fever; weight loss; posttussive crackles	Tuberculosis
Clubbing	Bronchogenic carcinoma; lung abscess; bronchiectasis
Telangiectases on skin and mucosae; continuous murmur over the lung fields	Hereditary hemorrhagic telangiectasia with pulmonary arteriovenous malformation

LABORATORY PROCEDURES PERTAINING TO HEMOPTYSIS[†]

Procedure	To Detect
Chest x-ray	Mass lesion: pulmonary neoplasm; pulmonary arteriovenous malformation; blood pneumonitis: aspiration of blood into contiguous areas
	Primary complex, apical infiltration, cavitary lesion: tuberculosis
	Cavitary lesion, air-fluid level: lung abscess

†See the appendix on Laboratory Reference Values for the associated normal laboratory values.

Procedure	To Detect
Chest x-ray *(continued)*	Lobar consolidation: bacterial pneumonia
	A mass within a cavity: aspergilloma
	Ring shadows, "tram lines", cyst formation: bronchiectasis
	Characteristic cardiac silhouette, Kerley B lines: mitral stenosis
Bronchoscopy	Rigid: visualization of the more central airway
	Fiberoptic: visualization of the smaller central airways
Blood	
Hematocrit	Anemia: underlying malignancy; Wegener's granulomatosis; iron-deficiency anemia: in Goodpasture's syndrome, idiopathic pulmonary hemosiderosis (hemoptysis is an uncommon cause of anemia)
BUN, creatinine	Uremia: in Goodpasture's syndrome, Wegener's granulomatosis
Hemostasis studies	Bleeding tendency
Sputum examination; culture, cytology	Tubercle bacilli; fungi; malignant cells

When indicated: thoracic computerized tomography; bronchography; ventilation-perfusion lung scans; pulmonary angiography

SELECTED BIBLIOGRAPHY

Adelman M, Haponik EF, Bleecker ER et al: Cryptogenic hemoptysis. *Ann Intern Med* 102:829–834, 1985.
Israel RH, Poe RH: Hemoptysis. *Clin Chest Med* 8(2):197–205, 1987.
Johnston H, Reisz G: Changing spectrum of hemoptysis. *Arch Intern Med* 149:1666–1668, 1989.

9
Hypertension

INTRODUCTION

Hypertension   Arterial pressure above 140/90 mmHg in a resting adult (which has been clearly established by repeated determinations).

The blood pressure is determined by the product of cardiac output and peripheral resistance. These factors are in turn modified by blood volume, stroke volume, pulse rate, blood viscosity, elasticity of blood vessels, neurogenic, and humoral stimuli (catecholamines, renin, angiotensin II, aldosterone, kinins, prostaglandins, arginine vasopressin, atrial natriuretic peptide). Essential hypertension (over 95 percent of cases) is arterial hypertension of unknown cause. Various pathogenic mechanisms have been implicated: increased peripheral vascular resistance, increased sympathetic stimulation, enhanced vascular responses to stress, deficient depressor activity, renal sodium retention, increased intracellular sodium and calcium, increased sodium intake, and genetic factors. If a defined cause of hypertension is found, the patient has secondary hypertension.

In most renal diseases, reduced perfusion of renal tissue activates the renin-angiotensin system. Angiotensin II is a potent vasoconstrictor and also causes the liberation of aldosterone, which acts at the renal tubule to facilitate sodium reabsorption and expansion of intravascular volume. Hypertension in renal parenchymal disease has also been attributed to failure by the kidney to destroy circulating vasopressor substances, failure to produce a vasodilator substance (? prostaglandin, ? bradykinin), production of an unidentified vasopressor substance other than renin, and retention of sodium.

Classification of Blood Pressure (BP)

Range, mmHg	Category

Diastolic

<85	Normal BP
85–89	High-normal BP
90–104	Mild hypertension
105–114	Moderate hypertension
≥115	Severe hypertension

Systolic, when diastolic BP is < 90 mmHg

<140	Normal BP
140–159	Borderline isolated systolic hypertension
≥160	Isolated systolic hypertension

ETIOLOGY

Systolic and Diastolic Hypertension

Primary: essential hypertension
Secondary
  Renal: chronic pyelonephritis; acute and chronic glomerulonephritis; diabetic
    nephropathy; polycystic renal disease; hydronephrosis; partial occlusion of renal
    artery; renal infarction; arteriolar nephrosclerosis; polyarteritis nodosa; systemic
    lupus erythematosus; renin-producing tumor
  Endocrine: adrenocortical hyperfunction (Cushing's syndrome, primary
    aldosteronism, adrenogenital syndromes); pheochromocytoma; acromegaly;
    hyperparathyroidism; hyperthyroidism; hypothyroidism
  Neurogenic: familial dysautonomia; acute porphyria, lead poisoning; acute in-
    creased intracranial pressure; sleep apnea; Guillain-Barré syndrome
  Miscellaneous: coarctation of the aorta; increased intravascular volume; psy-
    chogenic hyperventilation; acute stress; pregnancy-induced hypertension

Systolic Hypertension

Decreased compliance of aorta: arteriosclerosis
Increased cardiac output: arteriovenous fistula; aortic valvular regurgitation; thyro-
    toxicosis; fever; Paget's disease of bone; hyperkinetic heart syndrome; patent
    ductus arteriosus; beriberi

Iatrogenic Causes of Hypertension

Sympathomimetics; nasal decongestants; cold remedies; oral contraceptives; cortico-
    steroids; licorice; thyroid hormones; anorexigenics; cyclosporine; nonsteroidal
    anti-inflammatory agents; monoamine oxidase inhibitors; tricyclic antidepressants;
    clonidine withdrawal

HISTORY TAKING*

	Possible meaning of a positive response
1 Mode of Onset and Evolution	
1.1 At what time was high blood pressure first observed?	
• before age 35?	Secondary hypertension; acute glomerulonephritis
• between the ages of 35 and 55?	Essential hypertension
• after age 55?	Secondary hypertension; renovascular cause

*In this section, items in *italics* are characteristic clinical features, and items in **boldface** are
potentially life-threatening or urgent conditions.

1.2	How was your high blood pressure detected?	Many patients with hypertension are identified in the course of routine examination and have no symptoms referable to the high blood pressure
1.3	Is your blood pressure • variable?	Most patients with labile hypertension eventually develop sustained hypertension
	• constantly elevated?	
1.3a	What was the highest level of your elevated blood pressure?	Important in determining the approach to treatment
1.4	Has your blood pressure recently increased over previous high levels?	**Accelerated or malignant hypertension**

2   Precipitating or Aggravating Factors

2.1	What is your daily salt intake?	A high sodium intake may maintain the hypertension of some patients and limit the effectiveness of certain antihypertensive drugs
2.2	For female patients: Are you pregnant?	Pregnancy-induced hypertension: developing after the 20th week of gestation (preeclampsia if associated proteinuria or edema; eclampsia: the above, plus convulsions); chronic hypertension of whatever cause (usually essential hypertension)
2.2a	Do you take contraceptive pills?	May be the most common cause of secondary hypertension. Hypertension due to estrogen-containing oral contraceptives is attributed to activation of the renin-angiotensin-aldosterone system. It is often reversible within 3 to 6 months, but it may persist after the oral contraceptive is discontinued
2.3	Has your weight recently increased?	Hypertension is more common among obese individuals: (?) due to increased blood volume, stroke volume, and cardiac output

3   Accompanying Symptoms

Reflect the effects of hypertension on its target organs—the eyes, the heart, the brain, the kidneys. Uncomplicated hypertension is almost always asymptomatic

3.1 Do you have
   • headaches?

      Could be nonspecific; often psychogenic. Episodic: pheochromocytoma (a rare cause of hypertension: 1 in 1000 hypertensive patients)

   • *occipital? upon awakening in the morning?* wearing off after several hours?

      May occur in hypertension with diastolic pressure greater than 120 mmHg

   • severe headache? vomiting? visual disturbances? transient weakness?

      Manifestations of **hypertensive encephalopathy** with diastolic blood pressure usually > 140 mmHg

   • lightheadedness? vertigo? tinnitus?

      Possible CNS dysfunction in longstanding hypertension

   • syncope upon standing?

      Cerebrovascular insufficiency; diabetic neuropathy; postural hypotension in pheochromocytoma

   • episodes of weakness? dizziness?

      Transient cerebral ischemic attacks: develop more commonly on the background of hypertension

   • shortness of breath?

      Left ventricular failure complicating hypertension: rise in left atrial and pulmonary venous pressure

   • chest pain on exertion?

      Angina pectoris due to accelerated coronary artery sclerosis and increased myocardial oxygen requirements due to the increased myocardial mass. Vascular disease has progressed to dangerous stages

   • pain in the calves when walking?

      Arteriosclerotic involvement of the blood vessels of the legs with intermittent claudication; hypertension is a major risk factor for the development of arteriosclerosis obliterans

   • foot or ankle swelling?

      Congestive heart failure

   • pain on urination? blood in your urine?

      Renal cause of hypertension

   • an increased daily urine volume? an increased intake of fluids?

      Polyuria and polydipsia suggest renal or endocrine disease; hypokalemia with primary aldosteronism

   • frequent micturition during the night?

      Nocturia of renal or endocrine disease. Nocturnal frequency may occur when diastolic pressure is 120 mmHg or more

   • muscle cramps? weakness?

      Primary aldosteronism

   • blurred vision? a decrease in visual acuity?

      Indicates the presence of retinal cotton wool spots and/or macular edema; branch retinal vein occlusion

3.2 Do you have spells of headaches? sweating? palpitations? nervousness?

      Pheochromocytoma

4   **Iatrogenic Factors   See Etiology**

5 Personal and Social Profile

5.1 Do you smoke?

Cigarette smoking is not a risk factor for the development of hypertension; however, hypertensive smokers are at significantly greater risk to develop cardiovascular complications and appear to have a higher frequency of malignant hypertension and renal artery stenosis

5.2 What is your alcohol consumption?

Excess alcohol intake may lead to elevated blood pressure, poor adherence to antihypertensive therapy, and, occasionally, refractory hypertension

5.3 What is your fat intake?

The diet can contribute to hyperlipidemia or diabetes mellitus

5.4 Do you exercise regularly? Do you engage in sports?

Physical fitness may help prevent hypertension; hypertensive patients may lower their blood pressure by means of regular isotonic exercise

5.5 Are you under emotional stress at work? at home?

May influence blood pressure control

6 Personal Antecedents Pertaining to the Hypertension

6.1 Have you ever had a chest x-ray? an ECG? a urinalysis? an IV pyelogram? an eye examination? When? With what results?

6.2 Have you ever been treated for your high blood pressure? Name(s) of the drug(s)? Dosage? Duration of therapy? Results and side effects?

6.3 Do you have any of the following conditions:
- a heart disease? a heart murmur?

Coarctation of the aorta; aortic valvular regurgitation

- a kidney disease? repeated urinary infections? an episode of acute flank pain?

Renal parenchymal disease is one of the most common cause of secondary hypertension; volume excess is the predominant mechanism for hypertension in renal insufficiency. Primary hypertension is a common cause of progressive renal damage

- a previous stroke? transient ischemic attacks?

Involvement of the brain. Hypertension is the major risk factor for both thrombotic and hemorrhagic strokes

• diabetes?

Patients with hypertension and diabetes are very vulnerable to cardiovascular complications. Diabetes mellitus may be associated with accelerated arteriosclerosis, renal vascular disease, and diabetic nephropathy

• lipid abnormalities?

Hypercholesterolemia is a major cardiovascular risk factor

7 Family Medical History Pertaining to the Hypertension

7.1 Are there any members of your family who have
• hypertension?

Essential hypertension. Family diseases related to secondary causes of hypertension: pheochromocytoma; polycystic renal disease. A positive family history does not exclude the possibility of secondary causes

• a myocardial infarction? cerebrovascular disease? diabetes?

A family history of early deaths due to cardiovascular disease may justify a more aggressive treatment of the patient

PHYSICAL SIGNS PERTAINING TO HYPERTENSION

Possible significance

Response of diastolic blood pressure to standing:

orthostatic drop (in the absence of antihypertensive medications)

Secondary forms of hypertension; pheochromocytoma; autonomic dysfunction from diabetes

orthostatic rise

Essential hypertension

Cardiomegaly; left ventricular lift; accentuated aortic second sound; presystolic (atrial) gallop rhythm

Hypertensive heart disease with left ventricular hypertrophy: severe and/or long-standing hypertension

Significant bruit over carotid arteries

Atherosclerotic involvement of carotid arteries; stenosis of a carotid artery (may be associated with a renal arterial lesion)

Systolic murmur over the base of the heart; palpable collateral circulation on chest; decreased and/or delayed femoral pulses; blood pressure in legs 20 to 30 mmHg lower than in arms

Coarctation of the aorta

Bruits in the epigastrium or in the flanks

Renal artery narrowing

Renal mass	Polycystic renal disease; renal carcinoma
Tachycardia, orthostatic hypotension, sweating, pallor, hypertension triggered by abdominal palpation	Pheochromocytoma
Round plethoric facies; truncal obesity; purple striae; hirsutism	Cushing's syndrome
Abnormal neurologic examination	Previous cerebrovascular accident; intracranial pathologic change
Café au lait spots	Neurofibromatosis with associated pheochromocytoma
Funduscopic examination:	Indicates the duration and prognosis of hypertension
diffuse narrowing; arteriolar tortuosity	Grade I hypertensive retinopathy
arteriovenous nicking, segmental spasm	Grade II
linear hemorrhages; cotton-wool exudates	Grade III: progression or acceleration of hypertension
papilledema, hemorrhages, exudates; arterioles threadlike or invisible	Grade IV: malignant hypertension; often associated with arteriolar nephrosclerosis and a poor prognosis

LABORATORY TESTS PERTAINING TO HYPERTENSION[†]

Test	To Detect
For most patients: hemoglobin, hematocrit; urinalysis; blood: electrolytes, glucose, creatinine and/or BUN, cholesterol, uric acid; ECG, chest x-ray	To ascertain the degree of end-organ damage resulting from hypertension; to identify patients at high risk for cardiovascular complications; to screen for secondary, possibly reversible forms of hypertension; to provide baseline values for judging biochemical effects of therapy
For patients with features suggesting a secondary form of hypertension:	
24-h urine test for cortisol <100 μg/24 h	Rules out Cushing's syndrome
Vanillylmandelic acid (urine) >8 mg/24 h; free urinary catecholamines >110 μg/24 h	Pheochromocytoma

[†]See the appendix on Laboratory Reference Values for the associated normal laboratory values.

Test	To Detect
Hypokalemia; plasma aldosterone elevated	Primary or secondary aldosteronism
Plasma renin activity	
high	Secondary aldosteronism
low	Primary aldosteronism
Renal ultrasonography; IV pyelography; renal angiography	Chronic renal disease; renovascular disease

SELECTED BIBLIOGRAPHY

Frohlich ED (ed): Essential hypertension. *Med Clin North Am* 71(5):785–1049, 1987.

1988 Joint National Committee: The 1988 Report of the Joint National Committee on detection, evaluation, and treatment of high blood pressure. *Arch Intern Med* 148:1023–1038, 1988.

Prisant LM, Carr AA: Initial evaluation of the hypertensive patient. *Postgrad Med* 84(8):197–217, 1988.

10
Palpitations

INTRODUCTION

Palpitation   Unpleasant awareness of the heart's action, whether slow or fast, regular or irregular.

The healthy subject of average temperament is unaware of the beating of the heart under ordinary circumstances. Palpitation is a normal sensation when the force of the heartbeat and its rate are considerably elevated, as in strenuous physical effort or emotional stress. Certain pathologic conditions with hyperkinetic—high cardiac output—states (anemia, high fever, thyrotoxicosis) may be associated with increased contractility and tachycardia, and may give rise to palpitation.

Common causes of palpitations are ectopic tachycardias and unusual motion of the heart within the chest (ectopic beats, compensatory pause following extrasystoles). Heavy and regular palpitation is usually due to an augmented stroke volume (valvular regurgitation, ventricular septal defect). The onset of bradycardia (sudden development of heart block) may also give rise to palpitation. Palpitation is particularly prominent when the precipitating cause for increased heart rate or contractility or arrhythmia is recent, transient, and episodic.

In anxious patients the threshold of consciousness of the heart's beating may be so lowered that palpitation may occur with normal rhythm and rate.

ETIOLOGY

Anxiety states; neurocirculatory asthenia; mitral valve prolapse
Cardiac arrhythmias
   Premature contractions: ventricular, supraventricular
   Tachyarrhythmias
      Paroxysmal supraventricular tachycardia; atrial tachycardia with block; atrial flutter; atrial fibrillation; nonparoxysmal junctional tachycardia; ventricular tachycardia; preexcitation syndromes
   Bradyarrhythmias
      Sinus bradycardia; sino-atrial block; atrio-ventricular (AV) junctional rhythm; AV conduction blocks
   Sick-sinus syndrome
Palpitations not associated with arrhythmias
   Anemia; fever; hypotension; pulmonary emboli; shock; congestive heart failure; thyrotoxicosis; hypoglycemia; pheochromocytoma; arteriovenous fistula; aortic aneurysm; marked cardiomegaly (aortic valvular disease; hypertensive cardiovascular disease); alcohol; tobacco; coffee; tea; drugs

Iatrogenic Causes of Palpitation

Arrhythmias: sympathomimetics; atropine; thyroid hormone; digitalis; quinidine; procainamide; beta-adrenergic blockers; calcium channel antagonists; other antiarrhythmic drugs; guanethidine; emetine; propellants in aerosols; tricyclic anti depressants; phenothiazines; lithium; anticholinesterases; papaverine; daunomy- cine; adriamycine; lincomycin (intravenous)

HISTORY TAKING*

Possible meaning of a positive response

1 Duration of Palpitations

1.1 How long have you had palpita- tions?
   • from youth?

Ectopic tachycardia in preexcitation (Wolff-Parkinson-White) syndrome; idiopathic long Q-T syndrome

1.2 *Do you have recurrent attacks of pal- pitations?*

Paroxysmal supraventricular or ven- tricular tachycardia; paroxysmal atrial fibrillation or flutter; Wolff-Parkinson- White syndrome with recurrent epi- sodes of supraventricular tachycardia; pheochromocytoma

1.2a How frequently do these episodes occur?

1.2b How long do these attacks last?
   • an instant? about a minute?
   • a few minutes? an hour or more?

Extrasystoles
(Paroxysmal) ectopic tachycardia

2 Character of Palpitations

2.1 Do you feel
   • heart fluttering? beating rapidly?

Sensation of disturbed heartbeat: tachy- cardia

   • skipped beats? "flopping" sensa- tion? isolated "jumps"? "as if your heart is turning over"?

Extrasystoles and/or postpremature beats: the most common causes of pal- pitations; atrioventricular (AV) block with dropped beats

   • an unusually vigorous beat? "pounding"? "thudding"?
   • as if your heart stopped beating?

First ventricular contraction succeeding a compensatory pause
Compensatory pause following the pre- mature contraction

   • slow beating?

Atrio-ventricular block; sick-sinus syn- drome

2.2 Are onset and cessation of the attacks

*In this section, items in *italics* are characteristic clinical features.

• *abrupt? instantaneous?*

Paroxysmal supraventricular tachycardias (may appear to end gradually because of sinus tachycardia following them); atrial flutter; paroxysmal atrial fibrillation; paroxysmal AV junctional tachycardia; paroxysmal ventricular tachycardia (ventricular tachycardia is not usually associated with palpitations, perhaps because of the reduced cardiac output)

• gradual? (over minutes or seconds)

Sinus tachycardia; anxiety states; paroxysmal atrial tachycardia with block; multifocal atrial tachycardia; nonparoxysmal junctional tachycardia

2.3 Is the rapid heart action
• regular?

Anxiety state; sinus tachycardia; paroxysmal ectopic tachycardias

• irregular? chaotic?

Atrial fibrillation; fibrillo-flutter; atrial tachycardia with block

• fleeting and repetitive?

Multiple ectopic beats

2.4 How fast is your pulse rate during the palpitations?
• too fast to be counted?

Atrial fibrillation; ectopic tachycardia

2.5 Can you tap out with a finger what the rhythm feels like to you?

Assists the patient in describing what he/she means by "palpitations." Helps establish the rate and rhythm of the arrhythmia

3 Precipitating or Aggravating Factors

3.1 Do you have palpitations
• during or after strenuous physical activity?

Normal awareness of an overactive heart; paroxysmal atrial tachycardia

• during mild exertion?

Heart failure; atrial fibrillation; anemia; thyrotoxicosis; patient severely "out of condition"

• with effort? excitement?

Sinus tachycardia; underlying cardiac disease; paroxysmal atrial fibrillation

• on standing?

Postural hypotension resulting in reflex sinus tachycardia

• at rest? independently of exercise or excitement?

Atrial fibrillation; atrial flutter; thyrotoxicosis; febrile states; hypoglycemia; severe anemia; anxiety states

• when lying on your left side?

Occasionally in healthy subjects: better transmission of the heart sounds to the ear

• at night? during introspective moments?

Increased awareness of the heartbeat

- after a meal? after drinking coffee? tea? alcohol? after smoking?
- when tired? anxious? after a sudden emotional tension?

Precipitating factors in any arrhythmia; extrasystoles; sinus tachycardia
Anxiety state; an emotional upset may precipitate paroxysmal ectopic tachycardia; premature atrial complexes

4 Relieving Factors

4.1 Are your palpitations relieved or less marked by
- lying down?
- *breathholding? massaging the neck? stooping? inducing gagging or vomiting?*

- belching?
- activity?

- medications? which ones?

Paroxysmal ectopic tachycardia
Vagal stimulation (carotid sinus pressure, Valsalva maneuver) bringing to an end paroxysmal supraventricular tachycardia
Aerophagia; associated anxiety state
May bring about decreased awareness of the heartbeat in anxiety state

5 Accompanying Symptoms

5.1 Are your palpitations accompanied or followed by
- syncope? faintness?

- anxiety? a lump in your throat? dizziness? giddiness? tingling in the hands and face?
- a blurring of vision? buzzing in the ears?
- sweating? flushes? sweats?

- a sensation of hunger? trembling? weakness?
- headaches?

- breathing trouble?

- sighing?
- chest pain?

  - localized to the apex? lancinating? sticking? independently of your palpitations?

Syncope may occur during sinus node dysfunction, tachyarrhythmias; AV block; total cardiac asystole or severe bradycardia following the termination of a tachyarrhythmia; Stokes-Adams attack in AV block; hypoglycemia
Sinus tachycardia accompanying an anxiety state with hyperventilation

Decrease in cerebral circulation secondary to the tachycardia
Anxiety states; thyrotoxicosis; hypoglycemia; pheochromocytoma
Hypoglycemia

Pheochromocytoma; hypoglycemia; anxiety state
Anxiety state with hyperventilation; dyspnea in anemia; congestive heart failure
Anxiety state
Myocardial ischemia precipitated by increased oxygen demands induced by the rapid heart rate
Anxiety state; mitral valve prolapse

• fever?	Acute infections; acute rheumatic fever with carditis; thyrotoxicosis
• intolerance to heat?	Thyrotoxicosis

5.2 After your episodes of palpitations, do you
• urinate more than usual? — Polyuria following paroxysmal supraventricular tachycardia lasting over 20 minutes (due to increased plasma levels of atrial natriuretic peptide?)

• feel tired? for many hours? — Common with supraventricular tachycardias

6 Iatrogenic Factors   See Etiology

7 Personal and Social Profile

7.1 Age of the patient? — Older patients: sick-sinus syndrome; coronary artery disease
Young (women): mitral valve prolapse; anxiety

7.2 What is your daily intake of coffee? tea?

7.2a Do you have palpitations after unusual alcohol ingestion? — Cardiac arrhythmias, most commonly atrial, associated with acute alcoholic states

7.3 What is your occupation? — Cardiac arrhythmias due to solvents, fluorocarbone in: metal cleaning, solvents use, refrigerator maintenance

8 Personal Antecedents Pertaining to the Palpitations

8.1 Have you ever had an ECG? a thyroid examination? When? With what results?

8.2 Do you have any of the following conditions: a cardiac condition? high blood pressure? anemia? a thyroid condition? emotional problems? diabetes?

9 Family Medical History Pertaining to the Palpitations

9.1 Are there any members of your family who also have palpitations? a cardiac disease? sudden death? — Relatives of patients with preexcitation syndrome have an increased prevalence of preexcitation. Familial, congenital long Q-T syndrome; mitral valve prolapse

PHYSICAL SIGNS PERTAINING TO PALPITATIONS

	Possible significance
Normal heart rate with irregular rhythm	Frequent premature beats; atrial fibrillation with ventricular rate slowed by medication; sinus arrhythmia; partial heart block with dropped beats
Regular tachycardia (>100 beats per minute) with	
<150 beats per minute	Sinus tachycardia; anxiety state; ectopic tachycardia with AV block; nonparoxysmal junctional tachycardia
about 150 beats per minute	Atrial flutter with 2:1 AV conduction ratio
≥170 beats per minute	Ectopic tachycardia
Tachycardia with irregular rhythm	Atrial fibrillation; atrial flutter with varying block; paroxysmal supraventricular tachycardia with block; sinus tachycardia with numerous premature beats; sick-sinus syndrome
Irregular tachycardia with	
• a predictable basic cadence	"Regular irregularity": frequent premature beats
• an entirely unpredictable cadence	"Irregular irregularity": atrial fibrillation
Regular bradycardia (<60 beats per minute)	Sinus bradycardia; sick-sinus syndrome; AV junctional rhythm; complete AV block
Irregular bradycardia	Sinoatrial bradycardia with marked sinus arrhythmia or frequent premature beats; partial block with frequent dropped beats or changing degrees of block
Constant intensity of first heart sound and amplitude of peripheral pulse	Sinus, paroxysmal supraventricular, junctional tachycardia
Variable intensity of first heart sound and amplitude of peripheral pulse	Complete AV heart block; ventricular tachycardia; atrial fibrillation; atrial flutter
Inspection of jugular venous pulse:	
"cannon" a waves	Right atrium contracting against a closed tricuspid valve during ventricular systole: complete AV block; junctional or ventricular tachycardia
a waves at 250 to 350 beats per minute	Atrial flutter

Effect of exercise on an irregular rhythm:

disappearance of irregularity	Extrasystoles
increase of irregularity	Atrial fibrillation

Effect of carotid sinus massage on tachy-cardia:	This maneuver (not to be performed over a vessel with a bruit) elicits vagal efferent impulses influencing auto-maticity and conduction, slowing the rate of sinus nodal discharge and pro-longing AV nodal conduction time and refractoriness
no change in rate	Ventricular tachycardia; AV junctional rhythm; may also occur in supraven-tricular tachycardia
abrupt termination persisting after discontinuation of massage (or no change)	Paroxysmal supraventricular tachy-cardia
gradual slowing and return to former rate	Sinus tachycardia; atrial fibrillation
abrupt slowing and return to former rate	Atrial flutter
Enlarged thyroid; tremor; warm, moist skin	Thyrotoxicosis
Fever	The pulse rate in general rises about 9 beats per minute .for each degree Fahrenheit of temperature elevation

LABORATORY TESTS PERTAINING TO PALPITATIONS[†]

Procedure	To Detect
ECG; ECG exercise testing; ambulatory ECG monitoring; intracardiac electro-physiologic studies*	Cardiac arrhythmias; Wolff-Parkinson-White syndrome
Thyroid function tests	Thyrotoxicosis

[†]See the appendix on Laboratory Reference Values for the associated normal laboratory values.
*When indicated

SELECTED BIBLIOGRAPHY

Schmidt PJ, Ezri MD, Denes P: Cardiac arrhythmias-Update 1987. *DM* 33(7):365–432, 1987.
Zipes DP (ed): Symposium on cardiac arrhythmias, I and II. *Med Clin North Am* 68(4):795–1012; 68(5):1013–1390, 1984.

Digestive System

11
Abdominal Distention

INTRODUCTION

Abdominal Distention Sudden or gradual increase in the size of the abdomen.

Abdominal distention may be due to enlarged organs, masses, gaseous distention of the bowel, or accumulation of fluid in the peritoneal cavity (ascites).

In normal subjects, volumes of gas present in the intestine at any one time range from 30 to 200 mL. Gases are produced within the colon from bacterial fermentation of unabsorbed nutrients (especially dietary carbohydrates) or organic substances secreted into the lumen. Stomach gas has the composition of swallowed air. Increased amounts of gas in the intestinal tract may be due to aerophagia (excessive swallowing of air) or to increased intestinal gas production following the ingestion of certain foods containing nonabsorbable carbohydrates or in conditions associated with abnormal bacterial colonization of the small intestine. In acute intestinal obstruction, distention of the intestine is caused by the accumulation of gas and fluid proximal to, and within, the obstructed segment.

Subjective abdominal distention is usually transient and often due to a functional gastrointestinal disorder when it is not accompanied by objective physical findings of increased abdominal girth or local swelling.

The pathophysiologic mechanisms of ascites vary with the cause. Cirrhotic ascites results from increased portal venous hydrostatic pressure, increased renal sodium reabsorption, decreased portal venous colloid osmotic pressure, increased hepatic lymph formation, and decreased renal free-water excretion. Noncirrhotic ascites may be due to increased subperitoneal capillary permeability, decreased peritoneal lymphatic drainage, increased hydrostatic pressure within the hepatic sinusoids, leakage from disrupted abdominal viscera, and decreased renal sodium excretion.

ETIOLOGY

Localized

Hepatomegaly; splenomegaly; renal tumor or cyst; pancreatic cyst or tumor; uterine enlargement; ovarian mass; distended urinary bladder; abdominal wall hernia; inflammatory mass

Generalized Abdominal Distention Without Ascites (increased amounts of gas in the gastrointestinal tract)

Irritable bowel syndrome
Intestinal pseudo-obstruction
Adynamic ileus; mechanical intestinal obstruction
Aerophagia
Malabsorption; chronic pancreatic insufficiency
Following surgical procedures

Ascites

Transudative

Cirrhosis*
Right-sided cardiac valvular disease;* constrictive pericarditis
Hypoalbuminemia: nephrotic syndrome;* protein-losing gastroenteropathy
Hepatic vein thrombosis (Budd-Chiari syndrome)
Inferior vena cava obstruction; portal vein obstruction
Meigs's syndrome (ovarian fibroma with ascites and hydrothorax)

Exudative

Peritonitis: bacterial, tuberculous; ruptured viscus
Pancreatitis; leaking pseudocyst; bile peritonitis
Tumors; metastatic to the liver or peritoneum; disseminated carcinomatosis*
Myxedema

Chylous (lymphatic obstruction)

Abdominal neoplasm, lymphoma; mediastinal tumors
Trauma to the thoracic duct in the chest
Filariasis
Congenital lymphangiectasia
Occasionally: tuberculosis; cirrhosis; nephrotic syndrome

Iatrogenic Causes of Obstruction or Ileus

Aluminum hydroxide; calcium carbonate; barium sulfate; tricyclic antidepressants; phenothiazines; ion-exchange resins; ferrous sulfate; opiates; ganglionic blockers

HISTORY TAKING†

Possible meaning of a positive response

1   Mode of Onset and Duration

1.1   How long have you had a distended abdomen?

Considerable abdominal enlargement may go unnoticed for weeks or months, because of coexistent obesity or because the ascites formation has been insidious, without pain or localizing symptoms. Conditions that may mimic ascites: pregnancy, ovarian cyst, pancreatic cyst, mesenteric cyst, obesity

*Common cause of ascites
†In this section, items in *italics* are characteristic clinical features, and items in **boldface** are potentially life-threatening or urgent conditions.

1.2 Did you notice it because of
- a sensation of pressure or fullness in the abdomen? — Not specific; irritable bowel syndrome or ascites
- *a progressive increase in your belt or clothing size?* — Organic abdominal swelling; ascites
- the appearance of abdominal or inguinal hernias?
- the development of a localized swelling? — Neoplastic peritoneal involvement; metastatic liver

2 Character of the Abdominal Swelling

2.1 Is the abdominal distention
- intermittent? — Increased amounts of gas in the gastrointestinal tract; irritable bowel syndrome; intestinal pseudo-obstruction
- permanent? — Ascites; intraabdominal masses
- increasing? — Worsening of ascites in a cirrhotic patient suggests: hepatoma; portal vein thrombosis; spontaneous bacterial peritonitis; tuberculous peritonitis

2.2 Has the abdominal distention appeared
- rapidly? (days) — Rapid accumulation of ascites; rapidly expanding mass; intestinal obstruction
- gradually? (weeks) — Ascites formation may be insidious: cirrhosis of the liver

3 Precipitating and Relieving Factors

3.1 If the abdominal distention is intermittent, does it occur after eating?

3.1a Is it relieved by the passing of gas? belching? defecation? — Gaseous distention of the gastrointestinal tract

4 Accompanying Symptoms

4.1 Has your weight
- *increased?* — Ascites
- remained unchanged? — Increased amounts of gas in the gastrointestinal tract
- decreased? — Neoplastic intraabdominal process; cirrhosis of the liver; carcinomatosis with peritoneal involvement; tuberculous peritonitis; hepatoma

4.2 Do you have
- a sensation of "pulling" or "stretching" of the flanks or groins? a vague low back pain? — Progressive abdominal distention

• pain in the abdomen?

Patients complaining of bloating and "gas pains" have normal intestinal gas volume; abnormal intestinal motor activity usually accounts for their symptoms. Pain is uncommon in cirrhosis with ascites

  • localized?

Involvement of an abdominal organ, e.g., passively congestive liver, hepatoma, large spleen, colonic tumor

  • diffuse?

Peritonitis; pancreatitis; **intestinal obstruction**

4.3 Are your legs swollen?

Ascites with generalized edema

4.3a Were the legs swollen
  • *before the appearance of the abdominal distention?*

Dependent edema appears prior to ascites in right-sided congestive heart failure

  • after the appearance of the abdominal distention?

Ascites usually occurs early, prior to dependent edema, in cirrhosis, constrictive pericarditis

4.4 Do you have
  • heartburn? indigestion?

Gastroesophageal reflux due to tense ascites or abdominal tumors producing increased intraabdominal pressure

  • recent severe constipation? vomiting?

Intestinal obstruction; vomiting occurs earlier and is more severe, the higher the intestinal obstruction

  • shortness of breath?

Dyspnea, orthopnea, tachypnea, in combined congestive heart disease; elevation of the diaphragm due to ascites or abdominal tumor; coexistent pleural effusion (usually right-sided): presumably due to leakage of ascitic fluid through lymphatic channels in the diaphragm

  • puffiness of the face?

Generalized edema; nephrotic syndrome

  • a change in the volume of your urine?

Commonly decreased in ascites

  • bloody urine?

Acute glomerulonephritis

  • brown urine?

Hepatic disease with bilirubinuria

  • a loss of appetite?

Cirrhosis; peritoneal carcinomatosis; hepatoma

  • a change in your bowel habits?

Colonic tumor with peritoneal seeding

  • chronic diarrhea?

Malabsorption with abdominal distention

5 **Iatrogenic Factors   See Etiology**

6 **Personal and Social Profile**

6.1 What is your alcohol intake?

Cirrhosis with ascites

6.2 What is your occupation?

Bartenders, brewery workers: liable to alcoholism with cirrhosis and ascites

6.3   What is your usual diet?   May reveal malnutrition with hypoal-
                                                  buminemia and edema

7   Personal Antecedents Pertaining to the Abdominal Distention

7.1   Have you ever had liver or renal
      tests? When? With what results?

7.2   Do you have a liver condition?
      alcoholism? a cardiac disease? a re-
      nal disease?
      • a hernia?   **May become incarcerated and give
                                                  mechanical obstruction** with ab-
                                                  dominal distention
      • a past abdominal operation?   **Postoperative adhesions may give
                                                  intestinal obstruction**
      • a prior episode of jaundice?   Occult cirrhosis

PHYSICAL SIGNS PERTAINING TO ABDOMINAL DISTENTION*

	Possible significance
Abdominal inspection	To distinguish localized from general-ized swelling
Everted umbilicus; bulging flanks; shift-ing dullness, fluid wave; flank dullness	Ascites: peritoneal fluid
Abdominal percussion:	
Increased tympany	Gaseous distention
Localized dullness	Enlarged uterus, ovarian cyst, distended bladder
Prominent abdominal venous pattern with Blood flow away from the umbilicus	Caput medusae (rare): portal hyperten-sion
Flow upward toward the umbilicus	Inferior vena cava obstruction
Flow downward toward the umbilicus	Superior vena cava obstruction
"Doming" of the abdomen with visible ridges from underlying intestinal loops	**Intestinal obstruction or disten-tion**
Tympanites with high-pitched rushing bowel sounds; visible hyperperistalsis	Early intestinal obstruction
Tympanites with absent bowel sounds	Paralytic ileus
Venous hum at the umbilicus	Portal hypertension; increased col-lateral blood flow around the liver
Portal hypertension with	
A firm liver	Cirrhosis
A very hard or nodular liver	Tumor with neoplastic ascites
A soft liver	Extrahepatic obstruction to portal flow

*In this section, items in **boldface** are potentially life-threatening or urgent conditions.

Hard periumbilical lymph node	Sister Marie Joseph's nodule: metastatic disease from a pelvic or gastrointestinal primary tumor
Friction rub over the liver	Hepatoma
Ascites with palmar erythema, spider angiomas, jaundice, hepatosplenomegaly	Liver cirrhosis (with portal hypertension)
Ascites; distended jugular veins; hepatomegaly; peripheral edema	Congestive heart failure
Ascites; distended jugular veins; pulsus paradoxus; tender hepatomegaly; minimal peripheral edema	Constrictive pericarditis
Supraclavicular adenopathy	Virchow's node: underlying gastrointestinal malignancy
Ascites with pulsatile liver	Tricuspid insufficiency
Localized abdominal swelling	Neoplastic peritoneal involvement; metastatic liver
Rectal and pelvic examination	May reveal otherwise undetected masses due to tumor or infection

LABORATORY TESTS PERTAINING TO ABDOMINAL DISTENTION[†]

Test	Finding	Diagnostic Possibilities
Paracentesis		
Ascitic fluid: protein	<2.5 g/100 mL	Transudate: cirrhosis; hypoalbuminemic states (nephrotic syndrome, protein-losing enteropathy); congestive heart failure
	>2.5 g/100 mL	Exudate: neoplasm; tuberculous, pyogenic peritonitis; pancreatitis (occasionally congestive heart failure)
Protein ascites/ serum ratio	<0.5	Transudate
	>0.5	Exudate
LDH ascites/ serum ratio	<0.6	Transudate
	>0.6	Exudate
Serum albumin— ascites albumin	>1.1	Transudate
	<1.1	Exudate
WBC per cubic millimeter	<250	Transudate
	<1000 (predominantly mesothelial)	Congestive heart failure

[†]See the appendix on Laboratory Reference Values for the associated normal laboratory values.

Test	Finding	Diagnostic Possibilities
WBC per cubic millimeter	>1000 (variable cell type)	Neoplasm
	>1000 (predominantly lymphocytes)	Tuberculous peritonitis
	>1000 (predominantly PMNs)	Pyogenic peritonitis
Triglycerides	In excess of plasma concentration	Chylous ascites
Amylase	>500 U	Pancreatic ascites
Cytology	Abnormal	Intraabdominal malignancy
Gram's and acid-fast stains, and/or culture	Positive	Infection of peritoneum

LABORATORY PROCEDURES PERTAINING TO ABDOMINAL DISTENTION

Procedure	To Detect
Upright and recumbent abdominal films	Dilated intestinal loops; with fluid levels: intestinal obstruction
	Ascites with diffuse abdominal haziness and loss of psoas margins
	Size of liver and spleen
Ultrasonography; computerized tomography (CT) scanning	Ascites; presence of a mass; size of liver and spleen
Barium studies of the GI tract*	Esophageal and/or gastric varices: cirrhosis; malabsorption pattern; colonic obstruction
Laparoscopy; peritoneal biopsy; liver biopsy	Cirrhosis; hepatoma; intraabdominal neoplasm

*Upper GI series: contraindicated in complete intestinal obstruction. Barium enema: contraindicated in suspected perforation

SELECTED BIBLIOGRAPHY

Bender MD, Ockner RK: Ascites, in Sleisenger MH, Fordtran JS (eds). *Gastrointestinal Disease. Pathophysiology. Diagnosis. Management,* 4th ed., pp. 428–454, Philadelphia: Saunders, 1989.

Levitt MD, Bond JH: Intestinal gas, in Sleisenger MH, Fordtran JS (eds). *Gastrointestinal Disease. Pathophysiology. Diagnosis. Management,* 4th ed., pp. 257–263, Philadelphia: Saunders, 1989.

12

Acute Abdominal Pain

INTRODUCTION

Abdominal Pain   A sensation of malaise or discomfort related to the abdominal cavity.

Visceral Pain   Initiated by a stimulus acting upon sensory nerve endings in an abdominal viscus. True visceral abdominal pain is mediated over afferent visceral fibers accompanying the sympathetic trunks. The location of the pain corresponds generally to the segmental level of the affected organ. However, the pain originating in deep visceral structures cannot be localized closer than two to three sensory segments. The pain usually results from distention or exaggerated muscular contraction of a hollow viscus; the threshold to such stimuli may be lowered by inflammation. Acute stretching of the capsules of solid organs (liver, spleen, kidney, ovary) and tension on the mesentery also produce pain, presumably by acting on stretch receptors similar to those in muscle. Ischemia causes abdominal pain by increasing the concentration of tissue metabolites in the region of the sensory nerves.

Parietal (Somatic) Pain   Pain sensations which arise from noxious stimulation of the parietal peritoneum. Parietal pain is transmitted by cerebrospinal afferent nerves supplying the peritoneum and is located directly over the inflamed area.

Referred Pain   Pain not localized by the patient in the diseased viscus, but in remote areas supplied by the same neurosegment as the diseased organ, because of shared central pathways by afferent neurons from different sites.

ETIOLOGY

Intraabdominal Sources

Local peritoneal inflammation: acute appendicitis;* acute cholecystitis;* acute pancreatitis; acute diverticulitis; salpingitis, pelvic inflammatory disease; ruptured ovarian follicle (mittelschmerz); endometriosis; mesenteric lymphadenitis

Perforation of a hollow viscus:* lower esophagus, stomach, duodenum, small bowel, colon, gallbladder, urinary bladder

Intraperitoneal hemorrhage:* rupture of spleen; ruptured ectopic pregnancy; dissecting aortic aneurysm

Retroperitoneal hemorrhage:* laceration of kidney; fracture of spine; coagulation abnormality

Obstruction of a hollow viscus:* small or large intestine, biliary tree (gallstones), ureters (calculi, blood clots)

Vascular occlusion*
  Intestinal angina; mesenteric embolism or thrombosis; portal vein thrombosis; vascular rupture
  Torsional occlusion: ovarian cyst or tumor; undescended testes
  Sickle cell anemia

Abdominal wall: rectus sheath hematoma; trauma or infection of muscles; muscle strain

*Urgent condition

Acute stretching of visceral surfaces: hepatic, splenic, or renal capsules
Infectious diseases: enteric infections; hepatitis; acute pyelonephritis; peritonitis; abscess* (abdominal, hepatic, pancreatic)

Referred Pain from Extraabdominal Sources

Thoracic: diaphragmatic pleuritis: pneumonia, pulmonary infarction;* myocardial infarction;* pericarditis; esophageal disease
Neurologic: nerve root compression; spinal cord tumor or abscess
Genitalia: torsion of the testicle

Metabolic and Systemic Disorders

Diabetic ketoacidosis;* uremia; Addisonian crisis;* hyperlipidemia; hypercalcemia; hyperparathyroidism; acute porphyria; hereditary angioedema; familial Mediterranean fever; lactase deficiency; inflammatory bowel disease; systemic lupus erythematosus; polyarteritis nodosa; Henoch-Schönlein purpura; rheumatic fever
Neurogenic disorders: herpes zoster, tabes dorsalis, causalgia

Poisons and Toxins

Heavy metals (lead, arsenic, mercury); mushrooms; arachnoidism

Iatrogenic Causes of Abdominal Pain

Barbiturates in patients with porphyria
Enteric-coated potassium chloride tablets: intestinal mucosal ulceration
Anticoagulants: hemorrhage
Aspirin, indomethacin, phenylbutazone, corticosteroids, ethacrynic acid, reserpine (large doses): peptic ulceration
Calcium oxalate, aluminum hydroxide, ganglionic blockers, tricyclic antidepressants, phenothiazines, opiates, ion exchange resins: obstruction
Atropine-like drugs in prostatism: acute urinary retention
Corticosteroids, thiazides, azathioprine, oral contraceptives, sulfonamides, opiates, furosemide, ethacrynic acid: pancreatitis
Narcotic withdrawal

HISTORY TAKING†

		Possible meaning of a positive response
1	Location and Radiation of Pain	
1.1	Where do you have pain?	
1.1a	*Can you point to it?*	Epigastric pain of peptic ulcer

---

†In this section, items in *italics* are characteristic clinical features, and items in **boldface** are potentially life-threatening or urgent conditions.

1.2   Is the pain
      • *diffuse? difficult to localize?*   Visceral pain: inflammation; biliary col-
                                                   ic; colonic pain; acute hepatitis; **ob-
                                                   struction of small intestine;** vascu-
                                                   lar pain; diaphragmatic irritation

      • *well localized?*   **Parietal peritoneal inflammation;
                                                   appendicitis;** pain due to nerve root
                                                   stimulation: spinal cord tumor, herpes
                                                   zoster

1.3   Has the pain changed in its loca-   The shifting of pain to a localized site
      tion?   suggests a local inflammation of the
                                                   parietal peritoneum with a circum-
                                                   scribed inflammatory process: appendi-
                                                   citis; cholecystitis

1.4   In case of diffuse pain: At the onset,   Chronologic sequence of events may be
      where was the maximum intensity   more important than emphasis on the
      of the pain localized?   location of pain
      • upper part of the abdomen?   **Perforated duodenal ulcer**
      • lower part of the abdomen?   **Ruptured ectopic pregnancy**

1.5   Is the pain felt as being deep to the   Visceral pain; deep musculoskeletal
      surface?   pain; referred pain

1.6   Do you have pain in the
      • midline?   Unpaired structures
      • (mid)epigastrium?   Structures innervated by T6 to T8:
                                                   stomach, duodenum, pancreas, liver,
                                                   biliary tree; associated parietal per-
                                                   itoneum
      • periumbilical region?   Structures innervated by T9 to T10:
                                                   small intestine, appendix (early stages),
                                                   upper ureters, testes, ovaries. (Obstruc-
                                                   tion or distention of almost any hollow
                                                   viscera initially manifests as vague dis-
                                                   comfort in the central portion of the
                                                   abdomen)
      • hypogastrium?   Structures innervated by T11 to T12:
                                                   colon, bladder, lower ureters, uterus
      • right upper quadrant (RUQ)?   Liver: stretching of liver capsule in
                                                   acute congestive heart failure; in-
                                                   fectious hepatitis; gallbladder; bile tract;
                                                   duodenum; hepatic flexure; pancreas
                                                   (head); diaphragmatic pleuritis
      • left upper quadrant (LUQ)?   Pancreas (body and tail); spleen, peri-
                                                   splenitis; transverse colon; upper de-
                                                   scending colon; splenic flexure; di-
                                                   aphragmatic pleuritis
      • left lower quadrant (LLQ)?   Pelvic colon and rectosigmoid (func-
                                                   tional and organic lesion); diverticulitis;
                                                   left urinary tract; left adnexa

- right lower quadrant (RLQ)?
Appendix; terminal ileum; cecum; right urinary tract; right adnexa; subnephritic collection

- flank?
Acute obstruction of the intravesicular portion of the ureter

- costovertebral angle?
Obstruction of the ureteropelvic junction

- suprapubic region?
Obstruction of urinary bladder or of the intravesicular portion of the ureter; rectosigmoid distention

- widespread over the abdomen?
Perforated peptic ulcer; peritonitis; diabetic acidosis; lead colic

- *the entire abdomen, immediately or shortly after onset?*
Flooding of the peritoneal cavity with an irritating fluid: **perforated ulcus, ruptured ectopic pregnancy, ruptured pyosalpynx, ruptured aneurysm**

- upper part of the abdomen?
Acute pancreatitis; intrathoracic disease

1.7 Does the pain radiate
  - from the epigastrium to the
    - shoulder tips?
Perforated peptic ulcer; involvement of undersurface of the diaphragm by acute peritonitis; splenic rupture or infarct; liver abscess
    - tip of right shoulder?
Acute cholecystitis
    - upper part of the lumbar region?
Distention of the common bile duct
    - midline of the back?
Penetrating peptic ulcer; gallbladder disease; dissecting aortic aneurysm; pancreatitis; tumor of pancreas

  - from the RUQ to the
    - *right shoulder? tip of right scapula?*
Biliary colic, acute cholecystitis (acute distention of the extrahepatic biliary tree)
    - supraclavicular area?
Diaphragmatic pleuritis
  - from the LUQ to the left shoulder?
Splenic disorder; splenic flexure syndrome
  - from flank to hypochondrium? down to the groin? into the genitalia?
Ureteral stone, renal colic
  - from the infraumbilical area to the lumbar region?
Colonic obstruction
  - from the abdomen to the sacral region, flank or genitalia?
Rupturing abdominal aortic aneurysm
  - from suprapubic area to penis, scrotum, inner aspect of the upper region of the thigh?
Acute obstruction of the intravesicular portion of the ureter
  - (in female patient): from suprapubic area to the lumbosacral region?
Uterine pain

2   Mode of Onset, Duration, and Temporal Pattern

2.1   How long have you had pain in your abdomen?

Acute abdominal pain that has persisted for more than 6 hours usually indicates a surgical problem; acute appendicitis evolves steadily over 12 hours without remission

2.2   *Do you have recurrent episodes of abdominal pain?*

Medical diagnosis: peptic ulcer; pancreatic lesion; gallbladder disease; porphyria: Crohn's disease; ulcerative colitis; irritable bowel syndrome (see Chapter 15 "Dyspepsia")

2.3   Did the pain appear
• suddenly?

Perforation of a viscus: perforated peptic ulcer; **ruptured ectopic pregnancy; occlusion of the blood supply to an organ; strangulation** of a loop of intestine; mesenteric thrombosis; dissecting aneurysm; torsion of the pedicle of an ovarian cyst; occasionally acute pancreatitis; biliary colic

• gradually?

Inflammatory lesion: appendicitis; cholecystitis; salpingitis; intestinal obstruction

2.4   In case of severe pain: Did the pain reach a crescendo, followed by regression?

Perforation of a viscus

3   Character and Intensity of the Pain

3.1   Is the pain
• mild or moderate?

Peptic ulcer; small intestinal pain; appendicular pain; colonic pain; pelvic inflammatory disease, early stage; gradual dilatation of the biliary tree (carcinoma of the head of the pancreas); obstruction of the urinary bladder

• severe? intense?

Biliary colic; renal colic; perforated peptic ulcer; acute pancreatitis; dissecting aortic aneurysm; mesenteric occlusion; ruptured ectopic pregnancy

3.1a   Did the pain awaken you from sleep?

Pain often of serious import

3.2   Is the pain
• dull?

Epigastric: pain of peptic ulcer; suprapubic: obstruction of the urinary bladder; pyelonephritis

• burning?	Epigastric: psychogenic; duodenal ulcer; causalgic pain
• crushing?	Dissecting aortic aneurysm; peptic ulcer
• sticking in nature?	Crohn's disease; irritable bowel syndrome
• aching?	Visceral pain: peptic ulcer, cholecystitis; tumor; abdominal wall
• cramping?	Colic: colonic, renal, early stage of mesenteric vascular occlusion
• lancinating?	Pain arising from spinal nerves and roots: herpes zoster, arthritis, herniated nucleus pulposus

3.3 Is the pain

• steady? continuous?	Inflammatory process in an abdominal organ; parietal peritoneal inflammation; ischemia from strangulation obstruction (later stage); occlusion of the superior mesenteric artery; pain arising from the abdominal wall; sudden distention of the biliary tree (distention of a hollow viscus may produce steady pain with only very occasional exacerbations)
• crampy at the onset, becoming continuous later?	Strangulation obstruction; appendicitis
• persistent and mild or moderate?	Peptic ulcer; appendicular pain (later stage)
• persistent and severe?	Gallstone colic (sudden distention of the biliary tree)
• fluctuant and severe?	Ureteral colic
• intermittent? colicky?	Pain of obstruction of a hollow abdominal viscus: intestinal and colonic pain
• pulsatile?	Abdominal aneurysm of the aorta

3.4 Does the pain

• recur for several seconds, about three times a minute, with pain-free intervals of 4 to 5 min?	Proximal obstruction; intestinal colic
• last 1 to 5 min with pain-free intervals of 10 to 20 or 30 min?	Distal obstruction; colonic pain

4 Precipitating or Aggravating Factors

4.1 Is the pain worsened by

• coughing? sneezing? movement?	Peritoneal inflammation; pain arising from abdominal wall (e.g., hematoma of rectus sheath); referred pain from the spine (herniated nucleus pulposus)
• recumbency?	Pancreatic pain: distention of pancreatic ducts
• bending over?	Reflux esophagitis

• deep inspiration?

Involvement of diaphragm; acute cholecystitis, when the movement of the diaphragm brings the inflamed organ against the peritoneum

5   Relieving Factors

5.1   Is the pain relieved by
• *leaning forward?* sitting up?
• *lying still? avoiding motion?*

• *changing your position? moving about frequently?*
• vomiting?

Pancreatic pain
Peritoneal inflammation; perforation of peptic ulcer
Obstructed hollow organ: ureteral or biliary colic
Gastric outlet obstruction; pain due to an inflammatory lesion (appendicitis) is not relieved by vomiting

5.2   Have you received any drugs for your pain?

Analgesics may modify the clinical picture

6   Accompanying Symptoms

6.1   Is the pain associated with
• sweating? nausea? vomiting?

Severe abdominal pain: appendicitis; perforated ulcer; obstructive lesion; pancreatitis; cholecystitis; biliary colic; volvulus; intraperitoneal hemorrhage

• vomiting?
  • appearing at about the same time as the abdominal pain?
  • appearing some hours after the onset of the pain?
  • of gastric contents with bile staining?
  • of feculent material?
• severe constipation? (last bowel movement more than 24 h ago)
• black, tarry stools?

Peritonitis; acute cholecystitis; acute pancreatitis; high intestinal obstruction
Low intestinal obstruction; appendicitis

Biliary colic, ureteral colic, proximal bowel obstruction
Distal small bowel obstruction
Intestinal obstruction; appendicitis; cholecystitis; **volvulus**
Intussusception; mesenteric vascular occlusion; obstructing neoplastic or inflammatory lesion

• diarrhea?

Acute enteritis; unusual position of appendix

• bloody diarrhea?
• abdominal distention?
• decreased appetite?

Mesenteric arterial occlusion
Intestinal obstruction
Anorexia is the rule in acute intraabdominal disease

• fever? chills?
• jaundice?
• burning on urination? bloody urine?

Cholecystitis; acute pyelonephritis
Gallstone colic
Renal colic; dysuria in acute appendicitis if the appendix lies adjacent to the bladder

• dark urine?

Gallstone colic (bilirubinuria); porphyria

• purulent urine?

Urinary infection

- syncope?

Hypotension and severe blood volume loss: ruptured aortic aneurysm; ruptured spleen; ectopic pregnancy

6.2 For the female patient: What date did your last menstrual period begin?

6.2a Have you noticed any vaginal hemorrhage?

Last menstrual period more than 6 weeks previous: ectopic pregnancy. Pain in midcycle suggests midcycle follicular rupture (mittelschmerz)

7 Iatrogenic Factors   See Etiology

8 Personal and Social Profile

8.1 What is your occupation?

Abdominal pain due to lead in: battery making, enameling, smelting, painting, welding, ceramics, plumbing

8.2 What is your alcohol intake?

Alcohol abuse: pancreatitis; acute peptic ulcer; gastritis

8.3 Are there any other people in your immediate surroundings who also have abdominal pain?

Food poisoning

8.4 For the female patient: Are you sexually active?

Pelvic inflammatory disease in a woman with a history of sexual exposure

9 Personal Antecedents Pertaining to the Abdominal Pain

9.1 Have you ever had an x-ray of your stomach? gallbladder? intestine? kidneys? When? With what results?

9.2 Have you recently had a trauma to your abdomen?

Rupture of the spleen may occur after a minor injury

9.3 Do you have any of the following conditions:
- peptic ulcer?
- gallstone disease?
- kidney stones?
- any prior abdominal surgery?

Pain due to perforated ulcer
Biliary colic; pancreatitis

Postoperative adhesions causing intestinal obstruction; patients with porphyria frequently have abdominal operations

- a heart disease?

Acute congestive heart failure with stretching of liver capsule and pain in RUQ; embolic mesenteric arterial occlusion in atrial fibrillation or recent myocardial infarction

- diabetes?

Pain of impending diabetic coma

10 Family Medical History Pertaining to the Abdominal Pain

10.1 Is there a family history of similar attacks?

Medical diagnosis: familial Mediterranean fever; acute intermittent porphyria

PHYSICAL SIGNS PERTAINING TO ACUTE ABDOMINAL PAIN*

	Possible significance
Patient lying immobile in bed, resisting movement and change in position	Diffuse peritonitis
Restless patient, changing position frequently	Obstruction of ureter, bile ducts, or small bowel early in its course
Hypotension; rapid, weak pulse; cold, moist skin; restlessness	Shock: peritonitis; bowel infarction; intestinal obstruction; rupture of an abdominal aortic aneurysm
Fever	Infectious process: peritonitis, appendicitis, diverticulitis, tissue necrosis (the temperature is usually normal early with most causes of "surgical" abdomen)
Temperature over 103°F (39.5°C)	Acute urinary tract or pulmonary infection more likely than an acute surgical condition of the abdomen
Tenderness on abdominal palpation; **generalized rebound tenderness**	Diffuse peritonitis
Involuntary guarding	Reflex muscle spasm due to underlying peritoneal irritation; perforated intraabdominal viscus
Guarding, diminished during the inspiratory phase of respiration	Referred pain of thoracic origin
Localized direct and rebound tenderness	Surgical condition; localized peritonitis; vascular necrosis of an ischemic organ
Tenderness on palpation in RLQ	Acute appendicitis
Abdominal mass	Tumor; abscess; ruptured aortic aneurysm; distended loop of bowel; distended gallbladder
Auscultation of the abdomen Absent bowel sounds	Later stage of mechanical obstruction; paralytic ileus; severe chemical peritonitis; ischemia and strangulation of the bowel
Hyperactive high-pitched bowel sounds	Early stage of mechanical obstruction of the bowel (Auscultation of the abdomen may be misleading: active peristalsis often persists despite extensive peritonitis and peristaltic sounds may be absent when the proximal part of the intestine above an obstruction becomes markedly distended and edematous)

*In this section, items in *italics* are characteristic clinical features, and items in **boldface** are potentially life-threatening or urgent conditions.

Vascular bruit	Dissecting arterial aneurysm
Abdominal distention; absent bowel sounds; absence of liver dullness	Free intraperitoneal air: perforated viscus
Inspection of umbilicus and groin	May reveal an incarcerated hernia, a common cause of small-bowel obstruction; metastasizing intraabdominal malignancy at the umbilicus
Scars of previous surgery	Obstruction caused by adhesions; porphyria
Rectal examination	
Tenderness	Pelvic inflammation; appendicitis; etc.
Mass	Abscess; tumor; etc.
Abnormal pelvic examination	Masses of uterus or adnexae; pelvic inflammatory disease; twisted ovarian cyst; peritonitis; etc.

LABORATORY TESTS PERTAINING TO ACUTE ABDOMINAL PAIN†

Test	Finding	Diagnostic Possibilities
Urine		
Urinalysis	RBCs	Renal stone; tumor of the genitourinary tract
	Glycosuria	Diabetic acidosis
	Pyuria	Urinary tract infection
Porphobilinogen	Positive	Porphyria
Blood		
Hematocrit	Low	Mucosal ulceration; intestinal carcinoma; dissecting aortic aneurysm
	Elevated	Dehydration, usually caused by vomiting and deficient fluid intake
WBCs	Leukocytosis	Perforation of a viscus; appendicitis; acute cholecystitis; pancreatitis; intestinal infarction; pelvic inflammatory disease (a normal WBC count does not exclude perforation or strangulated intestinal obstruction)

†See the appendix on Laboratory Reference Values for the associated normal laboratory values.

Test	Finding	Diagnostic Possibilities
Electrolytes	Abnormal	Dehydration; imbalances needing correction prior to eventual surgery
BUN, creatinine	Elevated	Renal disease; dehydration secondary to vomiting and deficient fluid intake
Bilirubin	Elevated	Biliary tract or pancreas disorder
Amylase	Elevated	Pancreatitis; perforated ulcer; strangulating intestinal obstruction; acute cholecystitis; acute common duct obstruction (serum amylase may be normal in acute pancreatitis)

LABORATORY PROCEDURES PERTAINING TO ACUTE ABDOMINAL PAIN

Procedure	To Detect
Plain flat, upright, and lateral decubitus x-rays of the abdomen	Free air in the peritoneal cavity: perforation of a hollow viscus; acute small-bowel obstruction; calculus in biliary or urinary tract; soft-tissue masses; pancreatic calcifications; "sentinel loops": acute pancreatitis; absent psoas shadow: retroperitoneal mass or bleeding; displaced stomach or bowel shadows
Chest x-ray	Extraabdominal condition mimicking acute abdominal situation; pneumonia; free air under the diaphragm
Barium enema	Site and nature of colonic obstruction
ECG	Extraabdominal condition: myocardial infarction; acute pericarditis
Abdominal ultrasonography	Enlarged gallbladder or pancreas; gallstones; localized collection of fluid or pus; hydronephrotic kidneys; solid vs. cystic mass
Abdominal computerized tomography	Choledocholithiasis; enlarged pancreas; intraabdominal abscess; dissection of aorta; etc.

SELECTED BIBLIOGRAPHY

Eaves-Hill DM: Evaluation of the acute abdomen. *Postgrad Med* 81(4):125–135, 1987.

Phillips SL, Burns GP: Acute abdominal disease in the aged. *Med Clin North Am* 72:1213–1224, 1988.

Saclarides T, Hopkins W, Doolas A: Abdominal emergencies. *Med Clin North Am* 70:1093–1110, 1986.

Way LW: Abdominal pain, in Sleisenger MH, Fordtran JS (eds). *Gastrointestinal Disease. Pathophysiology. Diagnosis. Management,* 4th ed., pp. 238–250, Philadelphia: Saunders, 1989.

13

Constipation

INTRODUCTION

Constipation   Delay in the evacuation of feces, with passage of unduly hard and dry fecal material; less than three bowel movements per week.

Chyme passes through the small intestine rapidly, so that 5 or 6 h after a meal, the greater proportion is in the cecum. In the large bowel, the fecal mass progresses more slowly, about 12 h being required for a part of it to pass from the cecum to the sigmoid and descending colon. An additional 6 or 8 h usually elapses before evacuation of the residue of ingesta occurs. Normally the fecal mass does not pass beyond the sigmoid into the rectum until the act of defecation is about to occur. The mass peristaltic movement which propels the fecal matter into the rectum is usually initiated by the ingestion of food at breakfast time. The desire to defecate is initiated by distention of the rectum by the fecal mass as a result of the mass peristaltic movement.

Repeatedly ignoring the desire to defecate results in blunting of the "defecation sense of the rectum" and constitutes a frequent cause of constipation (rectal constipation or dyschezia). In rectal constipation, rectal examination discloses a rectum filled with feces. Patients with constipation may have a motility abnormality of the sigmoid and descending colon; transfer of feces into the rectum is delayed, and the rectum is relatively empty. Stools are small and excessively hard, owing to increased absorption of fluid as a result of prolonged contact of the luminal contents with the colonic mucosa consequent to delayed transit. Inadequate propulsion of feces may also result from mechanical obstruction (e.g., carcinoma of the sigmoid colon) or from diminished contraction of the proximal intestine (e.g., paralytic ileus).

ETIOLOGY

Impaired Motility

Inadequate dietary fiber; inactivity, bed rest; laxative abuse; irritable bowel syndrome; hypothyroidism; hypokalemia; diabetic enteropathy; hypercalcemia; pregnancy; scleroderma; drugs; intestinal pseudo-obstruction: collagen-vascular disease, amyloidosis, muscular dystrophy, hypothyroidism, hypoparathyroidism, chronic renal failure

Obstruction: Ileal, Colonic, Anal

Tumor; stricture; radiation; ischemia; volvulus; intussusception

Neurologic Disorders

Multiple sclerosis; Parkinson's disease; spinal cord lesions

Altered Defecation Reflex

Megacolon: aganglionic, chronic idiopathic, acquired
Secondary to painful rectal or anal lesions: hemorrhoids, fissures, strictures, abscess, proctitis
Inadequate evacuatory habits
Depression; psychoses

Iatrogenic Causes of Constipation or Ileus

Aluminum hydroxide, calcium carbonate; barium sulfate; ion exchange resins; ferrous sulfate; anticholinergics; ganglion-blockers; tricyclic antidepressants; phenothiazines; large amounts of sedatives; opiates; anticonvulsants; antiparkinsonian drugs; verapamil

HISTORY TAKING*

Possible meaning of a positive response

Acute Onset of Severe Obstipation

1   When did you have your last bowel movement?

1.1   Do you still pass gas?   Failure to pass gas suggests complete **intestinal obstruction**

2   Do you have

• abdominal pain? cramps?   **Mechanical intestinal obstruction** (see Chapter 11 "Abdominal Distention"); intestinal pseudo-obstruction

• abdominal distention?   Adynamic ileus; intestinal pseudo-obstruction; distention may be quite marked late in any form of obstruction

• nausea? *vomiting?*   **Intestinal obstruction;** ileus; intestinal pseudo-obstruction

3   Do you hear bowel sounds? abdominal rumbling?   Borborygmi: bowel sounds are active at the onset of mechanical ileus

4   What were your bowel habits before this episode?

• abnormal?   Chronic intestinal disorder progressing to complete obstruction

• constipation alternating with bouts of diarrhea?   Carcinoma of colon; irritable bowel syndrome; diabetic autonomic neuropathy; fecal impaction

*In this section, items in *italics* are characteristic clinical features, and items in **boldface** are potentially life-threatening or urgent conditions.

5   Have you taken any laxatives? enemas?

In high obstruction, the lower bowel may function well for a time, e.g., expelling an enema readily

6   Have you ever had an operation on the abdomen?

Postoperative adhesions or strictures interfering with the onward movement of the intestinal contents; intestinal pseudo-obstruction

Chronic Constipation

1   Mode of Onset and Duration

1.1   How long have you been constipated?

Of recent onset: psychological stress; organic disease: carcinoma of rectum or sigmoid colon; drug-related problem. A long history suggests: irritable bowel syndrome, chronic rectal constipation, megacolon

1.1a   Is the constipation
  • constant?

Poor bowel habits; insufficient dietary roughage; sedentarity

  • intermittent?

Irritable bowel syndrome (normal bowel habit may be present for variable periods of time between attacks of colonic dysfunction); intestinal pseudo-obstruction; voluntary suppression of the urge to defecate

1.2   How many stools do you have per day? or week?

Most normal people have more than 3 bowel movements per week. In constipation, stools are often described as infrequent, incomplete, or unduly hard

1.3   According to you, how many times a day should you have a movement?

Some patients are concerned because their bowel movements do not measure up to their expectations

1.3a   What do you regard as a normal defecatory pattern?

Defecatory habits are very varied among normal subjects. Bowel-conscious patients have an inordinate expectation of "regularity"

1.4   How many times a day, a week, do you feel the urge to defecate?

1.4a   Do you resist the defecatory urge?

Voluntary suppression of the urge to defecate, when abused, may lead to chronic rectal distention, reduced afferent signals, lax tone, and chronic constipation

1.4b Do you still feel a desire to defecate?

A decreasing desire is often due to repeated neglect to empty the colon when
the desire to defecate occurs

2 Character of the Stools

2.1 Are the stools
• excessively hard? like hard small
pellets?

Increased absorption of fluid resulting
from prolonged contact of the luminal
contents with the colonic mucosa due
to delayed transit

• accompanied by excessive mucus
and gas?

Irritable bowel syndrome (rare in constipation due to neglect of the bowels)

• like ribbons? (thin and narrow)

Organic narrowing of the distal colon or
sigmoid: rectal cancer; sigmoid colon
carcinoma; irritable bowel syndrome

• soft, semiformed? watery?

In an elderly, debilitated patient: fecal
impaction (liquid stool above the fecal
mass passing around the impaction)

• of variable consistency?

Malignant lesion of the colon; irritable
bowel syndrome

2.2 What is the color of the stools?
• mixed with mucus?

Irritable bowel syndrome

• streaked with blood?

Anal disease (hemorrhoids, fissures, ulcers)

• mixed with blood?

Neoplasm of the large bowel

• black, tarry?

Gastrointestinal bleeding

2.3 *Do you have periods of constipation
alternating with bouts of diarrhea?*

Neoplasm of large bowel; irritable
bowel syndrome

2.4 *Have you recently noticed a change in
your bowel habits?* a decrease in frequency of defecation?

Partial bowel obstruction (tumor)

3 Precipitating or Aggravating Factors

3.1 Have you recently
• been bedridden for a prolonged
period? admitted to a hospital?

May induce blunting of defecatory reflexes and diminished expulsive power

• had a recent psychological stress?

A major reason for altered bowel habits

3.2 Do you suppress defecatory urges
arising at inconvenient moments?

3.2a Do you take your time when you
have to move your bowels?

Inadequate allotment of time for full
defecation is a contributory cause of
chronic constipation. Social impropri-
ety, lack of toilet facilities, unaccustomed surroundings may lead to
voluntary suppression of the call to
stool

4   Accompanying Symptoms

4.1   Do you have

- abdominal pain? distress?

Irritable bowel syndrome; obstructive process: carcinoma of colon

- *relieved by defecation? passage of flatus?*

Colonic disease; irritable bowel syndrome

- painful defecation?

May be due to hard stools or perianal pathology: fissures, hemorrhoids. May reinforce the inhibitory impulses to defecation

- pain at the anus?

Thrombosis of external hemorrhoids

- an intense urge to defecate with unsuccessful straining? with a feeling of incomplete evacuation?

Tenesmus: carcinoma of the rectum or sigmoid colon; fecal impaction

- unusual straining required to achieve defecation?

Chronic constipation

- fecal incontinence?

Fecal impaction

4.2   Do you
- often pass gas?
- frequently hear rumbling from your abdomen? bowel sounds?

Irritable bowel syndrome; chronic constipation

4.3   Do you experience a sensation of fullness or pressure in the rectum?

Constipation of rectal type: fecal accumulation in the rectum

4.4   Do you have
- fatigue? malaise? headache? loss of appetite?

Underlying depression of which constipation is but one component

- bloating? belching?

Symptoms generally related to the anxiety aroused by the constipation and the attendant disturbance of intestinal motility

- anxiety?

May be produced by the bowel disturbance; irritable bowel syndrome often secondary to mental distress

4.5   Has your weight
- remained the same?

Chronic constipation; irritable bowel syndrome

- increased?

Hypothyroidism

- decreased?

Carcinoma of the colon

4.6   Have you recently noticed the appearance of
- frequent urination?

Carcinoma of pelvic colon or rectum invading, or pressing against, the lower urinary tract

- urinary retention?

Lesion in the cauda equina impairing the function of the parasympathetic innervation of the colon

5   Iatrogenic Factors   See Etiology

5.1	Do you take laxatives? enemas? Since when? which ones? every day?	Constipation is complicated by the use or abuse of laxatives in almost all patients with this disorder; abuse of laxatives induces a loss of the sensitivity of the rectal defecatory reflexes

6   Personal and Social Profile

6.1	What do you habitually eat?	Insufficient dietary roughage may induce constipation
6.1a	Did you recently modify your usual diet?	A marked change in dietary regime, particularly in combination with sedative drugs, may produce constipation
6.2	What is your occupation?	A sedentary occupation may produce constipation by blunting the defecatory reflex and diminishing expulsive power

7   Personal Antecedents Pertaining to the Constipation

7.1	Has an examination of your stool ever been performed? When? With what results?	
7.2	Have you ever had an x-ray examination of your intestine? a rectoscopy? When? With what results?	
7.3	Have you ever had any of the following conditions:	
	• an abdominal operation?	Postoperative adhesions or strictures
	• hemorrhoids? anal ulcers? fissure?	Often a result of the constipation; these lesions may also prevent adequate stool evacuation and induce a failure of relaxation of the anal sphincter
7.4	For the female patient: How many pregnancies have you had?	Multiple pregnancies may produce lax abdominal muscles and weaken the pelvic floor, resulting in rectal constipation

PHYSICAL SIGNS PERTAINING TO CONSTIPATION

	Possible significance
Hyperactive bowel sounds; visible peristalsis; abdominal mass	Mechanical ileus; intestinal obstructing lesion
Absent bowel sounds; distended abdomen	Adynamic ileus

Dry skin; delayed relaxation phase of the deep tendon reflexes	Myxedema

Rectal examination

Absence of stool	Primary disorder of defecation unlikely; point of obstruction at the rectosigmoid or above; irritable bowel syndrome
Presence of hard stool	Rules out significant obstruction. Chronic constipation with habitual neglect of afferent impulses, failure to initiate defecation and accumulation of large, dry fecal masses in the rectum
Fecal impaction	May be accompanied at first by constipation
Thrombosed hemorrhoids; anal ulcers	Disorders preventing the relaxation of the internal anal sphincter
Rectal mass	Carcinoma; fecal impaction

LABORATORY PROCEDURES PERTAINING TO CONSTIPATION[†]

Procedure	To Detect
Flat abdominal film	Megacolon; dilated loops of bowel; air-fluid levels in intestinal obstruction
Proctosigmoidoscopy	(Indicated if constipation of recent onset and/or blood in stool) Carcinoma of the rectum or descending colon; melanosis coli: pigmented colonic mucosa in anthraquinone laxatives abuse
Barium enema	(Indicated if constipation of recent onset) Neoplasm; megacolon
When indicated:	
Stool: occult blood tests	
Blood: electrolytes, calcium, thyroid function tests	

[†]See the appendix on Laboratory Reference Values for the associated normal laboratory values.

SELECTED BIBLIOGRAPHY

Devroede G: Constipation, in Sleisenger MH, Fordtran JS (eds). *Gastrointestinal Disease. Pathophysiology. Diagnosis. Management,* 4th ed., pp. 331–368, Philadelphia: Saunders, 1989.

Nivatvongs S, Hooks VH: Chronic constipation. *Postgrad Med* 74(5):313–323, 1983.

14
Diarrhea

INTRODUCTION

Diarrhea   Frequent passage of loose stools.

The absorptive surfaces of the intestinal tract are normally presented with 9 L of liquid (dietary and secretions) per day. In the healthy subject, all but 1000 mL is absorbed by the time the cecum is reached. Only 100 to 150 mL of that fluid volume remains unabsorbed and appears in the feces. Diarrhea is present when the stool weight exceeds 200 g per day. Increased fecal water can result from decreased water absorption, increased fluid secretion, or altered bowel motility.

Decreased reabsorption of fluid may be due to the presence of unabsorbable osmotically active solutes in the bowel lumen, abnormalities of the bowel mucosa, or loss of reabsorptive surface. Increased fluid secretion may be passive, in conditions with increased tissue hydrostatic pressure, as in obstruction of lymphatic drainage, or it can be triggered by inflammation, hormones, or enterotoxins. Altered bowel motility decreases the contact time with the bowel mucosa, limiting fluid reabsorption. At times, several mechanisms are involved.

Abnormalities of intestinal motility mediated by neurohumoral factors (serotonin, acetylcholine, prostaglandins) may also lead to diarrhea.

ETIOLOGY

Acute Diarrhea (of Less than 2 to 3 Weeks Duration)

Infection

Salmonella, Shigella, enteropathogenic *Escherichia coli, Campylobacter jejuni, Vibrio para-haemolyticus, Bacillus cereus, Staphylococcus, Vibrio cholerae, Clostridium perfringens, Proteus,* viral pathogens, helminths, protozoa *(Entamoeba, Giardia, Cryptosporidium)*

Toxic

Chemical poisons: arsenic, lead, cadmium, mercury; mushrooms; drugs

Dietary

Irritating foods

Acute Episode in a Patient with Chronic Disease Process

Ulcerative colitis; Crohn's disease; diverticulitis

Psychologic Stress

Miscellaneous

Fecal impaction; pericolic and perirectal abscess; retroiliac appendicitis; ischemic colitis; pellagra; gastrointestinal allergy; acute radiation sickness

Chronic Diarrhea (Persisting for at Least 3 Weeks)

Decreased Fluid Absorption

Oral intake of poorly absorbable solutes: habitual laxative abuse
Maldigestion and malabsorption*
  Pancreatic insufficiency: chronic pancreatitis, carcinoma of pancreas, pancreatic resection, cystic fibrosis
  Impaired mucosal absorption: sprue; Whipple's disease; lymphoma; amyloidosis; eosinophilic gastroenteritis; Crohn's disease; radiation enteritis and colitis; ischemia
  Enzyme deficiencies: lactase; other disaccharidase deficiencies
  Bile salt deficiency: biliary obstruction; bacterial overgrowth (scleroderma, diabetic visceral neuropathy, diverticula, fistulas, strictures, blind loops); ileal resection; Crohn's disease
Loss of reabsorptive surface: intestinal resection or bypass; enteroenteric fistulas (Crohn's disease)

Increased Fluid Secretion

Passive secretion: obstruction of lymphatic drainage
Active secretion
  Non-beta cell tumor of the pancreas; vasoactive intestinal polypeptides; medullary carcinoma of the thyroid (calcitonin, prostaglandins); Zollinger-Ellison syndrome (gastrin); carcinoid syndrome; villous adenoma
  Inflammatory bowel disease: ulcerative colitis; Crohn's disease; ischemic bowel disease

Motor Disturbances

Irritable bowel syndrome; diabetic enteropathy; scleroderma; carcinoid syndrome; hyperthyroidism; postgastrectomy

Iatrogenic Causes of Diarrhea (Partial List)

Antibiotics: broad-spectrum antibiotics; tetracycline; penicillins; lincomycin; clindamycin; ampicillin; may be associated with pseudomembranous enterocolitis caused by *Clostridium difficile*
Antimetabolites; ganglionic-blocking agents; gold, mercury; lactose excipients; laxatives, purgatives; magnesium-containing antacids; cholestyramine; sulfasalazine; cholinergic agents; phenformin; colchicine; diuretics; digitalis; quinine; quinidine; chenodeoxycholic acid; potassium supplements; prostaglandin analogues
Antihypertensive agents: methyldopa, beta-blockers, bethanidine, guanethidine, reserpine

*Multiple defects may be responsible.

HISTORY TAKING*

Acute Diarrhea: of Less than 2 to 3 Weeks Duration

Possible meaning of a positive response

1   Mode of Onset

1.1   How long have you had diarrhea?   Acute diarrhea lasting 1 to 3 days is usually presumed to be of viral etiology. Diarrhea due to *Salmonella* or *Shigella* may last 7 to 10 days

1.2   How many stools a day do you have?   Patients usually complain of diarrhea when they have abnormally frequent movements (more than 3 per day)

1.3   Did the diarrhea appear
        • abruptly?   Infectious cause: bacterial diarrhea, viral gastroenteritis; toxins; poisons; drugs; ulcerative colitis and Crohn's disease may begin as acute diarrhea

        • gradually?   Usual mode of onset of amebic colitis

1.4   Has the diarrhea appeared after a meal?
        • *almost immediately after ingestion?* < 2 hours?   Chemical food poisoning: cadmium, sodium fluoride
        • 2 to 6 hours after?   Staphylococcal food poisoning
        • 8 to 14 hours after?   *C. perfringens, B. cereus;* ingestion of a preformed toxin (e.g., staphylococcal exotoxin)

        • > 14 hours after?   *Salmonella, Shigella, V. cholerae; E. coli* (enterotoxic or invasive); *V. parahaemolyticus*

        • with a lag period of up to 3 days?   Can occur with salmonellosis
        • without relation to a meal?   Viral gastroenteritis

1.4a   What did you eat at this meal?
        • milk? prepared foods? creamed foods? pies? salad? filling? mayonnaise?   Poorly refrigerated: staphylococcal food poisoning. Foods containing staphylococcal enterotoxins have normal appearance, odor, and taste

        • egg products? poultry products?   (Of infected fowl): *Salmonella*
        • seafood?   *Vibrio parahaemolyticus*
        • meat that was warmed on steam tables?   *Clostridium perfringens*

In this section, items in *italics* are characteristic clinical features.

2   Character of the Stools

2.1   Do you have frequent expulsions of
       • watery stools?   Inflammatory disease of small intestine;
                                            viral gastroenteritis; giardiasis; fecal im-
                                            paction in elderly and debilitated
                                            patients: frequent expulsion of small
                                            amounts of liquid stools (due to colonic
                                            distention behind the impaction)

       • greenish stools?   Salmonellosis; giardiasis
       • small quantities of solid material Irritable bowel syndrome
         admixed with gas?

2.2   Do the stools contain
       • mucus and/or blood?   Shigellosis; diverticulitis; *Salmonella* en-
                                            teritis; amebiasis; *Campylobacter;* in-
                                            flammatory bowel disease

       • pus?   Acute enteritis; shigellosis
       • none of the above?   Functional disorder; viral gastroenteritis

2.3   What is the odor of the stool?
       • malodorous?   Salmonellosis; giardiasis
       • odorless?   Shigellosis

3   Accompanying Symptoms

3.1   Do you have
       • loss of appetite? nausea? vomit-   Foodborne diarrhea: *Staphylococcus au-
         ing?   reus, B. cereus, Salmonella, Shigella*
                                            (minimal vomiting with *Clostridium per-
                                            fringens*)

       • lower abdominal cramps?   Bacterial diarrhea: staphylococcal, shi-
                                            gellosis; viral gastroenteritis
       • epigastric or periumbilical pain? Inflammatory disease of small intestine
       • right lower quadrant pain?   Crohn's disease limited to the small
                                            bowel (regional enteritis)
       • left lower quadrant cramps?   Diverticulitis
       • *an intense urge to defecate, with* Tenesmus: suggests a lesion in the rec-
         straining, and a feeling of incom- tum near the anal sphincter: diverticuli-
         plete evacuation?   tis, bacillary dysentery; acute proctitis;
                                            amebic dysentery (not in inflammatory
                                            disease of small intestine)

       • fecal incontinence?   An embarrassing complaint infrequent-
                                            ly reported to the doctor. Diarrhea of
                                            any cause may contribute to in-
                                            continence
       • fever?   Infectious   origin: salmonellosis;
                                            shigellosis. Occasionally: ulcerative co-
                                            litis; Crohn's disease; diverticulitis
       • no fever?   Bacterial toxins (staphylococcal, *C. per-
                                            fringens*); viral gastroenteritis; psycho-
                                            genic diarrhea

• pain in your muscles? malaise? headache?	Myalgia may occur in acute infectious diarrhea

4   Iatrogenic Factors   See Etiology

5   Personal and Social Profile

5.1 *Are there other people in your family, at your job, at school, who became ill with diarrhea?*	Viral gastroenteritis; bacterial diarrhea
5.1a Did they eat the same food as you?	
5.2 Have you recently traveled to a tropical or a developing country?	Traveler's diarrhea: *Entamoeba histolytica; Giardia lamblia;* rotavirus; *Salmonella; E. coli; Shigella; V. cholerae:* Africa, Asia, Middle East
5.3 What is your sexual orientation?	Diarrhea in a homosexual man: *Shigella, Salmonella, Campylobacter, Giardia lamblia, E. histolytica.* Diarrhea in the AIDS patient: *Cryptosporidium, Isospora, Mycobacterium avium-intracellulare,* cytomegalovirus, herpes simplex virus
5.4 Have you recently had an acute psychological stress?	A major reason for altered bowel habits; can cause diarrhea at any age

Chronic Diarrhea (Lasting More Than 3 Weeks)

1   Mode of Onset, Frequency, and Duration

1.1 How long have you had diarrhea?	Diarrhea persisting for weeks or months may be a functional symptom or a manifestation of serious illness
• since adolescence or early adult life?	Inflammatory bowel disease; functional disorder
• in middle age? in the elderly?	Diverticulitis; carcinoma of the colon; pancreatic disease
1.2 Is the diarrhea	
• continuous? constant?	Crohn's disease; ulcerative colitis; fistulas; hyperthyroidism; gastric disorders; laxative abuse
• intermittent? recurrent?	Irritable bowel syndrome (emotional disorders); allergy; diverticulitis; malabsorption; inflammatory bowel disease; carcinoid syndrome (rare)
1.3 *Do you have bouts of diarrhea alternating with periods of constipation?*	Carcinoma of the colon; diverticulitis; irritable bowel syndrome; partial intestinal obstruction; diabetic autonomic neuropathy; fecal impaction; diarrhea of chronic constipation and laxative habit

2 Qualitative Aspects of the Diarrhea

2.1 Are the stools
- loose? pasty? soft?   Sigmoid hypomotility with poor water absorption
- watery?   Abnormal intestinal secretion: laxatives; bacterial toxins; polypeptide-secreting tumor: "pancreatic cholera"; medullary carcinoma of the thyroid; protein-losing enteropathy; rectal villous adenoma; Zollinger-Ellison syndrome; cathartics; diabetic visceral neuropathy; internal fistulas; fecal impaction; emotional disturbances
- foamy? frothy?   Small intestine: lactase or sucrase deficiency; monosaccharide malabsorption
- oily? floating? greasy? difficult to flush?   Small intestine: malabsorption syndrome; steatorrhea
- thin, fragmented, pelletlike? with excessive mucus and gas?   Irritable bowel syndrome
- narrow? pencil-like?   Irritable bowel syndrome; colorectal carcinoma

2.2 Do your stools contain
- mucus?   Irritable bowel syndrome; amebiasis; cathartics
- large amounts of mucus? (with solid stools)   Rectal villous adenoma
- blood?   Infammatory bowel disease; invasive infection: amebic or bacillary dysentery; diverticulitis; carcinoma; polyps; associated proctitis or anusitis; ischemic colitis (in the elderly or arteriopathic patient). The presence of blood excludes the diagnosis of irritable bowel syndrome
- pus?   Abscess; inflammatory bowel disease; ulcerating neoplasm
- undigested food?   Small intestine or colon; gastrocolic or gastroileal fistula

2.3 What is the color of your stools?
- pale? light in color?   Small intestine; steatorrhea
- black?   GI bleeding
- greenish?   Excessive amounts of bile: infection, laxative abuse

2.4 What is the odor of your stools?
- malodorous? foul smelling?   Small intestine; malabsorption
- odorless? (and large quantities of clear liquid)   Rectal villous adenoma

2.5 At what time in the day do you
     have diarrhea?
     - *in the early morning?*   Irritable bowel syndrome
     - only during the day?   Functional or organic
     - *also during the night?*   Favors organic disease over irritable
                                          bowel syndrome (but this is not always
                                          specific); severe inflammatory disease;
                                          hyperthyroidism; diabetic visceral
                                          neuropathy

3 Quantitative Aspects of the Diarrhea

3.1 How many bowel movements per
     day do you have?
     - *few? about six times (or less) daily?*   Small intestine, right colon: malabsorp-
       (without urgency)   tion
     - *many? exceeding six times per day?*   Left colon, rectum: ulcerative colitis,
       (with urgency)   amebiasis

3.2 What is the volume of your stools?
     - *large, bulky?*   More than 300 g/day: abnormal in-
                                          testinal secretion: small intestine, right
                                          colon: malabsorption; secretory di-
                                          arrhea; laxative abuse
     - *small?*   Less than 200 g/day: distal colon, rec-
                                          tum: infectious diarrhea, inflammatory
                                          bowel disease, diverticulitis, cancer;
                                          irritable bowel syndrome

4 Precipitating or Aggravating Factors

4.1 Do you have diarrhea
     - after meals?   A common finding: osmotic diarrhea;
                                          malabsorption; fistula; irritable bowel
                                          syndrome; Crohn's disease; ulcerative
                                          colitis
     - after eating cheese, ice cream,   Lactase deficiency
       yogurt, milk?
     - without any relation to meals?   Secretory diarrhea; infectious disease;
                                          hyperthyroidism
     - after emotional stress? anxiety?   Irritable bowel syndrome; ulcerative
       stressful events?   colitis

5 Relieving Factors

5.1 Does the diarrhea
     - *stop when you fast?*   Malabsorption syndromes; osmotic di-
                                          arrhea: lactase deficiency; food in-
                                          tolerance
     - *persist during fasting?*   Abnormal high intestinal secretion:
                                          laxative abuse, toxigenic bacteria,
                                          polypeptide-secreting tumor; Zollinger-
                                          Ellison syndrome; medullary carcinoma
                                          of the thyroid

6   Accompanying Symptoms

6.1   Do you have
- upper abdominal pain? radiating through to the back? relieved by sitting up?
- epigastric, ulcer-like pain?
- crampy central abdominal pain?

- left upper quadrant pain?
- left lower quadrant or lower abdominal pain?

Pancreatic disease

Zollinger-Ellison syndrome
Motor disorder in the small intestine, ileum, or right colon; Crohn's disease; ischemic colitis
Irritable bowel syndrome
Diverticulitis; disturbance in the rectosigmoid segment

6.1a   Is the abdominal pain
- relieved by defecation?

- not relieved by defecation?

Disorder of the left colon or rectum; diverticular disease; irritable bowel syndrome; neoplasm
Disease of small bowel

6.2   *Do you have painless diarrhea?*

Pseudomembranous colitis; small intestine disorder; hyperthyroidism; diabetes mellitus

6.3   Do you have
- abdominal distention?

- nausea? vomiting?

- *an intense urge to move the bowels, with straining but little or no results?*

- fecal incontinence?

- pain with defecation?

- excessive flatus?

Malabsorption; ingestion of large amounts of unabsorbable polysaccharides; chronic partial intestinal obstruction (due to adhesions or neoplasm)
Partial intestinal obstruction (e.g., due to adhesions); diabetic autonomic neuropathy
Tenesmus: involvement of distal colon, rectum: ulcerative colitis; amebiasis; carcinoma of rectum. Tenesmus is absent in disorders of small intestine, right colon: malabsorption; Crohn's disease
Potentially correctable anal sphincter abnormality. (Patients do not often report this information spontaneously)
Anus, rectum, colon; anal fissure; ulcerative colitis
Malabsorption: bacterial fermentation of unabsorbed carbohydrates; irritable bowel syndrome

6.4   Has your appetite
- remained the same?
- decreased?

Hyperthyroidism; malabsorption; allergy
Carcinoma

6.5   Has your weight
- remained the same?

Irritable bowel syndrome; bile salt enteropathy; allergy; lactase deficiency

• increased?	Edema due to malabsorption with hypoproteinemia
• decreased?	Organic disease: in malabsorption disorders (loss of calories): pancreatic insufficiency; cancer of pancreas; Crohn's disease; ulcerative colitis; hyperthyroidism; bacterial overgrowth in the small intestine; partial intestinal obstruction with postprandial pain and a resultant decrease in food intake

6.5a Did the weight loss
 • precede the onset of diarrhea?

Carcinoma of pancreas; hyperthyroidism; diabetes mellitus; malabsorption

 • appear late after the onset of diarrhea?

Carcinoma of the colon

6.6 Do you have
 • fatigue?

Anemia (in malabsorption: impaired absorption of iron, vitamin B_{12} and folic acid); hypokalemia

 • facial flushing?

Carcinoid syndrome

 • fever?

Organic disease; inflammatory bowel disease; lymphoma; amebiasis

 • no fever?

Absorptive defect of small intestine; chronic pancreatitis

 • pain, weakness in your limbs?

Avitaminotic neuropathies in malabsorptive disorders

 • pain in your joints?

Inflammatory bowel disease; amyloidosis; Whipple's disease; colchicine treatment of gout

 • bone pain?

Osteopenic bone disease in malabsorptive disorders: calcium, vitamin D, protein malabsorption

 • back pain?

Osteoporosis; osteomalacia; cancer of pancreas

 • easy bruising? bleeding?

Vitamin K malabsorption with hypoprothrombinemia

 • chronic cough? shortness of breath?

Cystic fibrosis with pancreatic insufficiency; scleroderma

 • urinary complaints?

Crohn's disease with fistula of the bladder

7   Iatrogenic Factors   See Etiology

The possibility of drug-induced diarrhea should be carefully considered

7.1 Do you take laxatives?

Habitual cathartic abuse must be suspected when the cause of prolonged diarrhea remains perplexing

8   Personal and Social Profile

8.1   What do you usually eat each day?

Overindulgence in beer or coffee; excessive intake of fruit, spicy food, curries, milk, vegetables, or bran may cause or exacerbate diarrhea

8.2   Have you ever lived in, or traveled to, tropical or developing countries?

Amebiasis; giardiasis; postdysentery lactase deficiency; tropical sprue (India, Far East, China, Central America)

8.3   What is your sexual orientation?

Diarrhea in a homosexual man: Shigellosis; *Campylobacter* enteritis; amebiasis; giardiasis; cryptosporidiosis

9   Personal Antecedents Pertaining to the Diarrhea

9.1   Have you ever had an examination of your stools? an x-ray of your intestines? a rectoscopy? When? With what results?

9.2   Have you ever been treated for your diarrhea? Did it respond to
   • corticosteroids?

Inflammatory bowel disease; Whipple's disease; sprue

   • *a gluten-free diet?*
Sprue
   • antibiotics?
Blind-loop syndrome; Whipple's disease; tropical sprue

9.3   Do you have any of the following conditions: pancreatitis? ulcerative colitis? Crohn's disease? diverticulosis?
   • diabetes?

Visceral neuropathy; exocrine pancreatic insufficiency; abnormal bacterial proliferation in proximal small bowel

   • a lung disease?
Carcinoid syndrome (asthma); cystic fibrosis

   • a liver disease?
Sclerosing cholangitis, cirrhosis in inflammatory bowel disease

   • anemia?
Malabsorption with vitamin B_{12}, folic acid, or iron deficiency

   • emotional problems?
Seem to be related to the onset or exacerbation of inflammatory bowel disease; irritable bowel syndrome

   • a recent attack of gastroenteritis?
Giardiasis, *Campylobacter, Yersinia* infection may linger several weeks

9.4   Have you ever had
   • GI surgery: vagotomy, cholecystectomy, gastric resection, intestinal resection, jejunoileal bypass?

Postgastrectomy diarrhea; blind-loop syndrome; gastrocolic fistula

10 Family History Pertaining to the Diarrhea

10.1 Is there any member of your family who has chronic diarrhea? a GI disorder?	Inflammatory bowel disease exhibits familial clustering. A strong family history is present in (rare) hereditary pancreatitis, medullary carcinoma of the thyroid

PHYSICAL SIGNS PERTAINING TO DIARRHEA

Possible significance

Acute Diarrhea

Shock; thready radial pulse; poor skin turgor; cold extremities; flat neck veins	Acute loss of 8 to 12 percent of body weight
Fever; diffuse abdominal tenderness; active bowel sounds	Acute infectious diarrhea

Chronic Diarrhea

Fever	Inflammatory bowel disease; amebiasis; lymphoma, pseudomembranous colitis; Whipple's disease
Edema; ascites	Protein-losing enteropathy with hypoalbuminemia; malabsorption of amino acids with hypoproteinemia; nephrotic syndrome with amyloidosis
Skin manifestations:	
Hyperpigmentation • generalized • sparing the mucosae • of oral mucosae	Addison's disease Whipple's disease Peutz-Jeghers syndrome
Erythema nodosum	Inflammatory bowel disease
Petechiae, ecchymoses	Vitamin K malabsorption with hypoprothrombinemia; Henoch-Schönlein purpura
Scleroderma	Stasis and bacterial overgrowth of the small intestine
Glossitis; cheilosis	Malabsorption syndromes with deficiency of iron, vitamin B_{12}, folate, other vitamins
Jaundice	Inflammatory bowel disease (sclerosing cholangitis); neoplasm
Lymphadenopathy	Whipple's disease; lymphoma
Enlarged thyroid; tremor; tachycardia	Thyrotoxicosis

Heart murmur; attacks of wheezing; loud bowel sounds; flushing; hepatomegaly	Carcinoid syndrome
Chronic pulmonary disease	Cystic fibrosis (may be observed in adults)
Abdominal mass, tenderness in RLQ	Carcinoma; Crohn's disease
Abdominal mass, tenderness in LLQ	Carcinoma; diverticulitis
Perianal fistula or abscess	Crohn's disease
Arthritis	Ulcerative colitis; Crohn's disease; Whipple's disease; amyloidosis
Peripheral neuropathy	Diabetes with autonomic neuropathy; Whipple's disease; amyloidosis; malabsorption syndromes with deficiency of vitamin B_{12}
Postural hypotension	Salt and water depletion in secretory diarrhea; diabetic diarrhea; Addison's disease
Stroke; atherosclerotic disease of large vessels	Ischemic injury to the gut: mesenteric arterial insufficiency
Abnormal rectal examination	Malignancy, etc.; decreased anal sphincter tone; impaction: usually associated with liquid feces

LABORATORY TESTS PERTAINING TO DIARRHEA[†]

Test	Finding	Diagnostic Possibilities
Acute Diarrhea		
Stool		
Examination for ova, parasites; culture	Positive	Salmonellosis; bacillary dysentery, amebiasis; giardiasis; etc.
Occult blood tests	Positive	Inflammatory bowel disease; bacterial infection; GI tumor
Fecal leukocytes	Positive	*Shigella; E. coli* (enteroinvasive strains); *Campylobacter; Salmonella; Yersinia; E. histolytica*
	Negative	*V. cholerae; E. coli* (enteropathic and enterotoxigenic strains); viruses; *Giardia; Cryptosporidium;* food poisoning: *C. perfringens; S. aureus; B. cerus*

[†]See the appendix on Laboratory Reference Values for the associated normal laboratory values.

Test	Finding	Diagnostic Possibilities
Proctosigmoid-oscopy		Indicated in acute bloody diarrhea or acute diarrhea not improved within 10 days. Inflammatory disease; parasitic disease; melanosis coli: chronic usage of anthraquinone laxatives; pseudomembranous colitis; rectal or colonic neoplasm

Chronic Diarrhea

Stool

Fat	More than 7 g/24 h	Steatorrhea; malabsorption, maldigestion (pancreatic insufficiency)
	Normal	Diarrhea of colonic origin
D-Xylose absorption	Normal	Pancreatic insufficiency
	Decreased	Malabsorption

Blood

Carotene	Decreased	Steatorrhea; malabsorption; maldigestion
Prothrombin time	Prolonged	Vitamin K deficiency; malabsorption; maldigestion
Iron	Normal	Maldigestion: pancreatic insufficiency
	Decreased	Chronic blood loss; impaired absorption
Vitamin B_{12} absorption (Schilling test)	Decreased	Bacterial overgrowth; exocrine pancreatic insufficiency; extensive ileal disease; pernicious anemia
Breath tests (with lactulose, ^{14}C-labeled bile acid, or ^{14}C-D-xylose)	Abnormal	Bacterial overgrowth in the small bowel
Secretin test	Normal	Malabsorption
	Abnormal	Pancreatic insufficiency

LABORATORY PROCEDURES PERTAINING TO DIARRHEA

Procedure	To Detect
Upper GI series; barium enema	Zollinger-Ellison syndrome; malabsorption pattern; inflammatory bowel disease; GI tumor; gastroileostomy; scleroderma; intestinal fistulas. (Normal small-bowel pattern: pancreatic insufficiency)
Fiberoptic colonoscopy	Inflammatory vs. neoplastic lesions; nature of localized lesions
Small-bowel biopsy	Sprue; Whipple's disease; amyloidosis; Crohn's disease; giardiasis; lymphoma; etc.

SELECTED BIBLIOGRAPHY

Fine KD, Krejs GJ, Fordtran JS: Diarrhea, in Sleisenger MH, Fordtran JS (eds). *Gastrointestinal Disease. Pathophysiology. Diagnosis. Management,* 4th ed., pp. 290–316, Philadelphia: Saunders, 1989.

Quinn TC, Bender BS, Bartlett JG: New developments in infectious diarrhea. *DM* 32:166–244, 1986.

Trier JS: Intestinal malabsorption: Differentiation of cause. *Hosp Pract* 23(5):195–211, 1988.

15

Dyspepsia (Indigestion, Chronic Abdominal Discomfort)

INTRODUCTION

Dyspepsia Abdominal distress associated with the intake of food.

Dyspepsia may result from disease of the GI tract or may be associated with pathologic conditions in other organ systems. Visceral abdominal pain of dyspepsia generally results from distention or exaggerated muscular contraction of a viscus and is mediated by visceral afferent nerves which accompany the abdominal sympathetic pathways. The pain of peptic ulcer is believed to be produced either directly by acid irritating exposed nerve endings in the ulcer or by alteration of the motor activity of the gastroduodenal segment that the patient appreciates as ulcer pain. Some patients with dyspepsia describe a sensation of abdominal distention and various complaints, some of which appear to be related to increased quantities of, or sensitivity to, gas in the gastrointestinal tract (flatulence).

Patients with dyspepsia may also complain of:

Belching Forceful regurgitation of air from the esophagus or stomach; usually due to aerophagia (excessive swallowing of air). Aerophagia is generally a compulsive habit and a manifestation of emotional tension.

Heartburn (pyrosis) A burning sensation located substernally or high in the epigastrium, with radiation into the neck and occasionally to the arms. Heartburn may result from abnormal motor activity of the esophagus, reflux of acid or bile into the esophagus, or direct esophageal mucosal irritation.

Regurgitation Effortless appearance of esophageal or gastric contents in the mouth. It may be due to an incompetent lower esophageal sphincter.

Dyspepsia with no clear etiologic explanation is often designated as "functional dyspepsia." However, some patients with functional indigestion also have other features of the irritable bowel syndrome, suggesting a diffuse disturbance of gastrointestinal motility.

ETIOLOGY

Irritable bowel syndrome
Anxiety and/or depression
Peptic ulcer (gastric, duodenal); carcinoma of stomach; gastritis
Gastroesophageal reflux
Chronic cholecystitis, cholelithiasis; choledocholithiasis
Chronic relapsing pancreatitis; carcinoma of the pancreas
Malabsorptive states; diverticulosis; inflammatory bowel disease; intermittent intestinal obstruction; ischemic disease of the intestine (intestinal angina)

Extraintestinal diseases and intoxications: polyarteritis nodosa; systemic lupus erythematosus; lead poisoning; hypercalcemia; porphyria; hyperlipidemia; uremia; congestive heart failure; pulmonary tuberculosis; neoplastic diseases

Iatrogenic Causes of Chronic Abdominal Discomfort

Nonsteroidal anti-inflammatory agents; potassium chloride; corticosteroids; ferrous salts; reserpine

HISTORY TAKING*

Possible meaning of a positive response

1   Location of Abdominal Distress

1.1	Where do you have discomfort? distress? pain?	The location of the discomfort corresponds generally to the segmental level of neural innervation of the affected organ

1.1   Where do you have discomfort? distress? pain?

The location of the discomfort corresponds generally to the segmental level of neural innervation of the affected organ

• in the epigastrium?

Esophageal, gastric, duodenal (first and second portions), biliary or pancreatic origin; also "functional" pain

• substernal?

Disorders of esophagus or cardia of stomach; cardiac disease

• right upper quadrant?

Biliary pain; cholelithiasis; cholecystitis; hepatitis; cirrhosis; passive congestion of liver; irritable bowel syndrome; lesion of head of pancreas

• periumbilical?

Small-bowel disease: regional enteritis; intestinal obstruction

• below the umbilicus?

Appendiceal, colonic: ulcerative colitis, carcinoma of colon, partial obstruction; pelvic origin of pain

• left upper quadrant?

Splenic flexure syndrome: swallowed air trapped in the splenic flexure of the colon; irritable bowel syndrome; tail of pancreas

• left lower quadrant? hypogastrium?

Irritable bowel syndrome; diverticulosis

1.2   Is the pain or discomfort
• diffuse?

Visceral pain

• localized?

Somatic pain; referred pain; if epigastric: large or penetrating peptic ulcer

1.3   Does the pain
• remain in the same place?

Gastric ulcer pain: usually no radiation in the absence of posterior penetration of the ulcer

*In this section, items in *italics* are characteristic clinical features.

- radiate from epigastrium
  - up into the middle of the chest? the neck?

    Esophageal dysfunction; gastroesophageal reflux
  - *through to the back?*

    Posterior penetration of an ulcer; pancreatic lesion
  - to the right upper quadrant?

    Involvement of gallbladder or biliary ducts; carcinoma of head of pancreas
  - to the left?

    Carcinoma of body and tail of pancreas
- radiate from the left upper quadrant to the left side of the chest? left shoulder?

  Splenic flexure syndrome

2 Mode of Onset, Duration, and Chronology

2.1 How long have you had pain in the abdomen?

For years: duodenal ulcer; functional dyspepsia

2.1a Was it precipitated by a stressful event?

Functional dyspepsia; irritable bowel syndrome

2.2 Is the pain or discomfort
- constant?

  Infiltrating gastric carcinoma
- intermittent? recurrent?

  May be associated with the use of certain drugs; chronic relapsing pancreatitis; acute gastritis; biliary colic; allergic reactions to food; irritable bowel syndrome: the most common cause of chronic or recurrent abdominal pain

2.3 If the pain is intermittent: What is the frequency, duration of the attacks?

2.4 *Does the pain occur in episodes of 2 to 10 weeks separated by pain-free periods lasting several months?*

Peptic ulcer disease

2.5 Do you experience more discomfort in the spring and autumn than at other times?

Seasonal pattern of peptic ulcer disease

3 Character of the Discomfort

3.1 Do you have abdominal pain? distress? discomfort? fullness? pressure? heartburn?

Most patients have difficulty in accurately describing chronic abdominal distress

3.2 Do you have
- a dull and aching distress?

  Visceral pain; peptic ulcer (if epigastric)
- epigastric hunger pain? gnawing, burning pain?

  Peptic ulcer disease
- vague, cramping pain or discomfort in the periumbilical area?

  Irritable bowel syndrome; intermittent intestinal obstruction; regional enteritis

• colicky (wavelike) pain?

Forceful peristaltic contractions attempting to overcome an obstruction: in small intestine, colon, biliary tract

• sharp? localized pain?

Acute abdominal process involving the peritoneum. This pain, mediated by cerebrospinal afferent nerves, must be distinguished from the visceral pain of dyspepsia

3.3   In case of epigastric pain: Does the pain
   • gradually increase in intensity? remain steady for 1/2 to 2 h before gradually subsiding?

Pain of peptic ulcer disease

   • reach a peak intensity within 15 to 45 min, subsiding over several hours?

Biliary "colic" (sudden distention of the biliary tree produces a steady type of pain)

4   Precipitating or Aggravating Factors

4.1   *Is the distress related to food?*

An important diagnostic feature

4.1a Does the distress occur or worsen
   • during, or shortly after, eating?

Early postprandial indigestion: esophageal disease; acute gastritis; gastric carcinoma; allergic reaction; biliary tract disease; abdominal angina (15 to 30 min after a meal)

   • *30 to 90 minutes after eating?*

Peptic ulcer disease

   • several hours after eating?

Late postprandial indigestion: gastric outlet obstruction or atony; duodenal ulcer; pancreatic insufficiency

   • *after drinking milk?*

Lactase deficiency, congenital or acquired (sprue, ulcerative colitis, Crohn's disease)

   • after eating
     • fatty foods?

Pancreatic or biliary tract disease (not specific for gallbladder dysfunction); functional GI disease more likely

     • gluten-containing foods? (wheat, barley, rye)

Celiac sprue

     • vegetables?

Fermentative action of bacteria on nonabsorbable sugars contained in vegetables, with increased gas production

     • citrus fruit?

Peptic ulcer disease; peptic esophagitis

     • fried foods?

Chronic cholecystitis; gallstones; nonulcer dyspepsia

     • large intake of alcohol?

Chronic relapsing pancreatitis; peptic ulcer; gastroesophageal reflux

     • others?

May initiate recurrent allergic reactions

   • before breakfast?

Functional: infrequent in peptic ulcer; may occur in carcinoma of stomach

4.2 Is the distress caused or worsened by
- certain drugs? — Porphyria, following use of barbiturates
- stress? — Irritable bowel syndrome
- when lying flat? — Carcinoma of pancreas
- *1 to 2 hours after retiring?* — Organic disease; duodenal ulcer (pain that occurs during the night should never be called "functional")

4.3 For the female patient: Is the pain related to your menstruations? — Intestinal endometriosis

5 Relieving Factors

5.1 Is the distress relieved by
- *food? antacids?* — Peptic ulceration: neutralization of the acid; acute gastritis
- vomiting? — Peptic ulcer (if not relieved: pancreatic or biliary tract disease)
- defecation? passing gas? — Functional or organic lesion likely in colon or distal ileum; irritable bowel syndrome; ulcerative colitis; splenic flexure syndrome
- belching? — Aerophagia
- standing? *leaning forward?* sitting upright? — Pancreatic pain: tumor, pancreatitis

6 Accompanying Symptoms

6.1 Do you have
- a substernal sensation of warmth or burning? — Heartburn (pyrosis): reflux of acid or bile into the esophagus, abnormal motor activity or distention of the esophagus, or direct esophageal mucosal irritation (esophagitis); may be psychogenic. When severe, may radiate to the sides of the chest and neck

6.1a Is your heartburn
- evoked or worsened by meals? citrus fruit juices? alcohol? aspirin? when lying down? bending? stooping?
- relieved by standing up? drinking milk? liquids? antacids?

Gastroesophageal reflux, with or without esophagitis

6.2 Do you have the spontaneous appearance in the mouth of
- salty or sour fluid? — Regurgitation often accompanies heartburn: severe gastroesophageal reflux of gastric contents
- bitter and green or yellow fluid? — Gastroesophageal reflux of bile

6.3   Do you have
      • frequent belching?

Results from aerophagia, not from excessive gas formation in the GI tract; in chronic anxiety; rapid eating, bad habit; drinking carbonated beverages; gum chewing; postnasal drip; poorly fitting dentures. Repeated belching also in gastric outlet obstruction

      • abdominal fullness? pressure?

Accumulation of swallowed air in the stomach may cause postprandial fullness and pressure ("magenblase syndrome"). Swallowed air trapped in the splenic flexure of the colon may cause LUQ fullness and pressure

         • after lying supine after a large meal?

Gastric (swallowed) air "trapped" below the gastroesophageal junction by overlying fluid cannot be eructated

         • relieved by belching? passing gas? defecation?

Aerophagia; irritable bowel syndrome

      • diffuse abdominal distention? bloating?

Abnormal intestinal motor activity rather than excessive intestinal gas causes bloating: irritable bowel syndrome. In malabsorption, fermentation of dietary carbohydrate may result in excessive gas production

      • frequent bowel sounds? gas?

Flatulence: aerophagia; irritable bowel syndrome; diet containing large quantities of nonabsorbable carbohydrates (some grains, vegetables); increased intraluminal gas production due to fermentative action of colonic bacteria on nondigestible carbohydrates in carbohydrate malabsorption states

      • difficulty swallowing?

Esophageal disease (see Chapter 16 "Dysphagia")

      • nausea? vomiting?

Peptic ulcer disease or nonulcer dyspepsia; biliary tract disease

      • a loss of appetite? of weight?

Excludes irritable bowel syndrome. Serious underlying disease; carcinoma of stomach; Crohn's disease; malabsorption

      • fever?

Chronic cholecystitis; Crohn's disease

      • lip swelling? urticaria? asthma? associated with the abdominal distress?

Allergic reaction to food

      • *a change in your bowel habits?*

Significant

         • constipation?

Obstructing lesion in the colon

         • watery diarrhea? small loose stools? with mucus?

Irritable bowel syndrome (some patients have "pencil-like" pasty stools rather than diarrhea)

- *alternating diarrhea and constipation?*

Carcinoma of left colon; irritable bowel syndrome; intermittent obstructive symptoms; Crohn's disease

- stools containing blood?

Inflammatory bowel disease; bleeding is not a feature of irritable bowel syndrome

7 Iatrogenic Factors   See Etiology

8 Personal and Social Profile

8.1 Do you smoke?

The incidence of peptic ulcer and the recurrence of ulcers are higher in smokers than in nonsmokers

8.2 What is your consumption of alcohol?

Acute alcohol intake can cause inflammation of the esophagus and stomach; alcoholism with chronic pancreatitis

9 Personal Antecedents Pertaining to the Dyspepsia

9.1 Have you ever had an x-ray of the stomach? intestine? gallbladder? When? With what results?

9.2 Do you have any of the following conditions: a peptic ulcer? alcoholism? colitis? diverticulosis? a liver disease (cirrhosis)?
- anxiety? depression?

Psychological factors often play an etiologic or contributing role in irritable bowel syndrome

PHYSICAL SIGNS PERTAINING TO DYSPEPSIA

	Possible significance
Abdominal distention; tenderness in the area of the colon; tender palpable sigmoid colon	Irritable bowel syndrome
Increased tympany in left lateral portion of the upper abdomen	Splenic flexure syndrome
Visible or palpable distended loops of bowel; visible peristalsis; hyperactive bowel sounds	Obstructive intestinal lesion; Crohn's disease; left carcinoma of colon
Abdominal masses	Neoplastic disease; inflammatory disease
Epigastric tenderness	Peptic ulcer; also observed in nonulcer dyspepsia: pancreatitis, cholecystitis, gastric cancer, functional dyspepsia

Jaundice; palpable gallbladder; hepatomegaly	Liver, bile ducts, or pancreas disorder
Fever	Inflammatory bowel disease; lymphoma; collagen-vascular disease
Fever; jaundice; RUQ tenderness	Biliary tract disease; chronic cholecystitis
Rectal and pelvic examination	May reveal: rectal mass; metastatic tumor; pelvic inflammatory disease; abnormalities of the uterus or adnexae; prostatic abnormalities

LABORATORY TESTS PERTAINING TO DYSPEPSIA[†]

Test	Finding	Diagnostic Possibilities
Blood		
Bilirubin, alkaline phosphatase	Elevated	Obstruction of the biliary tract
Amylase	Elevated	Pancreatitis
Stool		
Occult blood	Positive	Gastrointestinal mucosal lesion
Fat, muscle fibers	Present	Pancreatic disorders; malabsorption syndrome

[†]See the appendix on Laboratory Reference Values for the associated normal laboratory values.

LABORATORY PROCEDURES PERTAINING TO DYSPEPSIA

Procedure	To Detect
Plain abdominal film	Pancreatic, cholecystic calculi; large amounts of air in the splenic flexure of the colon
Upper GI barium series and/or endoscopy (for the patient with symptoms despite 6 to 8 weeks of therapy)	Reflux esophagitis; gastric or duodenal ulcers; atrophic gastritis; bile reflux gastritis; duodenitis
When indicated: ultrasonography of the gallbladder; barium enema; proctosigmoidoscopy; psychologic evaluation	

SELECTED BIBLIOGRAPHY

Drossman DA: Irritable bowel syndrome: A multifactorial disorder. *Hosp Pract* 23(9):119–133, 1988.

Health and Public Policy Committee, American College of Physicians: Endoscopy in the evaluation of dyspepsia. *Ann Intern Med* 102:266–269, 1985.

Levitt MD: Excessive gas: Patient perception versus reality. *Hosp Pract* 20(11):143–163, 1985.

Talley NJ, Phillips SF: Non-ulcer dyspepsia: Potential causes and pathophysiology. *Ann Intern Med* 108:865–879, 1988.

16
Dysphagia

INTRODUCTION

Dysphagia   A sensation of obstruction of the passage of food from the mouth to the
   stomach.

The esophagus is separated from the pharynx by the upper esophageal sphincter
(UES), which prevents air from filling the esophagus during inspiration, and from the
stomach by the lower esophageal sphincter (LES), which prevents the reflux of gastric
juice into the esophagus. The body of the esophagus, extending between these two
sphincters, contains predominantly striated muscle in the upper half and smooth
muscle in the lower half.
   When a subject swallows and transfers a bolus of food into the hypopharynx with
the tongue, the nasopharynx is closed by the soft palate to prevent the movement of
food into the nose; the larynx is elevated against the epiglottis, thereby preventing the
aspiration of food into the respiratory passages; the UES relaxes, thus permitting the
bolus to enter the esophagus from the hypopharynx; a peristaltic wave initiated in the
upper esophagus is propagated to the lower esophagus, propelling food along the body
of the esophagus; the LES relaxes and permits the esophageal contents to enter the
stomach. The movement of the bolus from the mouth to the pharynx is voluntary;
subsequent events are involuntary.
   In some patients, dysphagia is related to difficulty in initiating the voluntary act of
swallowing or to defects in the reflex coordination of oropharyngeal movements.
Neuromuscular diseases that affect striated muscle may cause dysphagia referable to
the upper half of the esophagus and the UES, where striated muscle is located.
Diseases involving smooth muscle (e.g., scleroderma) produce impaired peristalsis in
the lower half of the esophagus and decreased pressure and incompetence of the LES.
Achalasia is characterized by a hypertensive and poorly relaxing LES and absent distal
esophageal peristalsis. Dysphagia may also result from the narrowing of the lumen by
a tumor or an inflammatory stricture.
   Dysphagia is a most reliable symptom and indicates the presence of disease or
motor dysfunction; it should never be dismissed as an emotional disturbance.

ETIOLOGY

Oropharyngeal Disorders

Motility disorders
   Cerebral vascular accidents with pseudobulbar or bulbar paralysis; bulbar
      poliomyelitis; motor neuron disease; myasthenia gravis; myopathies; myotonic
      dystrophy; dermatomyositis-polymyositis; amyotrophic lateral sclerosis
Intrinsic obstructive disorders
   Inflammation: stomatitis; pharyngitis; epiglottitis; retropharyngeal abscess
   Pharyngeal web (Plummer-Vinson syndrome); diverticulum (Zenker's, lateral)
   Benign strictures: chemical-induced
   Tumor (benign or malignant); enlarged thyroid

Esophageal Dysphagia

Motility disorders: achalasia; diffuse esophageal spasm; collagen-vascular disease
   (scleroderma, systemic lupus erythematosus); chronic idiopathic intestinal pseudo-
   obstruction; metabolic neuromyopathy (alcoholism)
Intrinsic obstructive disorders
   Stricture* secondary to esophagitis (reflux, infectious, chemical)
   Tumor*: benign or malignant
   Lower esophageal (Schatzki) ring*
   Foreign body
Extrinsic obstructive disorders
   Mediastinal masses (glands, tumors)
   Vascular compression: aberrant right subclavian artery; aortic aneurysm; left atrial
      enlargement
   Cervical spondylitis

Iatrogenic Causes of Dysphagia

Antibiotics; immunosuppressive therapy: can cause dysphagia due to esophageal
   candidiasis, especially in patients weakened by prolonged illness and receiving
   corticosteroids
Tetracycline, ascorbic acid can cause esophageal ulcer

HISTORY TAKING†

Possible meaning of a positive response

1   Character of Complaint

1.1   Do you feel a lump in the throat, in
      the absence of food or fluid inges-
      tion?

1.1a Do you have a sensation of food   Pseudodysphagia: globus hystericus,
      stuck in the chest or throat 15 s to 2 with actually no dysphagia: depression;
      h after ingestion?   hysteria

1.1b Can you swallow foods and liquids
      without difficulty?

1.2   Do you fear or refuse to swallow?   Hysteria, rabies, tetanus, pharyngeal
                                             paralysis (fear of aspiration); painful in-
                                             flammatory lesions

1.3   Do you have difficulty
      • *at the beginning of a swallow?* in   Disorder of the voluntary phase of swal-
        initiating swallowing?   lowing; oropharyngeal dysphagia

*Common cause of dysphagia
†In this section, items in *italics* are characteristic clinical features.

- *after a swallow has begun?* 10 to 15 s after deglutition?

Esophageal dysphagia

1.4 Do you have difficulty swallowing
- liquids?

Motility disorder: achalasia; diffuse esophageal spasm

- solid foods?

Mechanical obstructing lesion with a lumen that is not severely narrowed

- solids, unrelated to posture? liquids, in the recumbent posture? (not in the upright posture)

Scleroderma

- solid and liquid foods?

Dysphagia due to motility disorder: achalasia, diffuse esophageal spasm (from the very onset); advanced obstruction dysphagia (esophageal tumor)

2 Location of Dysphagia

2.1 At what level do you feel the sticking sensation?

When described in the chest: fairly good correlation with the site of esophageal obstruction

- at the level of the lower part of the sternum?
- at the neck?

The most frequent site of esophageal disease
Of no diagnostic value: lesions of the pharynx, cervical esophagus, even lower esophagus may cause dysphagia to be perceived in the neck

2.2 How long after swallowing do you feel the sticking sensation?
- 2 to 5 s after swallowing?

Lesion in thoracic esophagus: carcinoma; cicatricial stenosis; midesophageal diverticulum

- 5 to 15 s after swallowing?

Lesion in lower thoracic or abdominal esophagus: carcinoma; reflux esophagitis; esophageal ulcer

3 Mode of Onset and Evolution

3.1 How long have you had difficulty swallowing?

The duration helps to indicate whether the lesion is benign (3 months or longer) or malignant. However, patients with potentially premalignant lesions (Barrett's esophagus, achalasia, stricture due to swallowing lye) may have a long history of dysphagia before carcinoma develops

3.2 Was the onset of dysphagia
- sudden?

Foreign body; ingestion of corrosive agent

- gradual?

Carcinoma; motor disorder: achalasia, scleroderma

3.3 Is the dysphagia
- transient? of short duration?   Inflammatory process
- intermittent? episodic?
  - to solids? of long duration?   Lower esophageal (Schatzki) ring
- present at every meal?   Fixed, mechanical lesion: carcinoma
- persistent, after having been at first intermittent?   Reflux esophagitis; esophageal ulcer; esophageal carcinoma (in some patients); achalasia

- *constant and progressively worse? first with solids? then with soft foods? then with liquids?*   Decreasing diameter of the esophageal lumen: in carcinoma, occasionally in esophageal stricture
  - over a period of a few weeks to a few months?   Esophageal carcinoma
  - over a period of several years?   Benign disease; achalasia; lower esophageal (Schatzki) ring

4 Relieving Factors

4.1 Is deglutition facilitated by
- tilting the head and neck a certain way?   Oropharyngeal dysphagia
- straightening or arching the back? repeated swallowing? drinking water?   Motor disorder

4.2 Is obstruction relieved by vomiting? regurgitation of the bolus?   Organic narrowing

4.3 Do you
- limit your diet to semiliquid or liquid foods?
- masticate your food longer than usual?
- drink liquids in order to be able to swallow solid foods?

May satisfactorily compensate esophageal dysphagia for a time; mechanical dysphagia (narrowing)

5 Accompanying Symptoms

5.1 Do you have pain on swallowing?   Odynophagia: occurs frequently with dysphagia. Nonreflux esophagitis, *Candida,* herpetic; peptic (Barrett's) ulcer of esophagus; carcinoma with periesophageal involvement; caustic damage; esophageal perforation. Unusual in uncomplicated reflux esophagitis

5.2 Do you have pain not concurrent with eating?   Any form of esophagitis, especially reflux esophagitis

5.3 Does fluid run out of your nose when you swallow liquids?   Nasal regurgitation: pharyngeal paralysis

5.4 Do you experience regurgitation of food
  • soon after swallowing? with neck bulge or gurgle when drinking?

Zenker's diverticulum

  • minutes or hours after a meal?

Achalasia, early stages; esophageal malignancy; esophageal diverticulum

  • particularly when lying down?

Regurgitation of retained material provoked by change in position: achalasia; also in Zenker's diverticulum

5.4a Did you experience regurgitation
  • before the appearance of dysphagia?

Regurgitation is often an early manifestation in Zenker's diverticulum: stagnant food in the diverticular sac

  • after the appearance of dysphagia?

Late manifestation of the other esophageal diseases

5.5 Do you sometimes choke, gag, cough, when trying to swallow?

In oropharyngeal dysphagia: aspiration into the trachea of material accumulating in the pharynx

5.5a Do you have coughing spells
  • with each swallow of food or drink?

Fistulous communication between esophagus and trachea: neoplastic erosion of the trachea

  • unrelated to swallowing? at bedtime?

Tracheobronchial aspiration secondary to achalasia, Zenker's diverticulum; incompetent lower esophageal sphincter causing nocturnal regurgitation and aspiration

5.6 Do you have
  • a sore throat?

Can make swallowing difficult

  • a painful tongue? a sore mouth?

Angular stomatitis, glossitis with iron-deficiency anemia and dysphagia (Plummer-Vinson syndrome): dysphagia due to hypopharyngeal webs

  • hoarseness preceding dysphagia?

Primary lesion in the larynx

  • hoarseness following dysphagia? after an interval of some duration?

Esophageal carcinoma with involvement of the recurrent laryngeal nerve; laryngitis secondary to gastroesophageal reflux; neuromuscular disorder with laryngeal and esophageal symptoms

  • heartburn?

Gastroesophageal reflux; esophagitis: peptic stricture

  • hiccups?

Lesion in the distal portion of the esophagus; carcinoma; achalasia

• a swelling in your neck?	Enlarged thyroid
• chest pain?	Diffuse esophageal spasm (excessive forceful contraction of esophageal muscle); periesophageal involvement caused by carcinoma
• *pain in your fingers when immersed in cold water?*	Raynaud's phenomenon: collagen-vascular disease with dysphagia; scleroderma (esophageal abnormalities may precede skin changes)
• any difficulty walking?	Pseudobulbar paralysis of diffuse cerebrovascular disease; spasticity of amyotrophic lateral sclerosis; myasthenia gravis
• speech difficulty?	Motor system disorder
• a loss of weight?	Common in most causes of dysphagia interfering with adequate food intake
• out of proportion to the degree of dysphagia?	Esophageal carcinoma
• no loss of weight?	Lower esophageal ring with intermittent dysphagia

6   Iatrogenic Factors   See Etiology

7   Personal and Social Profile

7.1	What is your sexual orientation?	Pain on swallowing in a homosexual man: *Candida* esophagitis; herpetic esophagitis

8   Personal Antecedents Pertaining to the Dysphagia

8.1	Have you ever had an x-ray examination of the esophagus? the stomach? an esophagoscopy? gastroscopy? chest x-ray? When? With what results?	
8.2	Do you remember having swallowed	
	• a caustic corrosive agent? a foreign body?	Dysphagia due to an esophageal stricture
8.3	Have you ever had	
	• a prolonged nasogastric intubation? previous radiation therapy?	Esophageal stricture
8.4	Do you have frequent bouts of pneumonitis?	Aspiration of regurgitated material; commonly observed in patients with achalasia

PHYSICAL SIGNS PERTAINING TO DYSPHAGIA

Possible significance

Ulcerative lesions of mouth and/or pharynx — Lesions interfering with passage of food because of pain

Pharyngeal swelling — Retropharyngeal abscess; peritonsillar abscess

Constricted skin around the mouth; joint deformities — Scleroderma

Neck: enlarged thyroid; spinal abnormality — Mechanical obstruction of the esophagus

Foul breath (halitosis) — Retained esophageal material; achalasia, Zenker's diverticulum

Abnormal neurologic examination; dysphonia; dysarthria; ptosis; tongue atrophy; hyperactive jaw reflex — Bulbar or pseudobulbar palsy: neuromuscular disorder

LABORATORY PROCEDURES PERTAINING TO DYSPHAGIA

Procedure	To Detect
Barium swallow, esophageal cineradiography	Mechanical obstruction; motor abnormality
Esophagogastroscopy with biopsy and/or exfoliative cytology	Superficial ulcers; esophagitis; inflammatory or neoplastic lesions; stricture
Esophageal motility study	Neuromuscular disorders of upper esophagus, pharynx; lower esophageal sphincter malfunction; diffuse esophageal spasm; achalasia; scleroderma

SELECTED BIBLIOGRAPHY

Kramer P: Dysphagia–Etiologic differentiation and therapy. *Hosp Pract* 23(3A):125–149, 1988.
Marshall, JB: Dysphagia. *Postgrad Med* 85(4):243–260, 1989.
Nelson JB, Castell DO: Esophageal motility disorders. *DM* 34(6):297–389, 1988.

17
Hematemesis and/or Melena

INTRODUCTION

Hematemesis Vomiting of blood, whether fresh and red or digested and black.
Melena Passage of black, tarry stools containing digested blood.

Hematemesis without melena is generally due to lesions proximal to the ligament of Treitz, since blood entering the gastrointestinal tract below the duodenum rarely enters the stomach. Melena without hematemesis is usually due to lesions distal to the pylorus. In general, the patient who presents with hematemesis is more likely to have bled greater amounts than the patient with melena.

  Approximately 60 mL of blood is required to produce a single black stool. Gaiac-impregnated slides detect approximately 5 mL of blood in a 24-hour sample of stool.

ETIOLOGY

Upper Gastrointestinal Bleeding

Common
  Peptic ulcer (gastric, duodenal); esophageal varices; esophagogastric mucosal tear (Mallory-Weiss syndrome); erosive gastritis
Unusual or rare
  Esophagitis; gastric or duodenal neoplasms; submucosal neoplasms; duodenitis; leaking aortic aneurysm or vascular graft; elastic tissue disorders; hereditary telangiectasia; bleeding disorders; vasculitis

Lower Gastrointestinal Bleeding

Common
  Inflammatory bowel disease; diverticulosis; ischemic colitis; angiodysplasia; hemorrhoids; proctitis
Unusual or rare
  Meckel's diverticulum; carcinoma of the colon; colonic or rectal polyps; radiation colitis; antibiotic-associated colitis; leaking aneurysm or vascular graft; amyloidosis; hereditary telangiectasia; bleeding disorders; vasculitis; infections (shigellosis, amebiasis, campylobacteriosis)

Iatrogenic Causes of Gastrointestinal Bleeding

Aspirin; other nonsteroidal anti-inflammatory drugs; alkylating agents; coumarin derivatives; heparin; antimetabolites; reserpine (large doses); ethacrynic acid; corticosteroids
Enteric-coated potassium chloride: intestinal ulceration
Oral contraceptives: ischemic colitis

HISTORY TAKING*

1 Mode of Onset of the Bleeding

1.1 When did the bleeding occur?

1.1a Have you
  • vomited blood?

Hematemesis: bleeding proximal to the ligament of Treitz

  • passed black, tarry stools?

Melena: usually denotes bleeding from the esophagus, stomach, or duodenum, but lesions in the jejunum, ileum, and even ascending colon may cause melena provided the gastrointestinal transit time is sufficiently prolonged. Melena alone occurs more often than hematemesis in patients with bleeding ulcer

  • had both hematemesis and melena?

Melena may occur independently of, or be associated with, hematemesis. Bleeding sufficient to produce hematemesis usually results in melena. Less than half of patients with melena have hematemesis

1.2 Have you had, prior to the hematemesis,
  • bleeding from the nose? bloody expectorations? a dental extraction?

Blood from these conditions may be swallowed and subsequently vomited, or resulting in melena

2 Character of the Bleeding

2.1 What is the color, the appearance of the vomited blood?

Depends on the concentration of hydrochloric acid in the stomach, its admixture with the blood, and the duration of contact of the blood with gastric acid in the stomach

  • red?

Vomiting occurring shortly after the onset of bleeding; bleeding site above the level of the pylorus; esophageal lesion

  • dark red? brown? black?

Delay in vomiting; blood converted to hematin in the stomach in the presence of hydrochloric acid

  • "coffee-ground" appearance?

Precipitated blood clots in the vomitus

  • bright red and frothy?

Blood coming from the lungs

*In this section, items in *italics* are characteristic clinical features, and items in **boldface** are potentially life-threatening or urgent conditions.

2.2   What is the color of the stool?
       • bright red?   Hematochezia: source of bleeding distal
                                                  to the ligament of Treitz: lesion in ter-
                                                  minal ileum, colon, rectosigmoid; may
                                                  result from rapid hemorrhage into the
                                                  esophagus, stomach, or duodenum (see
                                                  Chapter 20 "Rectal Bleeding")

       • black, tarry? ("sticky"?)   The altered color of the blood results
                                                  from prolonged contact with hydro-
                                                  chloric acid to produce hematin. Blood
                                                  must remain in the gut for approxi-
                                                  mately 8 h to produce melena

3   Extent and Rate of Bleeding

3.1   Have you vomited blood
       • only once? several times?   Patients with hematemesis have usually
                                                  bled greater amounts (often greater
                                                  than 1000 mL) than those who have
                                                  melena alone (usually 500 mL or less)

3.1a   Has the bleeding been abrupt?   **Variceal bleeding, peptic ulcer;** the
       massive?   patient should be considered to have
                                                  lost one-third to one-half of his or her
                                                  blood volume

3.2   In the case of melena: Have you   Usually associated with a loss of more
       had more than one black, tarry   than 25 percent of the blood volume
       stool within a 24-h period?

3.2a   For how long have the tarry stools   Acute blood loss greater than 60 mL
       persisted?   may produce melena for up to 3 days.
                                                 Stools may remain tarry for 48 to 72 h
                                                 after bleeding has stopped
       • for more than 3 days?   Severe hemorrhage

4   Accompanying Symptoms

4.1   *Have you had, prior to the hemateme-*   Mallory-Weiss syndrome: mucosal lac-
       sis, retching and severe nonbloody   eration at the esophagogastric junction
       vomiting?

4.2   Did you notice just before, during,
       or after, the hemorrhage:
       • *lightheadedness?* nausea? *thirst?*   Clinical manifestations of hypotension;
         sweating?   rapid hemorrhage of more than 500 mL
                                                 blood

       • faintness
         • *when lying down?*   **50 percent loss of blood volume**
                                                 should be assumed
         • *when standing?*   20 to 30 percent loss of blood volume
                                                 should be assumed
       • *syncope?*   Signifies a **blood loss of at least 1000
                                                  to 1500 mL**

4.3	Following the hemorrhage, did you have diarrhea?	Common in gastrointestinal bleeding: blood within the GI tract is irritating
4.4	Do you have any complaints?	Blood loss of less than 500 mL is rarely associated with systemic signs, except in the elderly or in the anemic patient
4.5	Have you noticed	
	• heartburn?	Esophageal lesion: inflammatory, ulcerous, or malignant
	• pain in the stomach?	
	• *relieved by food? antacids?*	Peptic ulcer (usually in the duodenum), the most common cause of upper GI bleeding. To be considered even when a characteristic history is not obtained: bleeding from duodenal or gastric ulcer occurs without prior symptoms in 20 percent of patients
	• a decrease of appetite? a weight loss? fatigue?	Carcinoma in upper or lower gastrointestinal tract
	• a change in the bowel habits? diarrhea?	Colonic neoplasm; inflammatory bowel disease; amebic colitis; diverticulosis
	• abdominal pain?	Aortoenteric fistula; vasculitis; inflammatory bowel disease; ischemic colitis; colonic neoplasm (diverticular hemorrhage is painless)
4.6	Do you bruise easily?	Hemorrhagic diathesis

5 Iatrogenic Factors   See Etiology

5.1	Do any of your medications contain aspirin?	Many patients do not consider aspirin a "medication." Aspirin and many other nonsteroidal anti-inflammatory drugs may cause erosive gastritis, gastroduodenitis, peptic ulceration, and bleeding
5.2	Do you receive anticoagulant therapy?	Consider an underlying gastrointestinal lesion (benign or malignant) as a possible cause of the intestinal bleeding
5.3	Do you receive iron? bismuth preparations? charcoal? licorice?	Impart a black or dark color to the stools, without a tarry consistency

6 Personal and Social Profile

| 6.1 | Age of the patient? | Common causes of lower gastrointestinal bleeding in patients aged 60 and over: angiodysplastic lesions (usually in the ascending colon); colonic neoplasm; ischemic colitis; colonic diverticulosis
In young adults: colonic polyps, inflammatory bowel disease, enteric bacterial and parasitic disease |

6.2   What is your alcohol intake?

GI bleeding in an alcoholic patient: variceal bleeding; alcoholic gastritis; peptic ulcer

7   Personal Antecedents Pertaining to the GI Bleeding

7.1   Have there been similar episodes in the past? When? Diagnosis?

7.1a Were you hospitalized on this occasion? Did you receive a transfusion?

7.2   Have you ever had an x-ray of your stomach? of your intestine? a gastroscopy? When? With what results?

7.3   Have you had, prior to the bleeding
      • a heavy alcohol intake?
      • a major trauma? surgery? a severe systemic disease?

Erosive gastritis
Erosive gastritis is frequently seen under such conditions

7.4   Do you have any of the following conditions:
      • peptic ulcer? bleeding tendency? ulcerative colitis? diverticulosis? polyposis?
      • liver disease? alcoholism? alcoholic cirrhosis?

Variceal bleeding, the result of portal hypertension; however, approximately half the patients with cirrhosis will be bleeding from other lesions (e.g., acute gastric erosions, gastritis, peptic ulcer)

      • aortic reconstructive surgery?
      • previous surgery for bleeding peptic ulcer?

Aortoenteric fistula
Possibility of recurrent ulcer

7.5   What was your blood pressure prior to the bleeding?

Knowledge of the previous blood pressure allows more accurate evaluation of the significance of the blood pressure immediately after the hemorrhage

8   Family Medical History Pertaining to the GI Bleeding

8.1   Are there any other members of your family who have
      • an intestinal disease?

Familial colonic polyposis; juvenile polyposis; Peutz-Jeghers syndrome

      • a bleeding tendency?

Congenital deficit of a coagulation factor; hereditary hemorrhagic telangiectasia

PHYSICAL SIGNS PERTAINING TO HEMATEMESIS AND/OR MELENA*

	Possible significance
Clinical shock: restlessness; acute hypotension; tachycardia; thready peripheral pulse; pallor; cold clammy skin	Acute blood loss of about 40 percent of the blood volume; blood loss in excess of 1500 mL usually leads to cardiovascular collapse
Systolic blood pressure below 100 mmHg	Blood volume probably less than 70 percent of normal
Pulse rate of 100 or more per minute	Blood volume probably less than 80 percent of normal
Postural signs: patient placed in the upright (from supine to sitting) position: • **pulse rate rises 25 percent or more** • **systolic blood pressure falls 20 mmHg or more**	**Significant hypovolemia; acute blood loss of more than 1000 mL**
Pallor of the palmar creases	Loss of more than 20 percent of the blood volume
Jaundice; spider angiomas; palmar erythema; hepatosplenomegaly; ascites	Cirrhosis with portal hypertension and varices, gastritis, or gastric ulceration
Abdominal tenderness or masses	Malignancy
Left supraclavicular (Virchow's) node	Metastatic intraabdominal malignancy
Epigastric tenderness	Peptic ulcer (not specific)
Arthritis	Possible salicylate and other drug ingestion causing gastritis; ulcerative colitis; vasculitis
Abdominal scars of previous surgery	Bleeding stomal ulcer; recurrent malignancy
Melanin pigmentation of the lips, buccal mucosae, distal extremities	Peutz-Jeghers syndrome: small intestinal polyps with recurrent melena
Telangiectases on upper trunk and oral pharynx	Hereditary hemorrhagic telangiectasia
Diffuse pigmentation; hepatomegaly	Hemochromatosis and liver impairment
Multiple sebaceous cysts; soft-tissue tumors; bony tumors	Colonic polyposis (Gardner's syndrome)
Palpable purpura	Vasculitis
Purpuric rash of the lower extremities	Henoch-Schönlein purpura

*In this section, items in *italics* are characteristic clinical features, and items in **boldface** are potentially life-threatening or urgent conditions.

Café au lait spots; dermal fibromas	Neurofibromatosis; may be associated with neurofibromas of the intestinal tract
Ecchymoses; petechiae; bleeding gums	Bleeding tendency
Lymphadenopathy	Malignancy; leukemia with bleeding tendency
Rectal examination	To observe the color of the stool. Malignancy; polyposis

LABORATORY TESTS PERTAINING TO HEMATEMESIS AND/OR MELENA[†]

Test	Finding	Diagnostic Possibilities
Blood		
Hemoglobin:	<11 g/100 mL	In an otherwise normal patient: blood loss greater than 1000 mL. The hematocrit, when determined immediately after the onset of bleeding, may not accurately reflect blood loss, since equilibration with extravascular fluid and hemodilution require several hours
RBC morphology	Hypochromic, microcytic anemia	Chronic blood loss
WBCs, platelets	Elevated	May develop within 6 h after the onset of bleeding
Prothrombin time, other coagulation studies	Abnormal	Primary or secondary clotting defects
BUN	Elevated	In upper GI bleeding: due to breakdown of blood proteins to urea by intestinal bacteria as well as from a mild reduction in the glomerular filtration rate
Liver function tests	Abnormal	Liver cirrhosis

[†]See the appendix on Laboratory Reference Values for the associated normal laboratory values.

LABORATORY PROCEDURES PERTAINING TO HEMATEMESIS AND/OR MELENA

Procedure	To Detect
Nasogastric tube	Amount and character of blood present
Esophagogastroduodenoscopy or upper GI x-ray series	Esophageal varices; peptic ulcer; superficial erosive gastritis; neoplastic ulcerative lesion; Mallory-Weiss tear
Sigmoidoscopy, fiberoptic colonoscopy	Site and nature of bleeding lesions proximal to the rectosigmoid area
Selective visceral arteriography	Site of bleeding; bleeding lesion in the small intestine
Radionuclide scanning	Site of bleeding (the rate of blood loss required to make a diagnosis is about 0.1 mL per min)

SELECTED BIBLIOGRAPHY

Isselbacher KJ, Richter JM: Hematemesis, melena, and hematochezia, in Wilson J, Braunwald E, Isselbacher KJ et al (eds). *Harrison's Principles of Internal Medicine*, 12th ed., p. 261, New York: McGraw-Hill, 1991.

Peterson WL: Gastrointestinal bleeding, in Sleisenger MH, Fordtran JS (eds). *Gastrointestinal Disease. Pathophysiology. Diagnosis. Management*, 4th ed., pp. 397–427, Philadelphia: Saunders, 1989.

Steer ML, Silen W: Diagnostic procedures in gastrointestinal hemorrhage. *N Engl J Med* 309:646–650, 1983.

18
Jaundice

INTRODUCTION

Jaundice Yellow pigmentation of the skin or sclerae by bilirubin.

In the normal adult, 80 to 90 percent of serum bilirubin is derived from the breakdown of hemoglobin from aged or injured red blood cells in the reticuloendothelial system. About 10 to 20 percent of serum bilirubin is derived from destruction of immature erythroid cells in the bone marrow (ineffective erythropoiesis) and from the breakdown of nonerythroid components (myoglobin, cytochromes, and heme-containing enzymes). Bilirubin is released from hemoglobin breakdown as a water-insoluble unconjugated compound (free bilirubin). It is transported in serum as a bilirubin-albumin complex which is not filtered by the renal glomeruli. At the hepatic cell membrane, bilirubin and albumin become dissociated, with selective uptake of the bilirubin. In the liver cell, bilirubin is conjugated to water-soluble mono- and di-glucuronides. The conjugated bilirubin is then secreted into the bile canaliculi by an active process. In the intestine, bacterial enzymes convert conjugated bilirubin to colorless urobilinogen, which is excreted in the feces. Some urobilinogen is reabsorbed in the ileum and colon and is either reexcreted in bile or excreted by the kidneys.

Hyperbilirubinemia with jaundice may be due to excessive bilirubin production resulting from accelerated red cell destruction, decreased uptake and conjugation of bilirubin, hepatocellular disease, or extrahepatic cholestasis (reduced bile flow with reduced excretion of bile constituents).

ETIOLOGY

Predominantly Unconjugated Hyperbilirubinemia

Overproduction of bilirubin
    Hemolytic disorders: intra- and extravascular
    Ineffective erythropoiesis
Decreased hepatic uptake of bilirubin
    Drugs; prolonged fasting; sepsis
Decreased bilirubin conjugation
    Decreased or absent glucuronyl transferase activity
        Gilbert's syndrome; Crigler-Najjar syndrome
    Acquired transferase deficiency: drug inhibition; hepatocellular disease: hepatitis; cirrhosis
    Sepsis

Predominantly Conjugated Hyperbilirubinemia

Decreased hepatic excretion of bilirubin into bile (intrahepatic defects)
    Hereditary or familial disorders: Dubin-Johnson syndrome; Rotor syndrome; recurrent (benign) intrahepatic cholestasis; cholestatic jaundice of pregnancy

Acquired disorders
  Hepatocellular disease: hepatitis, viral, bacterial (leptospirosis), or drug-induced;
    cirrhosis (alcoholic, postnecrotic, biliary, cardiac, hemochromatosis, Wilson's
    disease); hepatoma; metastatic tumor
  Drug-induced cholestasis
  Sepsis
Extrahepatic biliary obstruction (mechanical obstruction): stones, stricture, tumor of
  the bile duct, pancreas

Iatrogenic Causes of Jaundice (Partial List)

Hepatocellular Damage

Acetaminophen; methyldopa; aminosalicylic acid and salicylates; allopurinol; antidepressants; antimetabolites; ethionamide; phenytoin; sulfonamides; halothane;
  nitrofurantoin; isoniazid; ketoconazole; oxyphenisatin; phenylbutazone; propylthiouracil; propoxyphene; rifampin; sulfonamides; tetracyclines

Cholestasis

Erythromycin estolate; trimethoprim-sulfamethoxazole; phenothiazines; androgens;
  captopril; nifedipine; amiodarone; chlorpropamide; nitrofurantoin; anabolic steroids; oral contraceptives; gold salts; methimazole

Hepatic Tumors

Anabolic steroids and oral contraceptives (adenoma, carcinoma)

HISTORY TAKING*

		Possible meaning of a positive response
1	Mode of Onset and Duration	
		Jaundice can usually be recognized when the total serum bilirubin exceeds 2 to 2.5 mg/dL
1.1	How long have you been jaundiced?	Days to weeks: hepatitis; obstructive jaundice
		Months: cirrhosis; chronic active hepatitis; primary biliary cirrhosis (in middle-aged women)
1.2	Did the jaundice develop	
	• rapidly? (hours to days)	Hepatitis: viral, drug-induced; choledocholithiasis
	• gradually?	Cirrhosis; carcinoma; cholestasis; chronic active hepatitis; subacute hepatic necrosis; primary biliary cirrhosis

*In this section, items in *italics* are characteristic clinical features, and items in **boldface** are
potentially life-threatening or urgent conditions.

1.3 Was the jaundice preceded by the abrupt onset of

* *loss of appetite? malaise? nausea? vomiting? distaste for cigarettes and alcohol? arthralgias?*

Prodromal symptoms of acute viral hepatitis may precede jaundice by 1 to 2 weeks. Absent in posthepatic obstructive jaundice

* dark urine? light stools?

May be noted by the patient 1 to 5 days prior to the onset of jaundice. Because the renal threshold for conjugated bilirubin is less than 1.0 mg/dL, bilirubinuria may occur without clinically visible jaundice. Bilirubinuria may bring jaundice to clinical attention

* intermittent RUQ abdominal pain?

Gallstone disease with cholestatic jaundice

2 Character of Jaundice

2.1 Is the jaundice
* mild?

Cirrhosis; hemolytic jaundice: does not elevate the serum bilirubin level above 4 mg/100 mL, because of the ability of the normal liver to handle 6 times the usual 250 mg/day of bilirubin presented to it

* intense?

Obstructive jaundice, intra- or extrahepatic

* of varying intensity?

Incomplete extrahepatic obstruction: gallstone disease; hemolysis; cirrhosis

3 Precipitating or Aggravating Factors

3.1 *Have you had in the past 6 months any injections* (subcutaneous, intramuscular, intravenous)? blood tests? vaccinations? intradermal tests? blood or plasma transfusions? dental treatment? tattooing? acupuncture? ear-piercing?

Percutaneous route of transmission of hepatitis B, D, C (non-A, non-B): the major cause of post-transfusion hepatitis

3.2 Did you recently consume oysters? mussels? raw or steamed shellfish? contaminated water?

Viral hepatitis A

4 Accompanying Symptoms

4.1 *What is the color of your urine?*
* as usual?

Unconjugated hyperbilirubinemia (this pigment is not filtered by the glomerulus)

• *dark? like beer? Coca-Cola?*	Bilirubinuria in conjugated hyperbilirubinemia: hepatocellular or obstructive jaundice (if conjugated bilirubin is regurgitated into the serum, it can be filtered by the renal glomerulus). Dark urine is also observed in porphyria, hemoglobinuria, myoglobinuria, ochronosis (homogentisic acid), melanoma (melanin), drugs (e.g., pyridium)
• bloody?	Acute hepatic and renal disease: occupational or domestic exposure to halogenated hydrocarbons, to rats or dogs (leptospirosis)

4.2   *What is the color of your stools?*

• *pale? clay-colored?*	Conjugated hyperbilirubinemia; obstructive jaundice (intra- or posthepatic): failure of bile to reach the intestine resulting in disappearance of urobilinogen from the stool
• well colored?	Hemolytic jaundice
• black, tarry?	**Gastrointestinal hemorrhage**

4.3   Do you have

• fever?	Choledocholithiasis; alcoholic hepatitis; systemic or other extrahepatic infections. Low-grade fever (100–102°F): more often present in hepatitis A than in hepatitis B or C (non-A, non-B). Fever that persists after jaundice has appeared is rare in viral hepatitis, except cytomegalovirus infection or mononucleosis, and infrequent in drug-induced jaundice
• *with chills?*	Cholangitis (extrahepatic biliary obstruction). May occur in infectious mononucleosis. Unlikely in viral hepatitis

4.4   Do you have
• pain in your abdomen? intense? steady?

• in RUQ?	Gallstone obstruction; frank pain is rare in viral hepatitis
• epigastric or RUQ dull, dragging discomfort?	Hepatitis (viral, toxic); cirrhosis; tumor
• chronic dull, boring?	Carcinoma of pancreas

• epigastric pain radiating to the back?	Pancreas disease
• no abdominal pain?	Gradual onset of painless jaundice, with weight loss suggests tumor, such as carcinoma of the head of the pancreas
• loss of appetite? nausea? vomiting?	Viral hepatitis (anorexia at the onset of viral hepatitis improves with fully developed jaundice); cirrhosis (with splanchnic congestion and/or ascites)
• *pain in your joints?*	Hepatitis A, B (immune complex deposition), C (non-A, non-B); drug-induced hepatitis
• headaches?	Viral hepatitis; meningitis in leptospirosis
• *itching?*	Intra- or extrahepatic cholestasis; cholestatic drug reaction. In the female patient: primary biliary cirrhosis
• easy bruising?	Impaired hepatic production of coagulation proteins
• diarrhea?	May occur in viral hepatitis: due to the cathartic action of nonabsorbed fatty acids; pancreatic disease
• abdominal swelling?	Ascites: cirrhosis
• weight loss?	Underlying carcinoma; primary liver disease, tumor

4.5 Do you feel

• ill? sick?	Hepatocellular jaundice: hepatitis
• relatively well?	Cholestatic jaundice ("the patient with obstructive jaundice looks more yellow than sick"); Gilbert's syndrome

5 Iatrogenic Factors   See Etiology

6 Personal and Social Profile

6.1 Age of the patient?	Less than 40 years: viral hepatitis Over 60: anatomic obstruction of the biliary tree, carcinoma, choledocholithiasis At any age: drug-induced hepatic injury
6.2 *What is your alcohol intake?*	Cirrhosis; alcoholic hepatitis; pancreatitis. The alcoholic often denies or understates the amounts consumed; it is desirable to check the validity of the history with close friends or relatives of the patient

6.3   Have you recently had any contact with
      • a jaundiced person?   Hepatitis A is transmitted almost exclusively by the fecal-oral route; nonpercutaneous spread of hepatitis B infection, and hepatitis D infection in endemic areas, is related to intimate personal contact

      • rats? other animals?   Leptospirosis

6.4   Have you traveled to other countries in the past 6 months?   Hepatitis A virus is still widespread in developing countries; hepatitis D virus infection is endemic in Mediterranean countries and northern parts of South America

6.5   What is your occupation? What sort of work have you done in the past?   Hepatitis A more common in day care centers for toddlers. Health care workers in clinical laboratories, dialysis, transplantation, and oncology units are at increased risk for hepatitis B. Increased incidence of cirrhosis in bartenders, brewery workers; hepatitis due to halogenated hydrocarbons, e.g., carbon tetrachloride in: solvent use, lacquer use

6.5a What are your hobbies?   May reveal evidence of toxic exposure; carbon tetrachloride present in various solvents, spot removers, cleaning agents

6.6   What is your sexual orientation?   The prevalence of both hepatitis A and hepatitis B is increased in homosexual men; the prevalence of hepatitis C and D infection in homosexual men is probably increased

6.7   *Do you use intravenous drugs?*   Hepatitis B, D, non-A, non-B

7   Personal Antecedents Pertaining to the Jaundice

7.1   Have you ever had liver tests? a liver biopsy? an x-ray, an ultrasonography of your gallbladder? When? With what results?

7.2   Have you ever had
      • jaundice?   Cirrhosis; intrahepatic cholestasis; extrahepatic jaundice (stones); drug-induced hepatitis; chronic hepatitis B in relapse or with hepatitis D virus superinfection

      • a previous history of indigestion? recurrent RUQ pain?   Cholelithiasis; choledocholithiasis

   • an operation on the biliary tract?   Jaundice occurring shortly after operation: residual stone; within 6 months: hepatitis B, hepatitis C; after one or more years: stricture of the common bile duct

7.3   Do you have any of the following conditions: a liver disease (cirrhosis)? gallstones? GI bleeding? alcoholism?

8   Family Medical History Pertaining to the Jaundice

8.1   Does someone in your family have
   • a liver disease?   Wilson's disease; alpha-1-antitrypsin deficiency; hemochromatosis
   • jaundice?   Hemolytic jaundice; congenital or familial hyperbilirubinemia; gallstones; exposure to a common toxic agent
   • anemia? splenectomy? cholecystectomy?   Hemolytic jaundice; hereditary spherocytosis
   • a neurologic disease?   Wilson's disease (hepatolenticular degeneration)

PHYSICAL SIGNS PERTAINING TO JAUNDICE

	Possible significance
Jaundice	Conjugated bilirubin preferentially stains tissues with high elastin content such as the sclerae or mucous membranes. Unconjugated bilirubin accumulates predominantly in adipose tissue and is best seen in the subcutaneous fat of the abdomen or extremities
with a greenish hue	In pronounced jaundice: oxidation of conjugated bilirubin into biliverdin
Slate color to the skin	Increased melanin: hemochromatosis
Pallor	Anemia: hemolysis, malignancy, cirrhosis
Scratch marks over the body	Pruritus: chronic cholestasis: ascribed to retained bile acids, not related to the intensity of jaundice
Ecchymoses; purpura	Prothrombin deficiency: impaired hepatic synthesis of coagulation proteins; vitamin K malabsorption in obstructive jaundice; thrombocytopenia

Cachexia	Cancer; active cirrhosis
Normal liver size	Intrahepatic, not posthepatic, disorder; hemolytic jaundice
Hepatomegaly	Alcoholic cirrhosis, fibrosis with regeneration; fatty infiltration; cholestasis (intra- or extrahepatic); inflammation (hepatitis); venous congestion; malignancy
Large nodular and stony-hard liver	Hepatoma; hepatic metastases
Palpable liver nodules	Neoplasm; cysts; regeneration nodules; abscesses
Small liver	Acute and subacute hepatic necrosis; postnecrotic cirrhosis
Liver tenderness on palpation	Hepatitis; alcoholic hepatitis; congestive heart failure with acute liver enlargement
Friction rub over the liver	Neoplastic disease; hepatic abscess
Palpable enlarged gallbladder	Courvoisier's sign: extrahepatic biliary obstruction; pancreatic cancer
Tender gallbladder; positive Murphy's sign	Acute cholecystitis
Fever; chills	Suppurative cholangitis
Abdominal distention; shifting dullness; fluid wave	Ascites; in cirrhosis, due to portal hypertension, hypoalbuminemia, increased plasma aldosterone
Ascites, dilated periumbilical veins	Cirrhosis with portal collateral circulation
With venous hum at the umbilicus	In cirrhosis: significant portal hypertension
Spider angiomas; palmar erythema	Acute or chronic liver disease (local arteriovenous shunts?)
Dupuytren's contracture; parotid gland enlargement; gynecomastia; diminished axillary or pubic hair; testicular atrophy	In an alcoholic patient: cirrhosis
Splenomegaly	Medical nature of hepatic disease: cirrhosis; hepatitis; infectious mononucleosis; portal hypertension; hemolytic jaundice
Flapping tremor (asterixis); fetor hepaticus; altered mental state	Portal-systemic encephalopathy; impending hepatic coma
Extrapyramidal signs; Kayser-Fleischer corneal ring	Wilson's disease

LABORATORY TESTS PERTAINING TO JAUNDICE†

Test	Finding	Diagnostic Possibilities
Urine		
Bilirubin	Absent	Unconjugated hyperbilirubinemia: hemolysis; Gilbert's syndrome
	Present	Conjugated hyperbilirubinemia: hepatocellular jaundice, intrahepatic cholestasis; extrahepatic biliary obstruction
Blood		
Hyperbilirubinemia with conjugated-to-total bilirubin ratio	>0.4	Hepatic or obstructive jaundice
	<0.2	Hemolysis; Gilbert's syndrome; other causes of unconjugated hyperbilirubinemia
	Between 0.2 and 0.4	Combined mechanism
Alkaline phosphatase	<3 times normal	Hepatocellular jaundice: viral or toxic hepatitis; chronic active hepatitis; cirrhosis
	>3 times normal	Cholestatic jaundice; hepatic infiltrates; obstructive posthepatic jaundice
Aspartate (AST) and alanine (ALT) aminotransferases	>8 times normal	Acute hepatocellular jaundice: viral or toxic hepatitis
	<8 times normal	Chronic hepatocellular jaundice; chronic active hepatitis; nonalcoholic cirrhosis; intrahepatic cholestasis; posthepatic obstruction
	AST <8 times normal; ALT <3 times normal	Alcoholic hepatitis and cirrhosis
Serum albumin	Decreased	Hepatic necrosis; chronic active hepatitis; cirrhosis
Serum globulin	Elevated	Cirrhosis; chronic active hepatitis
Prothrombin time	Prolonged	Hepatitis; cirrhosis; chronic biliary obstruction

†See the appendix on Laboratory Reference Values for the associated normal laboratory values.

Test	Finding	Diagnostic Possibilities
Serum IgM anti-hepatitis A virus (HAV)	Present	Hepatitis A virus infection
Hepatitis B surface antigen (HBsAg)	Present	Acute or chronic hepatitis B infection
IgM anti-HBc	Present	Recent acute hepatitis B
Antimitochondrial antibodies*	Positive	In over 85 percent of patients with primary biliary cirrhosis
Hematocrit	Decreased	Hemolysis
Reticulocyte count	Elevated	

*When indicated

LABORATORY PROCEDURES PERTAINING TO JAUNDICE

Procedure	To Detect
Ultrasonography; computerized tomography	Gallstones; dilated intrahepatic ducts; tumors in liver, pancreas
Percutaneous transhepatic cholangiography; endoscopic retrograde cholangiopancreatography	Extrahepatic vs. intrahepatic cholestasis
Laparoscopy;* liver biopsy*	Cirrhosis; focal lesions (biopsy contraindicated in obstructive jaundice)

*When indicated

SELECTED BIBLIOGRAPHY

Frank BB, and Members of the Patient Care Committee of the American Gastroenterological Association: Clinical evaluation of jaundice. *JAMA* 262: 3031–3034, 1989.

Friedman LS, Dienstag JL: Recent developments in viral hepatitis. *DM* 32(6):313–385, 1986.

Scharschmidt BF: Jaundice, in Sleisenger MH, Fordtran JS (eds). *Gastrointestinal Disease. Pathophysiology. Diagnosis. Management,* 4th ed., pp. 454–467, Philadelphia: Saunders, 1989.

Zimmerman HJ, Deschner KW: Differential diagnosis of jaundice. *Hosp Pract* 22(5):99–122, 1987.

19

Nausea and Vomiting

INTRODUCTION

Nausea The feeling of the imminent desire to vomit, usually referred to the throat or epigastrium.

Vomiting Forceful expulsion of gastric contents through the mouth.

During nausea, gastric tone is reduced and peristalsis in the stomach is decreased or absent; duodenal tone is increased, with or without reflux of duodenal contents into the stomach. Nausea is followed by retching, which comprises spasmodic respiratory movements opposed by expiratory contractions of the abdominal muscles and raises the cardia of the stomach.

During vomiting, the gastric fundus and corpus are flaccid, the gastroesophageal sphincter is relaxed, the antrum and the proximal duodenum are strongly contracted. The glottis is closed, and respiration is inhibited, preventing pulmonary aspiration; the larynx and soft palate are elevated, preventing the entry of the gastric contents into the nasopharynx. Forceful contraction of the diaphragm and abdominal wall brings about a sharp increase in intraabdominal pressure; this results in the squeezing of the flaccid stomach and the ejection of its contents. The act of vomiting is controlled and integrated by the medullary vomiting center, which receives afferent stimuli from the intestinal tract and other parts of the body, from higher cortical centers, especially the labyrinthine apparatus, and from the chemoreceptor trigger zone. The efferent pathways in vomiting are the phrenic nerves (to the diaphragm), the spinal nerves (to the abdominal musculature), and visceral efferent nerves (to the stomach and esophagus). The chemoreceptor trigger zone, located in the medulla, is incapable of mediating the act of vomiting. Activation of this zone results in efferent impulses to the medullary vomiting center, which in turn initiates the act of vomiting. Emetic stimuli can lead to vomiting by acting directly on the vomiting center or by activation of the chemoreceptor trigger zone.

ETIOLOGY

Intraabdominal disorders
  Gastric outlet obstruction: chronic ulcer disease of pylorus or duodenum; antral carcinoma
  Intestinal obstruction; intestinal pseudo-obstruction
  Gastrointestinal infections: viral, bacterial; food poisoning; viral hepatitis
  Perforation of a viscus
  Peritonitis; abscess; systemic infection
  Acute appendicitis; acute pancreatitis; acute cholecystitis; acute cholangitis; acute pyelonephritis
  Acute ischemia
Intracranial disorders
  Increased intracranial pressure: brain tumor, hematoma

Acute meningitis
Acute labyrinthitis; Ménière's disease; migraine headache; motion sickness; autonomic epilepsy
Metabolic and endocrine diseases
Uremia; diabetic ketoacidosis; adrenal insufficiency; hyperparathyroidism; early pregnancy; thyrotoxicosis
Acute myocardial infarction; congestive heart failure; hypertensive crisis
Pregnancy
Drugs; drug withdrawal; chronic alcohol abuse; toxins; poisons
Psychogenic: rumination; bulimia; anorexia nervosa

Iatrogenic Causes of Nausea and/or Vomiting

Any medication, especially: digitalis; opiates; xanthine derivatives; potassium chloride; nonsteroidal anti-inflammatory agents; glucocorticosteroids; antibiotics; cytotoxics; levodopa; bromocriptine; x-ray treatment

HISTORY TAKING*

Possible meaning of a positive response

1   Duration of the Nausea and Vomiting

1.1   How long have you had nausea
      with vomiting?
      • for a brief period of time? (hours   Acute infection of the GI tract; ingestion
        or days)   of a toxin, poison, medication; appendicitis; pregnancy

      • for weeks or months?   Partial mechanical obstruction of the
                                                     stomach or small intestine; carcinoma
                                                     of stomach or pancreas; brain tumor

      • for years?   Psychogenic vomiting (especially in
                                                     young females)

1.2   Is the vomiting recurrent?   Metabolic disorder (uremia, adrenal insufficiency); in patients with bulimia,
                                                     with conscious and voluntary vomiting
                                                     to control their weight; gastric retention; psychogenic vomiting; gastroduodenitis; drug intolerance (e.g., to
                                                     digitalis or antibiotics); pregnancy; intestinal pseudo-obstruction

*In this section, items in *italics* are characteristic clinical features, and items in **boldface** are potentially life-threatening or urgent conditions.

2   Character of Vomiting

2.1   Does the vomitus contain
　　　• yellow-greenish material?

Bile: often present whenever vomiting is prolonged; open connection between the proximal duodenum and the stomach. When constantly present in large quantities: may signify an obstructive lesion below the ampulla of Vater (Vomitus without bile: prepyloric problem)

　　　• mucus?

(In the morning): pregnancy

　　　• undigested food?

Gastric outlet obstruction. Regurgitation: expulsion of food not preceded by nausea and without the abdominal diaphragmatic contraction which is part of vomiting: in esophageal stricture or diverticula (regurgitation of esophageal contents); gastroesophageal sphincter incompetence; peptic ulcer (regurgitation of gastric contents); psychogenic vomiting

　　　• *food ingested more than 12 h previously?*

Gastric outlet obstruction or atony; rarely, if ever, seen in patients with psychogenic vomiting

　　　• blood?

Bleeding from esophagus, stomach, or duodenum: ulcer, neoplasm, varices. Vomiting of any cause may lead to a mucosal tear at the gastroesophageal junction with hematemesis (Mallory-Weiss syndrome); **acute abdominal emergency**

2.2   Does the substance that you vomit have
　　　• a particular odor?

Might indicate the ingestion of toxic substances, such as alcohol

　　　• *a fecal odor? a putrid odor?*

The result of bacterial action on the intestinal contents: **low-intestinal obstruction;** gastrocolic fistula; **peritonitis with ileus;** ischemic injury to the intestine; long-standing gastric outlet obstruction with bacterial overgrowth caused by stasis

　　　• no odor?

Regurgitation; vomitus from an achylic stomach

2.3   Can you estimate the quantity of vomit produced at any time?

Useful in judging replacement therapy; the volume lost may be very large when pyloric obstruction is present

2.4   Do you vomit
     • every day?   Peptic ulcer with obstruction; pyloro-
                                                     spasm with hypersecretion; psycho-
                                                     genic vomiting

     • *in the early morning?*   Pregnancy; uremia; alcoholism; alka-
                                                     line reflux gastritis after peptic ulcer
                                                     gastric surgery; brain tumor (often be-
                                                     fore breakfast; projectile vomiting of in-
                                                     creased intracranial pressure)

     • late in the day?   Pyloric obstruction
     • during the night?   Duodenal ulcer

2.5   Is the vomiting
     • *forceful?* ("projectile"), *without*   Increased intracranial pressure: brain
      any associated nausea or retching?   tumor

2.6   Do you have nausea without   Obstructive and hepatocellular jaun-
     vomiting?   dice; alcoholism; carcinoma of the
                                                     stomach; early stages of cardiac failure;
                                                     chronic renal failure; pregnancy; (in a
                                                     cardiac patient): digitalis intoxication

3   Precipitating or Aggravating Factors

3.1   Do you vomit after meals?
     • during or shortly after a meal?   Psychogenic vomiting; pyloric channel
                                                     ulcer; gastritis; esophageal disorder
                                                     (stricture, Zenker's diverticulum, acha-
                                                     lasia)

     • 1 hour or more after a meal?   Gastric outlet obstruction; motility dis-
                                                     order of the stomach: diabetic neuropa-
                                                     thy, postvagotomy gastroparesis; bowel
                                                     obstruction

3.1a   Is vomiting unrelated to meals?   Drug reaction; metabolic disorder; in-
     spontaneous?   creased intracranial pressure (in-
                                                     tracranial tumor); delayed gastric
                                                     emptying, diabetic gastroparesis. Reflex
                                                     vomiting secondary to lesions of the
                                                     gut, biliary tree, peritoneum, other
                                                     organs distal to the stomach. In a car-
                                                     diac patient: digitalis intoxication

3.2   Is vomiting self-induced?   Psychogenic vomiting: bulimia; an-
                                                     orexia nervosa

3.3   Do you vomit only
     • in certain places? under stress?   Psychogenic vomiting (rarely in public
      fear? depression?   or at the dinner table)
     • as a passenger in a car? aircraft?   Motion sickness
      ship?

3.4   For the female patient: When did   Possibility of early pregnancy if last
     you last have your menstruation?   menstruation more than 6 weeks ago

4 Accompanying Symptoms

4.1 Is the (severe) nausea associated with increased perspiration? hypersalivation? pallor of the skin?

Evidence of altered autonomic (parasympathetic) activity

4.2 Do you have
- pain in the abdomen?

Peptic ulcer disease; biliary tract disease; gastroenteritis; **intestinal obstruction; acute appendicitis; acute peritonitis;** pancreatitis; **abdominal emergency**

- diarrhea?

Acute gastroenteritis; drug toxicity

- constipation?

Intestinal obstruction

- a loss of appetite?

Organic cause of vomiting

- weight loss?

Loss of ingested nutrients by vomiting. Organic cause of vomiting: carcinoma of the stomach; concealed vomiting in anorexia nervosa or bulimia

- light stools? dark urine? jaundice?

Hepatitis

- acute chest pain?

Acute myocardial infarction accompanied by vomiting

- fever?

Infectious process

- trouble with hearing? vertigo? an unsteady gait?

Disorders of the labyrinthine apparatus and its central connections; Ménière's disease

- headaches?

Migraine; brain tumor

5 Iatrogenic Factors   See Etiology

6 Personal and Social Profile

6.1 Are you concerned about your (chronic intermittent) vomiting?

The patient with psychogenic vomiting does not consider vomiting a pathologic phenomenon and is not concerned about the problem

7 Personal Antecedents Pertaining to the Nausea and Vomiting

7.1 Have you ever had an x-ray of your stomach? gallbladder? When? With what results?

7.2 Do you have any of the following conditions: a peptic ulcer? a renal disease?
- diabetes?

Onset of diabetic ketoacidosis

- a cardiac disease?

In congestive heart failure: congestion of liver with nausea and vomiting; digitalis intoxication

- prior abdominal surgery?

Bile reflux gastritis following peptic ulcer surgery

8   Family Medical History Pertaining to the Nausea and Vomiting

8.1   Is there someone in your family with recurrent vomiting?   Psychogenic vomiting has a strong familial incidence

PHYSICAL SIGNS PERTAINING TO NAUSEA AND VOMITING*

	Possible significance
Hypotension; soft eyeballs; dry skin	Dehydration: acute prolonged vomiting
Fever	Acute gastroenteritis; viral hepatitis; systemic infection; meningitis
Abdominal mass	Intraabdominal neoplasm; intussusception; abscess with intestinal obstruction
Distended abdomen; abdominal tenderness; hyperactive high-pitched bowel sounds	Intestinal obstruction
Abdominal direct and rebound tenderness; guarding; absent bowel sounds	Peritonitis; adynamic ileus
Fever; jaundice; liver tenderness; hepatomegaly	Viral hepatitis; biliary tract disorder
Stiff neck; fever	Meningitis
Neurologic abnormalities	Central nervous system disorder with increased intracranial pressure
Nystagmus; disturbances of gait	Labyrinthine disorder
Pigmentation of skin and mucosae; hypotension; orthostatic hypotension	Adrenal insufficiency
Funduscopic examination	To detect papilledema

LABORATORY TESTS PERTAINING TO NAUSEA AND VOMITING†

Test	Finding	Diagnostic Possibilities
Blood		
Electrolytes	Metabolic alkalosis, hypokalemia	Prolonged vomiting; loss of gastric secretions. May document concealed vomiting: anorexia nervosa; bulimia
Glucose	Elevated	(With metabolic acidosis): diabetic ketoacidosis
BUN	Elevated	Dehydration; chronic renal failure

*In this section, items in **boldface** are potentially life-threatening or urgent conditions.
†See the appendix on Laboratory Reference Values for the associated normal laboratory values.

LABORATORY PROCEDURES PERTAINING TO
NAUSEA AND VOMITING

Procedure	To Detect
Plain abdominal film	Intestinal obstruction
Barium studies of GI tract	Peptic ulcer; gastric carcinoma
Biliary tract ultrasound	Biliary system disorder; cholelithiasis
EEG, brain CT scan	Intracranial mass lesions
ECG	Acute myocardial infarction
Pregnancy test	Pregnancy
Labyrinthine examination	Disorder of the vestibular system; Ménière's disease; acute labyrinthitis

SELECTED BIBLIOGRAPHY

Feldman M: Nausea and vomiting, in Sleisenger MH, Fordtran JS (eds). *Gastrointestinal Disease. Pathophysiology. Diagnosis. Management,* 4th ed., pp. 222–238, Philadelphia: Saunders, 1989.

Malagelada JR, Camilleri M: Unexplained vomiting: A diagnostic challenge. *Ann Intern Med* 101:211–218, 1984.

Meerof JC: Evaluation of patients with nausea and vomiting. *Hosp Pract* 20(10):177–180, 1985.

20
Rectal Bleeding

INTRODUCTION

Rectal Bleeding (Hematochezia)   Passage of bright red blood per rectum.

Bright red blood, either by itself or coating the stools, may originate from any portion of the lower ileum as well as from the colon (hemorrhage from the right colon may result in darker maroon-colored blood). Red blood may also appear per rectum from an upper intestinal or gastric lesion with massive bleeding and hypermotility. Thus, the appearance of blood in the stool depends largely on the site of the lesion and the rate of blood loss.

ETIOLOGY

Anal and Rectal Lesions

Hemorrhoids; anal fissures; anal fistulas
Proctitis: idiopathic; gonorrheal or mycoplasmal infections
Rectal trauma; foreign objects

Colonic Lesions

Carcinoma; polyps
Angiodysplastic lesions (usually ascending colon); other vascular anomalies; leaking
    aneurysm or vascular graft
Ulcerative colitis
Infections: shigellosis, amebiasis, campylobacteriosis, salmonellosis
Ischemic colitis
Colonic diverticula; Meckel's diverticulum

Iatrogenic Causes of Rectal Bleeding

Clindamycin, lincomycin; anticoagulants; enteric-coated potassium chloride tablets;
    oral contraceptive agents (ischemic colitis)

HISTORY TAKING*

Possible meaning of a positive response

1   Onset and Duration of the
    Bleeding

1.1   How long have you noticed red
      blood in your stools?

*In this section, items in *italics* are characteristic clinical features, and items in **boldface** are potentially life-threatening or urgent conditions.

| 1.2 | Has the onset of bloody diarrhea been acute? | May indicate the presence of inflammatory bowel disease or an infectious colitis |

2 Character and Intensity of Rectal Bleeding

| 2.1 | Do you see streaks of bright red blood
• on the surface of the stools?
• on the toilet paper?
• in toilet water? | Lesion in anal canal or rectum; commonly bleeding from hemorrhoidal veins, anal fissures, anal fistula (rare in rectal carcinoma). An anal lesion does not preclude other sources of bleeding |

| 2.2 | Do you pass per rectum
• small quantities of bright red blood?

• large quantities of bright red blood? | Lesion of the sigmoid colon or rectum (brisk hemorrhage is uncommon in colonic neoplasm). Stools may appear red in some patients after ingestion of beets
Aortoenteric fistula; bleeding from angiodysplastic lesion or colonic diverticula; occasionally massive hemorrhage from an upper gastrointestinal source with rapid bowel transit |

| 2.3 | Is the bleeding dark, associated with clots, well mixed with mucus, or adherent to the stool? | Colonic bleeding; also in rectal carcinoma |

3 Accompanying Symptoms

| 3.1 | Have you vomited blood? | Bleeding site usually above the ligament of Treitz |

| 3.2 | Did you notice after your bloody stool weakness? syncope? | **Massive rectal bleeding: losses of at least 1000 to 1500 mL of blood (greater than 20 percent of the blood volume)** |

| 3.3 | Have you recently noticed
• *a change in your bowel habits?*
• *a change in the caliber of the stools?*
• painful straining at stool, with a sensation that evacuation is incomplete?
• diarrhea?

• abdominal pain? | Carcinoma of the left colon

Tenesmus: rectal disease: retention of stool in the rectum; rectal tumor; colonic inflammation
Bloody diarrhea: acute inflammation of the colon; amebic colitis; ulcerative colitis; ischemic colitis; rectal and colonic carcinoma; shigellosis
Carcinoma of the colon; ischemic colitis (in an elderly patient); ulcerative colitis; amebic colitis |

• no abdominal pain?	Painless bleeding from colonic diverticula, colonic angiodysplastic lesion; malignant lesions arising in the rectal ampulla
• anal pain?	External hemorrhoids; anal fissure
• fever?	Infectious colitis (amebiasis, shigellosis); ulcerative colitis
3.4 *Is defecation painful?*	Anal ulcer; fissure; external hemorrhoids
3.5 Is the bleeding associated with straining? with passage of hard stools?	Hemorrhoids; anal fissure or fistula (with small amounts of bright red blood on the surface of the stool and toilet tissue)
3.6 Have you noticed bleeding from other sites?	Bleeding diathesis with gastrointestinal hemorrhage (does not preclude an underlying local lesion)

4   Iatrogenic Causes   See Etiology

5   Personal and Social Profile

5.1 Age of the patient?	Common causes of colonic bleeding in the elderly: carcinoma of the colon; angiodysplastic lesion (usually in the ascending colon); ischemic colitis; diverticulosis In the young adult: ulcerative colitis; enteric bacterial and parasitic disease; Meckel's diverticulum
5.2 Have you ever lived in, or traveled to, foreign countries?	Amebiasis (Mexico, western South America; south Asia; west and southwestern Africa)
5.3 What is your sexual orientation?	Rectal bleeding in a homosexual man may be due to gonorrhea, chlamydial proctitis, syphilis, herpetic proctitis, amebic proctitis, trauma, foreign body, condylomata acuminatum, malignancy

6   Personal Antecedents Pertaining to the Rectal Bleeding

6.1   Have you ever had an x-ray of your intestine? a rectosigmoidoscopy? When? With what results?

6.2   Do you have hemorrhoids? diverticulosis? ulcerative colitis? polyps?

PHYSICAL SIGNS PERTAINING TO RECTAL BLEEDING*

	Possible significance
Shock; acute hypotension; tachycardia; pallor; cold clammy skin; restlessness	Losses of about 40 percent of blood volume
Systolic blood pressure below 100 mmHg; pulse rate above 110 beats per min	At least 20 percent volume depletion
Abdominal mass	Malignancy
Hepatomegaly; jaundice	Cirrhosis
Epigastric tenderness	Peptic ulcer (not specific)
Fever; abdominal muscle spasm; guarding; rebound tenderness	Acute diverticulitis with peritoneal irritation
Arthritis	Ulcerative colitis; ingestion of salicylates and other drugs causing gastritis
Arthritis; purpura	Henoch-Schönlein purpura
Erythema nodosum; uveitis	Ulcerative colitis
In a patient over 60 years of age: evidence of atherosclerotic disease	Ischemic colitis
Rectal examination	May reveal: internal or external hemorrhoids; anal fissures, fistulas; rectal polyps; carcinoma

LABORATORY PROCEDURES PERTAINING TO RECTAL BLEEDING

Procedure	To Detect
Proctosigmoidoscopy	Anal diseases; proctitis; tumor (approximately half of all colorectal neoplasms lie in the distal 25 cm of the large bowel and within reach of the flexible sigmoidoscope); ulcerative colitis
Arteriography	Detects actively bleeding lesions only when blood loss exceeds 0.5 mL/min
Radiolabeled erythrocyte scanning	Detects blood loss of 0.1 mL/min
Colonoscopy	Site and nature of bleeding lesions proximal to the rectosigmoid area: tumor; polyps; diverticulitis; ulcerative colitis; angiodysplasia

*In this section, items in **boldface** are potentially life-threatening or urgent conditions.

Procedure	To Detect
Stool examination: polymorphonuclear leukocytes	Ulcerative colitis; amebic colitis; bacillary dysentery
Ova, parasites; culture	Infectious origin of bleeding; amebic colitis

SELECTED BIBLIOGRAPHY

Johnson DA: Fecal occult blood testing. *Postgrad Med* 85(5):287–299, 1989.

Lawrence MA, Hooks VH, 3d, Bowden TA Jr: Lower gastrointestinal bleeding. *Postgrad Med* 85(1):89–100, 1989.

Lieberman DA: Common anorectal disorders. *Ann Intern Med* 101:837–846, 1984.

Peterson WL: Obscure gastrointestinal bleeding. *Med Clin North Am* 72(5):1169–1176, 1988.

Genitourinary System

21
Acute Renal Failure

INTRODUCTION

Acute Renal Failure (ARF)   Rapid decline in renal function resulting in accumulation of nitrogenous wastes in the body.

There is an obligation to excrete an osmotic load of at least 400 to 500 mOsm daily, which represents the products of normal metabolism (urea, creatinine, uric acid, and ammonium). As the maximum urine osmolality achievable by the normal human is approximately 1200 mOsm per kg, a urine volume of at least 400 mL is necessary to excrete the daily osmotic load.

A urine volume of less than 400 mL/day—oliguria—may be associated with inadequate renal perfusion due to depletion of total salt and water or to intravascular volume depletion (prerenal failure). Under these circumstances, oliguria results from a reduced glomerular filtration rate (GFR). The renal tubule responds to the deficit of effective extracellular fluid volume with enhanced salt and water reabsorption. Urine has a high specific gravity (over 1015 to 1020), a low sodium concentration (less than 10 to 20 meq/L), and an unremarkable sediment.

Various intrinsic renal diseases producing sufficient renal parenchymal damage result in acute oliguria. Acute interstitial nephritis is associated with an inflammation of the interstitium resulting in alterations in tubular and glomerular function. Acute tubular necrosis causes a decrease in glomerular filtration rate mediated by hemodynamic alterations, tubular obstruction, back-leak of filtrate through damaged tubules, and decreased glomerular capillary permeability. Oliguria associated with glomerulopathies is due predominantly to a drastic reduction in filtration rate. In the patient with chronic or end-stage renal insufficiency, oliguria results from the destruction of renal cell mass. The oliguria of renal parenchymal disease is generally accompanied by both diminished GFR and impaired tubular reabsorption of water and salt. Urinary sodium concentration is greater than 30 to 40 meq/L, specific gravity is fixed at 1010 to 1012, and the creatinine urine to plasma (U/P) ratio is less than 10.

In postrenal obstructive failure, the increase in tubular pressure causes a decrease in renal blood flow and glomerular filtration rate.

ETIOLOGY

Prerenal Causes of Acute Renal Failure (ARF)

Volume depletion: hemorrhage; gastrointestinal losses (diarrhea, vomiting); **urinary** losses (diuretics, salt wasting); losses from third space—burns, pancreatitis, **perito-**nitis; decreased "effective" volume: nephrosis, cirrhosis; peripheral vasodilatation; sepsis, drugs

Reduced cardiac output: congestive heart failure; myocardial infarction; arrhythmias; pericardial tamponade; acute pulmonary embolism

Vascular obstruction: bilateral renal artery occlusion-thrombosis; dissecting aneurysm

Intrarenal Causes of Acute Renal Failure

Postinfectious glomerulonephritis: poststreptococcal, pneumococcal, viral, etc.

Noninfectious glomerulonephritis: rapidly progressive, membranoproliferative, Good-pasture's syndrome

Vasculitis: SLE, hypersensitivity angiitis, polyarteritis nodosa, Wegener's granuloma-tosis, Henoch-Schönlein purpura, mixed cryoglobulinemia

Vasoconstrictive diseases: malignant hypertension, hemolytic-uremic syndrome, thrombotic thrombocytopenic purpura, scleroderma

Acute interstitial nephritis

    Drug-related

    Systemic infections; primary renal infections

    Papillary necrosis: diabetes mellitus, sickle cell diseases, analgesic abuse, alcoholism

    Miscellaneous: leukemia, lymphoma, sarcoidosis

Intratubular obstruction: uric acid, oxalates, sulfadiazine, Bence-Jones protein

Acute tubular necrosis (ATN)

    Nephrotoxins: drugs, radiocontrast dyes, heavy metals, endotoxins, poisons (ethylene glycol, methanol, carbon tetrachloride)

    Ischemia: hypotension, hemorrhage, sepsis, burns, renal infarction, postaortic surg-ery

    Pigment release: hemolysis, rhabdomyolysis

    Obstetric accidents: septic abortion, eclampsia

Postrenal Causes of Acute Renal Failure

Ureteral and pelvic obstruction: stones, blood clots, tumor, sloughed papillae, retro-peritoneal fibrosis, anomalies of the ureteropelvic junction, surgical (inadvertent ligation of the ureters)

Obstruction of the bladder outlet: stones; blood clots; prostatic hypertrophy or carci-noma; bladder carcinoma; neuropathic

Urethral obstruction: strictures, phimosis

Iatrogenic Causes of Acute Renal Failure (Partial List)

Prerenal Form

Angiotensin-converting enzyme inhibitors in patients with bilateral renal artery stenosis

Acute Interstital Nephritis

Penicillins (methicillin); cephalosporins; erythromycin; sulfonamides; phenytoin; furosemide; thiazides; allopurinol; nonsteroidal anti-inflammatory agents; cimetidine; captopril; phenindione

Acute Tubular Necrosis

Amphotericin B; cephalosporins; sulfonamides; colistin; tetracyclines; aminoglycosides; polymyxins; radioiodinated contrast media; methoxyflurane

Obstructive Uropathy

Cytotoxics (intrarenal uric acid crystals); methysergide (retroperitoneal fibrosis)

Acute Urinary Retention (in Patients with Prostatic Hypertrophy)

Ganglionic-blocking agents and/or antihistamines

HISTORY TAKING*

Possible meaning of a positive response

1   Mode of Onset and Evolution

Obvious causes of prerenal failure such as dehydration, diarrhea, vomiting, shock, sepsis, injury, hemorrhage, surgery are not discussed.

1.1   How long have you been urinating
   • less than usual?

Oliguria: urine output of less than 400 mL/day: prenal or renal causes. The oliguric stage of acute tubular necrosis usually lasts for 8 to 16 days (the period of diminished urine flow may be so short as to pass unrecognized)

   • *not at all?*

Total anuria: urine volume <50 mL/day: relatively uncommon. **Obstructive uropathy.** Complete anuria (for more than 48 hours) also in: acute overwhelming glomerulonephritis; bilateral occlusion of the renal arteries or veins. (Complete anuria is rare in ARF due to parenchymal damage or to prerenal causes)

*In this section, items in *italics* are characteristic clinical features, and items in **boldface** are potentially life-threatening or urgent conditions.

1.2	Do you have varying urine volumes?	Polyuria alternating with oliguria: can be present in partial urinary tract obstruction. Urine flow fluctuating widely from day to day: intermittent obstruction. 30% to 60% of patients with ARF may have nonoliguric ARF (urine volume in excess of 400 mL/day) due to less severe tubular damage; most often seen in patients who are receiving nephrotoxic antibiotics or have had open heart surgery
1.3	Presently, how many times a day do you urinate?	Normal frequency of micturition: five to six times a day
1.4	Can you estimate the amount of urine passed • at each voiding? per day?	The persistence of urine flow of less than 15 mL/hour in the face of adequate hydration is strong presumptive evidence of acute renal failure

2   Character of the Urine

2.1	What is the appearance of your urine, if you are passing any? • smoky?	Acute glomerulonephritis; nephritic syndromes
	• cloudy?	Urinary infection; papillary necrosis
	• dark, reddish, bloody?	Gross hematuria: calculi, clots, or tumor; acute vasoocclusion of renal arteries or veins; glomerular disease

3   Precipitating or Aggravating Factors

3.1	Have you recently had • a sore throat?	Group A beta-hemolytic streptococcal infection preceding acute glomerulonephritis by 2 to 3 weeks
	• a viral infection? hematuria?	Glomerular disease
	• a urinary infection?	May precipitate acute retention in a patient with prostatism
	• an x-ray of your gallbladder? kidneys? aorta? a CT scan?	Acute tubular necrosis may follow administration of high-osmolar contrast media. Patients at risk: diabetics, patients with multiple myeloma, heart or liver disease, or previous renal insufficiency
	• an angiography?	Renal atheromatous emboli or contrast-induced acute tubular necrosis
	• a recent aortic catheterization?	Cholesterol or atheromatous emboli

3.2 How much fluid do you drink a day?

Oliguria may occur in individuals with normal renal function as a result of water restriction

4 Accompanying Symptoms

Severe systemic symptoms during the first days of oliguria usually result from associated conditions, not from renal failure.

4.1 Do you have
  - a constant urge to urinate? pain on urination? a slow stream?

Obstructive uropathy: urethral obstruction somewhere between the prostate and the meatus

  - no desire to urinate?

Obstruction to the outflow of urine from the kidneys; failure of secretion by the kidneys

  - pain in your abdomen?

Obstructive uropathy with distended bladder; Henoch-Schönlein purpura; acute renal artery embolism

  - pain in the lumbar regions?

May occur in acute glomerulonephritis; papillary necrosis

  - acute flank pain?

Renal stone (anuria if contralateral kidney has previously been destroyed by obstruction or infection)

  - fever? chills?

Urinary infection: may precipitate acute retention in a patient with prostatism; subacute bacterial endocarditis with glomerulonephritis; systemic infection with acute tubular necrosis (ATN) from endotoxin, prerenal failure from vasodilatation, or acute interstitial necrosis associated with infection

  - headaches? nausea? vomiting?

In untreated patients symptoms of uremia generally develop during the second week of oliguria; end-stage of chronic renal disease with oligoanuria

  - sinusitis? nosebleeds?

Wegener's granulomatosis: granulomatous vasculitis of the upper and lower respiratory tract together with glomerulonephritis

  - bloody expectorations?

Goodpasture's syndrome: pulmonary hemorrhage, glomerulonephritis, and antibody to basement membrane antigens

  - pain in your joints? a rash?

Collagen-vascular disease; acute interstitial nephritis

  - puffiness of your eyelids? face? swollen legs?

Retention of water of acute glomerulonephritis or chronic renal disease

5   Iatrogenic Factors   See Etiology

A drug history is critical; all drugs should be considered to have at least the potential to provoke acute interstitial nephritis

5.1 Do you regularly take
     • diuretics?

Prerenal failure (extracellular fluid volume depletion); acute interstitial nephritis

     • antibiotics?

Acute tubular necrosis or acute interstitial nephritis as the basis of the oliguria

6   Personal and Social Profile

6.1 What is your profession?

6.1a Do you have any hobbies?

} Possible nephrotoxic acute tubular necrosis

6.2 Have you recently used a cleaning agent? a spot remover?

Inhalation of carbon tetrachloride present in various solvents

6.3 Do you use drugs?

Heroin, intravenous amphetamines, marijuana, cocaine may cause rhabdomyolysis with myoglobinuria and acute renal failure

7   Personal Antecedents Pertaining to the Acute Renal Failure

7.1 Do you have

     • a kidney disease? recurrent urinary infections?

Oliguria of end-stage chronic renal disease

     • renal stones?

Bilateral ureteral calculi

     • a prostate disease?

Acute retention: obstruction of the bladder outlet

     • arterial hypertension?

Oliguria in malignant hypertension

     • gout?

Gouty nephropathy, obstructive uropathy

     • angina? congestive heart failure? rheumatic heart disease?

Reduced cardiac output; intrinsic heart disease

     • recent surgery in the lower part of the abdomen?

Immediate anuria following surgery suggests bilateral ureteral injury

8   Family Medical History Pertaining to the Acute Renal Failure

8.1 Does someone in your family have a renal disease?

Polycystic disease; Alport's syndrome

PHYSICAL SIGNS PERTAINING TO ACUTE RENAL FAILURE

	Possible significance
Skin	
purpura	Systemic vasculitis; collagen-vascular disease; thrombotic thrombocytopenic purpura
rash	Drug sensitivity: in acute interstitial nephritis; collagen-vascular disease
livedo reticularis	May be associated with atheromatous emboli
"skin popping"	Heroin abuse
Dry skin and mucosae; sunken eyeballs; flat neck veins; hypotension	Dehydration: severe fluid and electrolyte imbalance with diminished renal blood flow
Peripheral edema	Overhydration due to administration of excess fluid; acute glomerulonephritis
Pulmonary edema	Acute left ventricular failure; possibly due to overhydration
Suprapubic cystic swelling	Distended bladder: urinary retention; obstruction of the lower part of the urinary tract; prostatic enlargement
Abnormal abdominal palpation	Renal mass; hydronephrosis in obstructive uropathy
Diastolic hypertension	Observed in about 25 percent of patients during the second week of oligoanuria; hypervolemia; malignant hypertension with oliguria
Abnormal cardiac status	Prerenal failure; subacute bacterial endocarditis
Cardiac arrhythmias	Prerenal failure; potassium intoxication
Abnormal rectal, pelvic examination	May reveal enlargement of the prostate, a large pelvic mass compressing the ureters

LABORATORY TESTS PERTAINING TO ACUTE RENAL FAILURE[†]

Test	Finding	Diagnostic Possibilities
Urine		
Specific gravity	>1020	Prerenal basis for the acute renal failure
	<1020	Tubular dysfunction: acute tubular necrosis, glomerulonephritis with tubule injury
Sediment	RBCs	Calculi, tumor, or glomerular disease
	WBCs	Inflammation: acute interstitial nephritis; infection
	Renal tubular cells	Acute tubular necrosis
	Erythrocyte casts	Active glomerulonephritis
	Heme granular ("muddy brown") casts	Glomerulonephritis; acute tubular necrosis
	Granular casts	Intrarenal disease; prerenal failure unlikely
Sodium (meq/L)	<20	Prerenal acute renal failure; volume depletion
	>40	Oliguric acute tubular necrosis
	20 to 40	Combined hypoperfusion and acute tubular necrosis
Osmolality (mOsmol/kg of water)	>500	Prerenal disorder
	<350	Acute tubular necrosis
Urine/plasma (U/P) creatinine	<20	Acute tubular necrosis; postrenal failure
	>40	Prerenal failure: extracellular fluid volume depletion; acute glomerulonephritis
Fractional excretion of sodium; renal failure index	<1 percent	Prerenal failure; glomerulonephritis
	>2 percent	ATN; postrenal cause of acute renal failure
Blood		
BUN: creatinine ratio	10 to 15:1	Renal parenchymal disorder
	>15 to 20:1	Prerenal disorder

[†]See the appendix on Laboratory Reference Values for the associated normal laboratory values.

LABORATORY PROCEDURES PERTAINING TO ACUTE RENAL FAILURE

Procedure	To Detect
Bladder catheterization	Residual bladder urine; suspected urethral obstruction
Plain abdominal film	Kidney size, shape; radiopaque stones
Ultrasound	To rule out obstructive uropathy; to assess kidney size and shape
IV or retrograde pyelography*	Obstructive uropathy
Renal arteriography*, venography*	Vascular occlusion
Renal biopsy*	Specific forms of parenchymal renal diseases

*When indicated

SELECTED BIBLIOGRAPHY

Badr KF, Ichikawa I: Prerenal failure: A deleterious shift from renal compensation to decompensation. *N Engl J Med* 319:623–629, 1988.

Corwin HL, Bonventre JV: Acute renal failure. *Med Clin North Am* 70(5):1037–1054, 1986.

Epstein FH, Brown RS: Acute renal failure: A collection of paradoxes. *Hosp Pract* 23(1):171–194, 1988.

Spiegel DM, Burnier M, Schrier RW: Acute renal failure. *Postgrad Med* 82(4):97–105, 1987.

22
Dysuria

INTRODUCTION

Dysuria   Difficulty or pain associated with voiding.

Micturition is normally a voluntary, painless act. The commonest cause of dysuria is infection in the bladder, urethra, or prostate. Dysuria is often accompanied by frequency and urgency. In acute inflammatory lesions of the bladder, the loss of elasticity that results from edema and the pain induced by even mild stretching of the bladder decrease the capacity of the organ (normal capacity of the adult bladder: 400 to 500 mL). Under these circumstances, frequency—voiding at abnormally brief intervals—will occur when only a small quantity of urine is present in the bladder. Extrinsic compression or distortion of the lower part of the urinary tract may also cause dysuria. Urgency—an exaggerated sense of needing to urinate—occurs as a result of trigonal or posterior urethral irritation by inflammation, stones, or tumor. Urgency may occur with acute cystitis, particularly in women, or in tense, anxious women even in the absence of infection. Overflow incontinence is a loss of urine due to chronic urinary retention or secondary to a flaccid bladder. Small involuntary voidings occur as the intravesical pressure of accumulating urine overcomes the urethral resistance. Incontinence may also be related to detrusor instability, sphincter or pelvic incompetence (stress incontinence), spinal cord damage, or peripheral neuropathy. When incontinence results from upper and lower motor neuron lesions, associated neurologic signs are present in the lower extremities.

ETIOLOGY

Difficulty in Voiding, with Pain on Urination

Acute urinary tract infection: acute urethritis, cystitis, or prostatitis; acute pyelonephritis with cystitis
Chronic infection: chronic prostatitis; prostatodynia; chronic interstitial cystitis; chronic posterior urethrotrigonitis (in women)
Vesical calculi; urethral calculi
Urethral caruncle; meatal stenosis
Vaginitis: fungi, bacterial, protozoa
Genital infections
Atrophic vaginitis (estrogen deficiency); chemical irritants: contraceptive jellies, douches
The conditions under "Difficulty in voiding, without pain" when complicated by infection or vesical calculi

Difficulty in Voiding, without Pain

Obstructive uropathy
   Benign prostatic hypertrophy; carcinoma of prostate; urethral stricture; bladder-neck contracture; bladder cancer

Expanding masses in the pelvis: pregnancy, large ovarian cyst, uterine or rectal tumor

Incontinence

Urge incontinence
    Decreased cortical inhibition of detrusor contractions: strokes, brain tumor, dementia, lesions of the spinal cord above the sacral level
    Hyperexcitability of sensory pathways: bladder or pelvic infection or tumor, fecal impaction
Stress incontinence: weakened urethral sphincter in women: childbirth, surgery; postmenopausal atrophy of the mucosa; urethral infection
Overflow incontinence
    Obstruction of the bladder outlet: prostatic hypertrophy or tumor
    Weakness of the detrusor muscle: lower motor neuron disease at the sacral level
    Impaired bladder sensation: autonomic peripheral neuropathy: diabetes mellitus, Guillain-Barré syndrome; collagen-vascular diseases
    Drugs
Mechanical incontinence
    Congenital anomalies
    Acquired: following transurethral resection of the prostate; vesicovaginal, ureterovaginal, vesicoperineal, ureteroperineal fistulas following pelvic surgery or irradiation of the uterus or rectum
Functional incontinence (inability to reach a toilet in time)
    Impaired health or environmental conditions: weakness, arthritis, poor vision, unfamiliar settings, distant bathroom facilities, bedrails, physical restraints

Iatrogenic Causes of Urinary Dysfunction

Bladder dysfunction and difficulty in urination: anticholinergics; monoamine oxidase inhibitors, tricyclic antidepressants; disopyramide; antihistaminics; hydralazine
Diuretics: frequency with polyuria; incontinence

HISTORY TAKING*

Possible meaning of a positive response

1   Mode of Onset and Duration

1.1   How long have you had pain or difficulty in urinating?
      • 1–2 days?   Bacterial cystitis
      • 2–7 days?   Female urethral syndrome: dysuria, frequency without bacteriuria; a longer duration suggests a chlamydial infection

---

*In this section, items in *italics* are characteristic clinical features, and items in **boldface** are potentially life-threatening or urgent conditions.

1.2   Was the onset of painful urination
      • sudden?   Bacterial infection
      • gradual?   Chlamydial infection

1.3   When did you last void?   If no urination in the last 12 h: exclude
                                            acute urinary retention

2   Character of the Dysuria

2.1   *When urinating, do you have a burn-*   Dysuria: usually related to inflamma-
      ing sensation, as if passing hot water?   tion of the lower urinary tract: cystitis,
                                            urethritis, urethral calculus; foreign
                                            bodies or tumor in the bladder; acute
                                            prostatitis

      • (in men) in or proximal to the
        glans penis?   Urinary tract infection: cystitis
      • (in women): as an internal
        urethral discomfort? pressure?
        • as an external burning sensa-   Urine flowing over irritated or inflamed
          tion caused by urine?   vaginal labia: dysuria associated with
                                            vaginitis
      • worse at the beginning of the   Urethritis
        stream?
      • worse at the end of the stream?   Cystitis; prostatitis
      • persisting a few seconds or min-   Terminal tenesmus: acute cystitis
        utes after urination?

3   Accompanying Symptoms

3.1   How many times a day do you   The normal adult urinates 5 to 6 times a
      urinate?   day and no more than once a night,
                                            with an average volume of 300 mL

3.2   Do you urinate more frequently   Frequency: may be due to an increased
      than usual? at abnormally brief in-   volume of urine (polyuria) or to a de-
      tervals?   creased capacity of the bladder
      • only during the day?   Daytime frequency without nocturia in
                                            functional bladder syndrome ("psy-
                                            chosomatic cystitis"): common in mid-
                                            dle-aged and older women; polyp in
                                            posterior urethra (frequency relieved by
                                            recumbency)
      • also at night? more than once?   Nocturia: frequency with decreased
                                            ability of the bladder to expand. One of
                                            the first symptoms of benign prostatic
                                            hypertrophy. Polyuria with increased
                                            amount of urine formed at night: di-
                                            uretics; congestive heart failure

3.2a Do you void while up at night   "Pseudo frequency"; insomnia
      without a real urge?

3.3   In case of frequent micturitions: Do
      you pass

- relatively small amounts of urine with each voiding?

  Frequency: the sense of bladder fullness is due not to a full bladder but to a bladder that is irritable and feels full even when it is not

  - *without pain on urination?*

    Decreased capacity of the bladder due to bladder outlet obstruction: benign prostatic hypertrophy, neurogenic bladder; anxiety

  - *with pain on urination?*

    Increased bladder sensitivity due to inflammatory condition: infection of lower urinary tract

- high volumes of urine with each voiding? without pain on urination?

  Polyuria: diabetes mellitus; chronic renal insufficiency; diabetes insipidus; psychogenic water drinking; diuretics

3.4 Do you have at times an exaggerated sense of needing to urinate?

Urgency: due to an irritable or inflamed bladder with a decreased ability of the bladder to expand: infection; radiation; chemicals; bladder cancer (carcinoma in situ); CNS disorder with neurogenic bladder dysfunction

3.5 (In men) Do you have pain on urination without frequency or urgency?

Urethritis

3.6 Are you at times unable to initiate urination in spite of an urgent desire to do so?

Episodes of urinary retention (often painful if acute): prostatic obstruction, neurogenic bladder, occasionally urethral stricture

3.7 Is the urge at times so severe that you void involuntarily?

Urge incontinence: too strong detrusor contractions: acute cystitis; in upper motor neuron lesion; bladder tumor; recent prostatectomy; also in tense, anxious women

3.8 Do you ever leak any urine or wet yourself
- intermittently?

  Incontinence: inability to retain urine in the bladder. Can be psychologically devastating for both the patient and family

- with a strong desire to void?

  Urge incontinence (in the elderly male or female)

- on straining? stooping? coughing? sneezing? laughing? bending over? lifting heavy objects?

  Stress incontinence: sudden leakage of a small amount of urine with rapid increases in intravesical pressure and partial incompetence of the urinary sphincter due to poor muscular support (common in women). The incontinence does not occur when the patient is recumbent

- with urine dribbling out in small amounts at frequent intervals? without warning?
- continuously? with dripping of urine? especially when standing or sitting?

Overflow incontinence, when bladder is overfilled

Overflow incontinence: detrusor contractions are insufficient to overcome urethral resistance; the bladder is dilated. In: obstruction of the bladder outlet (prostatic hypertrophy or tumor); weakness of the detrusor muscle associated with spinal cord disease; hypotonic neurogenic bladder (diabetic neuropathy). Vesicovaginal fistula; ectopic ureter

3.9   Do you have to wait more than a few seconds before your urine begins to flow?

Hesitancy: delay in the initiation of urination: reflects the latency period required by the detrusor muscle to generate enough pressure to overcome the bladder outlet resistance; usually accompanied by decreased size and force of the urinary stream; bladder outlet obstruction: prostatic obstruction, urethral stricture; neurogenic bladder (may be one of the earliest signs of multiple sclerosis)

3.10 In middle-aged or elderly men: Is the stream of urine decreased in caliber? slow? weak? split? sprayed? varying in intensity? intermittent?

3.10a Do you have to stand closer to the toilet than you used to?

Bladder outlet obstruction: early stage of prostatic hypertrophy, urethral stricture; neurogenic bladder

3.10b Do you dribble after you have completed voiding?

Postvoiding dribbling: detrusor musculature hypertrophy and secondary bladder contraction; further bladder decompensation and increased outlet resistance

3.10c Do you feel that
- your urinations last longer than usual?
- you still have urine in your bladder when you have finished urinating?

Prostatic obstruction

3.11 Do you have
- difficulty in maintaining the stream?
- to strain down to initiate urination? at the end of urination?

Increasing severity of obstructive uropathy; obstruction of the bladder outlet due to prostatic hypertrophy

3.12 After having apparently emptied your bladder, are you still able, a few minutes later, to pass several milliliters or ounces more?

Significant vesical residuum; bladder diverticulum

3.13 Is your urine
• clear?

May occur in chronic urinary tract infection

• cloudy?

Pyuria; precipitation of phosphate in alkaline urine

• dark or bloody?

Hematuria, occasionally in cystitis; benign prostatic hypertrophy; urothelial and renal malignancy

3.14 Does your urine have an ammoniacal odor?

Urinary tract infection with urea-splitting *Proteus*

3.15 (In men) Do you have a urethral discharge?
• scant? clear? whitish? (mucoid)

Acute anterior nongonococcal urethritis: chlamydial, *Ureaplasma urealyticum*

• moderate to heavy? thick? purulent?

Gonococcal urethritis

3.16 (In women): Do you have a vaginal discharge? vulvar itching? pain on intercourse?

Dysuria may be associated with a vaginal rather than a urinary tract infection

3.17 Do you have
• severe pain in the bladder area?

Acute urinary retention with distended bladder (the patient with a chronically overdistended bladder may experience little or no pain)

• a dull suprapubic pain?

Bladder pain: infection, obstruction (if not related to the micturition: usually not of urologic origin)

• with pain at the tip of the penis?

Vesical calculus (referred pain to the distal urethra)

• a fullness, a vague discomfort in the perineal and rectal areas?

Prostatitis; prostatic cancer; cystitis; bladder cancer

• flank pain?

Nephrolithiasis with urinary tract infection

• fever? chills?

Acute infectious process: pyelonephritis, cystitis

• pain in your joints? eyes? a skin rash?

Reiter's syndrome

3.18 For the patient with incontinence: Do you have a loss of power in your lower limb(s)? a change in bowel habits? impaired sexual function? fecal incontinence?

Sacral or distal spinal cord neuropathy as a cause of incontinence

3.18a Do you lack any sensation of blad-
      der fullness? of voiding?

Unawareness of a full bladder or of
wetness suggests a sensory or mental
deficit. Overflow incontinence: flaccid
neurogenic bladder

3.18b *Do you have to strain or apply manual
      pressure on the bladder during all the
      micturition?*

Overflow incontinence: flaccid neurogenic bladder

3.19 For the female patient: Do you lose
      urine from the vagina?

Ureterovaginal or vesicovaginal fistula

4   Iatrogenic Factors   See Etiology

5   Personal and Social Profile

5.1   Have you recently had (multiple)
      sexual contact(s)? a vacation with
      increased frequency of intercourse?

Sexually transmitted disease: gonorrheal, or nongonorrheal urethritis or
cervicitis

5.2   (In women): Do you use vaginal
      sprays, douches, bubble baths?

May induce a chemical vaginitis presenting with dysuria

5.3   What is your sexual orientation?

In a homosexual male:
  • urinary hesitancy: bacterial prosta-
    titis, traumatic prostatitis, urethral
    condylomata acuminata, traumatic
    urethritis from penile rings or
    urethral instrumentation
  • urethral discharge: gonorrhea,
    nongonococcal chlamydial urethri-
    tis, bacterial prostatitis

6   Personal Antecedents Pertaining to the Dysuria

6.1   Have you ever had an examination
      of your urine? blood? an x-ray
      of your kidneys? a cystoscopy?
      When? With what results?

6.2   Have you ever had
      • a urologic operation? a trauma
        during parturition?

May cause partial or total incompetence
of the urinary sphincter

6.3   Do you have
      • kidney stones? urinary tract in-
        fections?

A history of recurrent urinary tract infection suggests underlying anatomic or
physiologic abnormality of the urinary
tract

      • a sexually transmitted disease?

Gonorrhea; nongonococcal urethritis;
syphilis: neurogenic bladder in tabes

      • a neurologic disorder or surgery?

Neurogenic bladder dysfunction

      • a prostate condition?

Obstructive uropathy

PHYSICAL SIGNS PERTAINING TO DYSURIA

	Possible significance
Fever; suprapubic tenderness	Cystitis; acute prostatitis
Fever; costovertebral angle tenderness	Acute pyelonephritis
Distended bladder	Overflow incontinence: urinary retention; obstruction of the lower part of the urinary tract; prostatic hypertrophy
Incontinence with small, undetectable bladder	Urge incontinence; stress incontinence
Rectal examination	May reveal: benign prostatic hypertrophy; prostatic carcinoma; prostatitis
Pelvic examination	May reveal: uterine fibroids, pelvic masses reducing the bladder capacity by external compression
Neurologic abnormalities in the legs: upper or lower motor neuron lesions	Neurogenic bladder dysfunction with incontinence

LABORATORY TESTS PERTAINING TO DYSURIA

Test	Finding	Diagnostic Possibilities
Urine		
Sediment	Pyuria: >2 to 5 WBCs/high power field (HPF)	Urinary tract infection, calculi, tumors, tuberculosis
	Sterile, abacterial pyuria	Renal tuberculosis
Culture	>100,000 colonies of bacteria per milliliter of urine	Urinary tract infection
Urethral discharge: Gram's strain, culture	Positive	Gonorrhea; nongonococcal urethritis
Prostatic fluid (obtained by prostatic massage)	>10 leukocytes/HPF	Prostatitis
Serum acid phosphatase	Elevated	Metastatic prostatic cancer (does not screen patients for localized prostate cancer)

LABORATORY PROCEDURES PERTAINING TO DYSURIA

Procedure	To Detect
Pelvic ultrasonography	To estimate the prostate size; the amount of postvoid residual urine
Excretory urography; cystoscopy	Anatomic or functional abnormalities of the urinary tract
Voiding cystourethrography	Ureteral reflux; posterior urethral valves; urethral stricture
Urodynamic studies	Types of nervous system lesions causing neurogenic vesical dysfunction

SELECTED BIBLIOGRAPHY

Coe FL: Alterations in urinary function, in Wilson J, Braunwald E, Isselbacher KJ et al (eds). *Harrison's Principles of Internal Medicine*, 12th ed., pp. 271–278, New York: McGraw-Hill, 1991.

Komaroff AL: Acute dysuria in women. *N Engl J Med* 310:368–375, 1984.

Office of medical application of research, National Institutes of Health: Consensus Conference: Urinary incontinence in adults. *JAMA* 261:2685–2690, 1989.

Smith RA, Wake R, Soloway MS: Benign prostatic hyperplasia. *Postgrad Med* 83(6):79–85, 1988.

23
Hematuria

INTRODUCTION

Hematuria   Bleeding from the urinary tract. Hematuria may be gross (more than 1 million red cells are excreted per minute) or microscopic (more than 2 red blood cells per high power field).

Vigorous exercise and certain febrile diseases may increase the number of red cells in the urinary sediment of otherwise normal subjects without implying serious renal disease. Microscopic or macroscopic hematuria generally results from diseases of the renal parenchyma or of the genitourinary tract. The presence of red blood cell casts is pathologic and identifies the nephron as the source of bleeding.

Red urine is not necessarily indicative of hematuria (presence of red blood cells); it may also be produced by hemoglobinuria (intravascular hemolysis) and myoglobinuria (skeletal muscle damage). In the latter two conditions, occult blood tests in urine are positive. Nonheme pigments (liver diseases, rare diseases such as acute porphyria, ochronosis, malignant melanoma) may impart a red to brown to black color to the urine (occult blood tests negative).

The actual color of the urine that contains heme pigments depends on the concentration of the blood red cells or pigment, the pH of the urine, and the duration of contact between the pigment and the urine. In an acid urine, the color is dark or smoky, while in an alkaline urine, the color will be more nearly red.

ETIOLOGY

Renal (Glomerular)

Glomerulonephritis:* acute proliferative, primary mesangiopathic, focal proliferative, rapidly progressive, membranoproliferative; lupus nephritis; Alport's syndrome; benign familial hematuria

Renal (Nonglomerular)

Renal cell carcinoma;* renal infarct; tuberculosis; pyelonephritis;* polycystic kidney disease; medullary sponge kidney; interstitial nephritis; vascular malformations; trauma;* papillary necrosis; sickle cell anemia or trait; coagulation disorders

Postrenal

Stones;* periureteritis secondary to extraurinary pathology; tumors of lower urinary tract;* cystitis; prostatitis; epididymitis; meatal ulceration; urethral stenosis; foreign body in bladder or urethra (including Foley catheter); strenuous exercise; urethritis;* phimosis; prostate: hypertrophy,* prostatitis, carcinoma; vascular malformations; endometriosis; vesicoureteral reflux

*Common cause of hematuria

Iatrogenic Causes of Hematuria

Penicillins, cephalosporins, phenytoin: allergic interstitial nephritis
Phenacetin, nonsteroidal anti-inflammatory agents: papillary necrosis
Cyclophosphamide, mitotane: chemical hemorrhagic cystitis
Sulfonamides, 6-mercaptopurine: promote crystalluria
Cyclophosphamide, phenacetin: malignant neoplasm of uroepithelium
Anticoagulants: spontaneous bleeding or induction of bleeding from an occult lesion

False Hematuria

Vaginal bleeding; pigmenturia: porphyria; hemoglobinuria; myoglobinuria; food (beets, blackberries, rhubarb); drugs: phenazopyridine (Pyridium); rifampin; laxatives containing phenolphthalein, cascara, senna; levodopa

Iatrogenic Causes of False Hematuria (Pigmenturia)

Hemoglobinuria (in glucose-6-phosphate dehydrogenase deficiency): nitrofurantoin, primaquine, sulfonamides, aspirin, phenacetin, cotrimoxazole

HISTORY TAKING*

Possible meaning of a positive response

1 Mode of Onset and Duration

1.1 How long have you had reddish, dark, urine?

1.2 Is this the first time that you have had red urine?
Even a single episode of hematuria requires a complete urologic investigation

1.3 Do you have repeated episodes of gross hematuria?
In a young patient: IgA nephropathy

In a black patient: sickle cell trait; combined hemoglobinopathy

2 Character of the Hematoma

2.1 What is the color of your urine?
• bright red?
Alkaline urine; renal stone; tumor; bladder source; prostatic hypertrophy

• reddish-brown? smoky brown? like Coca-Cola?
Small amounts of blood, acid urine: diffuse renal parenchymal disease; acute glomerulonephritis; hemoglobinuria, myoglobinuria

• dark brown?
Upper tract source

*In this section, items in *italics* are characteristic clinical features.

• grayish-green?	Hematuria less prominent: color due to the mixture of small amounts of pigments from red cell destruction with the normal urochrome pigmentation of concentrated urine

2.2   Is blood present
- *at the beginning of the micturition?* — Initial hematuria: bleeding lesion in the urethra, distal to the bladder neck
- *only at the conclusion of voiding?* in the last few drops? — Terminal hematuria: lesion in the posterior urethra, bladder neck, or prostate; trigonitis
- *throughout the urinary stream?* — Total hematuria: the bleeding originates from either the kidney or the ureter; may also occur in diffuse bladder inflammation: hemorrhagic cystitis
- independently of micturition? — Bleeding from the distal urethra

2.3   *Does the urine contain clots?* — Postglomerular source of bleeding
- large bulky clots? — Bleeding from the bladder
- wormlike? long shoestring-shaped clots? — Bleeding from the ureter: casts of the ureter. Excludes glomerular bleeding, i.e., glomerulonephritis

3   Precipitating or Aggravating Factors

3.1   Does the dark urine appear
- only in the morning? — Paroxysmal nocturnal hemoglobinuria (in 25 percent of cases)
- following
  - prolonged walking or running? other activities? — March hemoglobinuria; does not preclude further urologic evaluation. Hematuria occurs in about 18 percent of otherwise normal subjects after very strenuous exercise
  - exposure to cold? — Paroxysmal cold hemoglobinuria (rare): urine dark brownish

3.1a   *Does the urine, of normal coloration when freshly passed, darken on standing?* — Hepatic porphyria

3.2   Have you recently had
- *a sore throat?* an acute upper respiratory infection? — Acute glomerulonephritis with preceding infection of group A beta-hemolytic streptococcus. Upper respiratory infection may precede hematuria associated with Berger's disease; other mesangial glomerulonephropathies; Henoch-Schönlein purpura, rapidly progressive glomerulonephritis, membranoproliferative glomerulonephritis

- a trauma to the lower part of the back? the abdomen? a renal biopsy?
- a urologic manipulation?

Hematuria due to trauma to the kidney (hematuria often painless); contusion of the bladder with hematuria

Traumatic hematuria; urinary tract infection

3.3 In case of recurrent hematuria for months or years, does the hematuria occur
- immediately (within a few hours) after a respiratory infection? a febrile illness?
- following exercise?

Focal glomerulonephritis with recurrent hematuria (Berger's disease, IgA nephropathy or idiopathic renal hematuria): affects young adults, mostly males

3.4 For the female patient: Do your episodes of hematuria occur simultaneously with your menstruations?

Endometriosis of the urinary tract; bleeding perhaps vaginal in origin, not from the urinary tract

4 Accompanying Symptoms

4.1 Do you have
- *back pain? flank pain? abdominal pain?*

Nephrolithiasis; embolic phenomena (may be painless in subacute bacterial endocarditis); urinary tract infection; renal or ureteral tumor; papillary necrosis; renal infarction; cyst rupture in polycystic disease

- a dull loin pain?

Acute glomerulonephritis

- difficulty, burning on urination?

Probable source of bleeding: lower urinary tract: infection, passage of stone in urethra

- vague suprapubic discomfort? frequent urination? a constant urge to urinate?

Bleeding due to lower urinary tract infection; urethritis, urethrotrigonitis; hemorrhagic cystitis secondary to bacterial infection

- hesitancy? straining to void? decreased force and caliber of the urinary stream?

In the older male: bladder outlet obstruction due to benign prostatic hypertrophy

- no pain?

Painless total hematuria in: urinary tract cancer; bladder tumor; diffuse kidney disease; acute glomerulonephritis; polycystic disease; infection, tuberculosis; staghorn calculus; solitary renal cyst; sickle cell disease; hydronephrosis

4.2 Do you have
- fever? (and/or chills?)

Urinary tract infection; renal cell carcinoma; papillary necrosis; acute glomerulonephritis; bacterial endocarditis with focal glomerulonephritis; prostatitis; prostatic abscess

• a decreased volume of urine?	Papillary necrosis; acute glomerulonephritis; obstructive lesion; chronic renal failure, late stage
• a loss of weight?	Renal tumor; chronic renal failure
• swelling of your eyelids? face? feet?	Edema in acute glomerulonephritis
• a loss of appetite? nausea? vomiting?	Uremia: acute or chronic glomerulonephritis
• deafness?	Alport's syndrome
• bloody expectorations?	Goodpasture's syndrome; Wegener's granulomatosis
• chronic sinusitis?	Wegener's granulomatosis
• pain in your joints? a skin rash?	Glomerular lesion: secondary to a collagen-vascular disease (systemic lupus erythematosus; polyarteritis nodosa) or as a manifestation of a drug reaction
• easy bruising?	Bleeding tendency; thrombocytopenia with hematuria
• pale stool?	Liver disease with bilirubinuria

5   Iatrogenic Factors   See Etiology

5.1   Do you take

• any medications?	Drug-induced nephritis has become one of the most common kidney disorders seen by nephrologists
• anticoagulants?	Hematuria in a patient taking an anticoagulant should not routinely be ascribed to the drug. Other causes, such as an occult tumor or vascular anomaly, should be ruled out

6   Personal and Social Profile

6.1 Age of the patient?	In patients 20 years of age and younger: glomerulonephritis (IgA nephropathy); urinary tract infection 20 to 40 age range and women aged 40 to 60: urinary tract infection; kidney stones; trauma; cancer of the kidney or urinary tract Men aged 40 to 60: cancer of the bladder; kidney stones; urinary tract infection; kidney tumors Men over 60: same causes plus prostatic disease Women over 60: bladder cancer (more prevalent than in younger women)
6.2 What is (was) your occupation?	Bladder cancer due to β-naphthylamine, benzidine dyes: in dye industry, leather, rubber-working, chemists

6.3   Do you smoke?   Cigarette smoking has been linked to
                                       bladder cancer

6.4   What is your sexual orientation? Dark urine in a homosexual man: hepa-
                                       titis; side effect of metronidazole used
                                       for amebiasis

7   Personal Antecedents Pertaining to the Hematuria

7.1   Have you ever had an examination
      of your urine? blood? an x-ray of
      your kidneys? any operation for a
      stone? When? With what results?

7.2   Have you ever had any of the
      following conditions: a kidney dis-
      ease? a stone passed in your urine?
      a prostate disease? a urinary infec-
      tion?

7.3   Do you have
      • a cardiac condition?   Atrial fibrillation, mitral stenosis: he-
                                       maturia due to embolic phenomenon
      • gout?   Uric acid urolithiasis
      • a blood disease?   Sickle cell anemia or trait: papillary in-
                                       farct; aplastic anemia, leukemia, with
                                       thrombocytopenia
      • a bleeding tendency?

8   Family Medical History Pertaining to the Hematuria

8.1   Does someone else in your family
      have
      • hematuria? a renal disease?   Polycystic kidney disease; Alport's syn-
                                       drome (with deafness); benign familial
                                       hematuria; cystine stones
      • a blood disease?   Hemoglobinopathies (sickle cell ane-
                                       mia); hereditary hemorrhagic telangiec-
                                       tasia

PHYSICAL SIGNS PERTAINING TO HEMATURIA

	Possible significance
Abdominal mass	Renal tumor, cyst
Bilaterally enlarged kidneys	Polycystic renal disease
Costovertebral angle tenderness	Nephrolithiasis; renal inflammation
Fever	Urinary tract infection; collagen-vascular disease
Hypertension, edema	Acute glomerulonephritis

Arthritis	Systemic lupus erythematosus; Henoch-Schönlein purpura
Atrial fibrillation; mitral stenosis	Renal embolism and infarction
Ecchymoses; petechiae	Bleeding tendency
Lymphadenopathy; splenomegaly	Lymphoma, leukemia, with bleeding tendency
Jaundice	Hemolytic disease; sickle cell trait; bilirubinuria rather than hematuria
Abnormal rectal examination	Prostatic hypertrophy or carcinoma; prostatitis

LABORATORY TESTS PERTAINING TO HEMATURIA[†]

Test	Finding	Diagnostic Possibilities
Urine		
Proteinuria	Present	Glomerulonephropathy (proteinuria may be absent at the onset); diffuse renal lesion
	Absent	Localized lesion of the collecting system; bleeding disturbance; abnormal hemoglobin; does not exclude glomerulonephritis
Sediment	RBCs, WBCs	Stone; tumor; cystitis
	RBCs, WBCs; bacteria; culture: positive	Urinary tract infection; cystitis
Morphology of red cells in the urine	>80 percent of red cells dysmorphic (wide range of morphologic variation)	Glomerular bleeding
	>80 percent isomorphic (similar in shape and size to red cells in peripheral blood)	Source of bleeding is likely to be postglomerular
	RBC casts	Glomerular bleeding: glomerulonephritis

[†]See the appendix on Laboratory Reference Values for the associated normal laboratory values.

Test	Finding	Diagnostic Possibilities

Blood

RBCs	Anemia	Chronic renal failure; systemic illness; hematologic disorder
	Polycythemia	Hypernephroma; polycystic disease (erythropoietin-secreting mass)
Platelet count	Thrombocy-topenia	Bleeding tendency
Prothrombin time	Prolonged	Bleeding tendency
BUN, serum creatinine level	Increased	Renal parenchymal disease
Sickle cell preparation; hemoglobin electrophoresis*	Abnormal	Sickle cell disease

*When indicated

LABORATORY PROCEDURES PERTAINING TO HEMATURIA

Procedure	To Detect
Plain abdominal film	Radiopaque stones
IV pyelogram	Renal masses; polycystic disease; hydronephrosis
Renal ultrasound	Size and shape of the kidneys; renal masses and obstruction; renal tumor vs. cyst
Cystoscopy	Site of bleeding; urethral or bladder lesions; cystitis; bladder tumor; vesical calculi; prostatic bladder disease; diverticula
Arteriography	Tumors; cysts; renal infarction; arteriovenous malformations
Renal biopsy*	Specific forms of renal parenchymal disease

*When indicated

SELECTED BIBLIOGRAPHY

Abuello JG: The diagnosis of hematuria. *Arch Intern Med* 143:967–970, 1983.

Finney J, Baum N: Evaluation of hematuria. *Postgrad Med* 85(8):44–53, 1989.

Schoolwerth AC: Hematuria and proteinuria: Their causes and consequences. *Hosp Pract* 22(10A):45–62, 1987.

24
Pain in the Flank

INTRODUCTION

Pain in the flank commonly originates in urinary organs. A diseased kidney gives rise to local pain (T10 to T12, L1) in the costovertebral angle and in the flank, in the region of and below the twelfth rib. The pain is associated with renal diseases which cause sudden distention of the renal capsule (acute pyelonephritis, acute ureteral obstruction, hematoma) or renal ischemia (infarction from an embolus or thrombus). Renal diseases with a slow progression are not associated with sudden capsular distention and are painless (cancer, chronic pyelonephritis, tuberculosis, staghorn calculus, mild ureteral obstruction with hydronephrosis).

Ureteral pain is due to acute obstruction (stone, blood clot). This produces capsular distention with back pain, and renal pelvic and ureteral muscle spasm with severe pain that radiates along the course of the ureter.

ETIOLOGY

Flank Pain of Urologic Origin

Nephrolithiasis
  Hypercalciuria: hyperparathyroidism, hypervitaminosis D, milk-alkali syndrome, sarcoidosis, malignancy, bone disease, renal tubular acidosis, hyperthyroidism, idiopathic hypercalciuria
  Uric acid lithiasis: gout, myeloproliferative disorders, chronic diarrheal states, ileostomy, chemotherapy
  Hyperoxaluria: primary; acquired (small-bowel disease); pyridoxine deficiency
  Xanthinuria; cystinuria
  Magnesium ammonium phosphate stones: recurrent renal infections due to urea-splitting microorganisms
Upper urinary infection; papillary necrosis; renal abscess
Renal arterial embolism or thrombosis; renal vein thrombosis
Bleeding into: renal tumor, polycystic disease, renal tuberculosis; renal hematoma
Retroperitoneal fibrosis

Flank Pain in Nonurologic Disease

Cardiovascular: abdominal aortic aneurysm; bacterial endocarditis with splenic embolism
Irritation of diaphragm: pleural effusion; pneumonia; pulmonary embolism; perinephric and subphrenic abscess
Gastrointestinal: colonic obstruction; irritable bowel syndrome; splenic flexure syndrome; acute gallbladder disease; acute appendicitis; diverticulitis
Neurologic: herpes zoster; cord tumor; radiculitis syndrome (spondylosis; compression fracture; vertebral body)

Retroperitoneal: lymphoma; metastatic carcinoma; pancreatic carcinoma; pancreatitis; psoas abscess; lumbar abscess; torsion, undescended testis
Trauma: fracture of transverse process, lumbar spine
Psychogenic: depression; anxiety reaction; malingering

Iatrogenic Causes of Renal Stones

Antacids with absorbable alkali
Allopurinol: may cause hyperxanthinuria
Chronic use of acetazolamide (persistently alkaline urine with calcium phosphate stone formation)
Vitamin D abuse
Ascorbic acid abuse: hyperoxaluria

Iatrogenic Causes of Hyperuricemia

Thiazides, chlorthalidone; furosemide; ethacrynic acid; cytotoxic drugs; aspirin (small doses); cyclosporine

HISTORY TAKING*

		Possible meaning of a positive response
1	Location and Radiation of the Pain	
1.1	Where did the pain begin?	
	• in the back? (costovertebral angle?)	Renal pain: stone; acute pyelonephritis; renal tumor, pelvis or calyx (blood clot causing obstruction); papillary necrosis; obstruction of the ureteropelvic junction
	• in the side? flank?	Renal pain; obstruction of the remainder of the ureter
	• in the right hypochondrium?	Gallbladder disease; acute pancreatitis; penetrating duodenal ulcer
	• in the right flank?	Right colon; acute appendicitis; renal pain
	• in the left hypochondrium?	Splenic infarction; penetrating gastric ulcer; acute pancreatitis; splenic flexure syndrome
	• in the left flank?	Diverticulitis; renal pain
1.2	Does the pain radiate from the costovertebral angle	

*In this section, items in *italics* are characteristic clinical features, and items in **boldface** are potentially life-threatening or urgent conditions.

• along the subcostal area toward the umbilicus?	Sudden distention of the renal capsule; acute ureteral obstruction with sudden renal back pressure; acute pyelonephritis with sudden edema
• *down toward the lower anterior abdominal quadrant?*	Ureteral pain
• into the ipsilateral testicle? (labia?)	Ureteropelvic stone; stone lodged in the upper ureter (the nerve supply to the testis and to the kidney and upper ureter is the same: T11 and T12)
• with pain in the lower abdominal quadrant? the inguinal area?	Stone in midportion of ureter (T12–L1)
• in the suprapubic area? distal urethra? scrotum? (vulva?)	Lower ureteral stone (common innervation of the lower ureter and bladder, scrotum, or vulva)

1.3	*Does the pain radiate from the right hypochondrium to the back? right shoulder?*	Gallbladder colic
1.4	Does the pain radiate from the left hypochondrium to the precordium?	Splenic flexure syndrome

2 Mode of Onset and Evolution of the Pain

2.1	How long have you had pain in the flank?	
2.2	Has the pain appeared	
	• suddenly?	Stone colic; vascular pain (dissecting aortic aneurysm); blood clot causing urinary tract obstruction
	• gradually?	Inflammatory pain: acute pyelonephritis; renal abscess, lumbar abscess
2.2a	Did the pain disappear abruptly?	Renal colic
2.3	How long did the pain last?	The duration of a renal colic is variable; it may subside within a few minutes or last for hours
2.4	Have you experienced in the past similar episodes?	Renal stones tend to recur (the patient usually can identify an attack of recurrent renal colic); gallbladder stones
2.4a	When did the first episode occur?	Hyperoxaluria, cystinuria, xanthinuria and renal tubular acidosis are often associated with stones at an early age; idiopathic calcareous nephrolithiasis and primary hyperparathyroidism commonly occur after age 30

3   Character and Intensity of the Pain

3.1   Is the flank pain
      • dull? aching? steady? low-grade?   Dull flank pain due to chronic distention of the renal capsule: chronic obstructive nephropathy; stone in the renal pelvis; acute pyelonephritis; hydronephrosis; renal tumor; polycystic disease; nonurologic condition

      • excruciating? with a steady crescendo? (and radiating to the groin, the testicles, or the labia)   Acute ureteral obstruction ("renal colic"): sudden distention of the ureter and associated distention of the renal pelvis. The severity of pain is related to the rapidity rather than the degree of distention.

4   Precipitating or Aggravating Factors

4.1   In case of chronic discomfort in the flank: Is it increased by
      • exertion?   May occur with steady pain due to renal lithiasis or stone impacted in the ureter; polycystic disease

      • movements of the spine? straining?   Radicular pain: compression vertebral fracture; cord tumor
4.2   *Does the flank pain come on only with micturition?*   Vesicoureteral reflux

5   Relieving Factors

5.1   In case of acute flank pain, do you prefer, in order to relieve the pain, to
      • *remain immobile or lie quietly in bed?*   Inflammatory type of pain; peritoneal irritation
      • *pace the floor, move constantly,* in an attempt to find a position that could give some relief?   Characteristic of renal colic
5.2   In case of chronic discomfort: Is it relieved by
      • lying down?   Polycystic disease
      • passage of gas?   Irritable bowel syndrome; splenic flexure syndrome; incomplete obstruction of the large bowel

6   Accompanying Symptoms

6.1   During or after the attack, did you pass
      • urine of normal color?   Probably nonrenal disorder
      • dark urine?   Acute gallbladder disorder with bilirubinuria

• *bloody urine?*	Hematuria, almost always present in renal colic; renal or ureteral calculus; renal tumor; massive infarction of the kidney
• cloudy urine?	Acute pyelonephritis; infection complicating a renal stone; papillary necrosis

6.2   During the attack, did you pass

• a decreased amount of urine?	Renal colic
• a normal amount of urine?	Probably nonrenal disorder

6.3   After the attack, did you

• urinate more than usual?	Polyuria frequently appears after a renal colic
• stop urinating?	**Anuria** associated with bilateral ureteral calculi; papillary necrosis

6.4   Do you have

• a frequent desire to urinate? burning on urination?	Urgency, frequency, dysuria: stone at the ureterovesical junction with inflammation and edema of the ureteral orifice (may mimic bladder infection); urinary tract infection
• fever? chills?	Urinary tract infection; renal or perinephric abscess; infection in other system(s)
• nausea? vomiting? abdominal distention?	Gastrointestinal symptoms may result from renointestinal reflexes (common autonomic and sensory innervation of the two systems), the proximity of the pancreas, duodenum, or colon to the kidney, or peritoneal irritation; paralytic ileus may accompany renal colic. Nausea and vomiting in intestinal obstruction; hyperparathyroidism; chronic renal insufficiency
• pain in your joints? toes?	Gout with uric acid lithiasis
• pain in your bones?	Multiple myeloma, hyperparathyroidism with hypercalcemia and nephrolithiasis
• increased intake of fluid? increased urinary output?	Hypercalcemia with polyuria and polydipsia; chronic renal failure
• chronic diarrhea?	The incidence of hyperoxaluria with calcium oxalate kidney stone is significantly higher in patients with inflammatory bowel disease, malabsorption, ileal resection, jejunoileal anastomosis

7   **Iatrogenic Factors   See Etiology**

8   Personal and Social Profile

8.1 What is your daily intake of fluids?	A low fluid intake may produce an increased urinary concentration of salts and organic compounds and promote saturation of the urine with stone constituents; the type of water may give relevant information as to calcium content
• your diet?	May reveal excessive calcium intake (milk, cheese), oxalate intake (leafy green vegetables, strong tea)

9   Personal Antecedents Pertaining to Pain in the Flank

9.1 Have you ever had an examination of your urine? blood? an x-ray of your kidneys? a treatment for renal stones? When? With what results?	
9.2 Have you ever had • previous kidney stone? gravel? • a stone ("gravel") passed in your urine? a chemical analysis of a stone?	About 80 percent of stones which reach the ureter can pass spontaneously (sites of impaction of a ureteral stone: the ureteropelvic junction and the uretero-vesical zone)
• recurrent urinary infections?	Suggests infection as an etiologic or complicating factor of renal calculus
• gout?	Uric and lithiasis
• a long period of immobilization?	May cause hypercalciuria

10   Family Medical History Pertaining to Pain in the Flank

10.1 Is there someone in your family who has (had) renal stones?	Idiopathic uric acid lithiasis; hereditary hyperoxaluria, cystinuria, xanthinuria; primary hyperparathyroidism; renal tubular acidosis

PHYSICAL SIGNS PERTAINING TO PAIN IN THE FLANK

	Possible significance
Restless patient changing position frequently	Renal colic
Tenderness in the costovertebral angle and flank	Ureteral stone; blood clot obstructing the ureter
Fever; costovertebral angle tenderness on deep pressure	Acute pyelonephritis; infection complicating urinary lithiasis; renal abscess
Palpable kidney	Acute hydronephrosis; renal tumor
Fever; tenderness of flank; palpable mass moving with respiration	Perinephric abscess

Left pleural effusion; splenic friction rub	Splenic abscess
Fever; tenderness along the costal margin; basilar crackles	Subphrenic abscess; pleurisy with pain referred to the abdomen
Jaundice	Gallbladder disease; sickle cell disease with renal infarction
Abdominal distention; diminished peristalsis	Often present in acute renal colic
Atrial fibrillation; cardiac lesion	Renal or splenic embolic episode
Tophi; gouty arthritis	Uric acid nephrolithiasis

LABORATORY TESTS PERTAINING TO PAIN IN THE FLANK[†]

Finding	Diagnostic Possibilities
Urine	
Alkaline pH	Infection with urea-splitting organisms and struvite formation; renal tubular disorder
Sediment: RBCs	Renal calculus
Culture positive	Renal infection with urea-splitting bacteria: may promote the formation of magnesium ammonium phosphate (struvite) stones
Hypercalciuria	In most patients with calcareous calculi: hyperparathyroidism; hypervitaminosis D, sarcoidosis, idiopathic hypercalciuria, etc.
Qualitative test for cystine positive	Cystinuria
Analysis of stone	Oxalosis, primary or secondary; uric acid stones, etc. Provides the basis for rational therapy
Blood	
Calcium; phosphorus; alkaline phosphatase abnormal	High calcium, low phosphate in hyperparathyroidism (with high alkaline phosphatase when there is significant bone disease)
Electrolytes abnormal	Metabolic acidosis in renal tubular acidosis
Uric acid elevated	Gouty nephropathy
Parathormone assay* elevated	Hyperparathyroidism

[†]See the appendix on Laboratory Reference Values for the associated normal laboratory values.
*When indicated

LABORATORY PROCEDURES PERTAINING TO PAIN IN THE FLANK

Procedure	To Detect
Plain abdominal film	Radiopaque stones : calcium phosphate, calcium oxalate, magnesium ammonium phosphate stones; slightly opaque: cystine stones (nonopaque: uric acid and xanthine stones)
IV pyelography	Radiopaque or radiolucent stones; obstruction; nephrocalcinosis; anatomic abnormalities predisposing to calculus formation; obstruction, medullary sponge kidney, localized deformity
X-rays of hands, lateral heads of clavicles, skull, long bones, pelvis*	Subperiosteal bone resorption in hyperparathyroidism

*When indicated

SELECTED BIBLIOGRAPHY

Coe FL, Favus MJ: Disorders of stone formation, in Brenner BM, Rector FC (eds). *The Kidney*, 3rd ed., pp. 1403–1442, Philadelphia: Saunders, 1986.

25
Polyuria

INTRODUCTION

Polyuria A urine volume above 3 liters per day.

The normal daily urine output in adults varies between 700 and 2000 mL. When a normal subject ingests an appreciable volume of water, plasma solute concentration decreases. Hypothalamic osmoreceptors sense the fall in plasma osmolality and inhibit both thirst and release of vasopressin, the neurohypophyseal antidiuretic hormone (ADH). In the absence of ADH, the distal convoluted tubule and the collecting duct become impermeable to water and an increased volume of dilute urine is formed. With the loss of free water, osmolality of plasma increases, stimulating ADH secretion and thus preventing further water loss. Vasopressin secretion can also be influenced by alterations in blood volume (an increased plasma volume inhibits ADH release and produces a diuresis that corrects the hypervolemia, whereas hypovolemia stimulates the secretion of ADH), blood pressure (hypotension produces antidiuresis), and stress, either physical or emotional, which stimulates ADH release. The failure of the kidney to concentrate urine in the presence of increased plasma solute concentration results in the syndrome of diabetes insipidus (DI) with polyuria.

Diabetes insipidus due to vasopressin deficiency may be caused by any type of lesion in the hypothalamus or pituitary region. Patients with central DI cannot concentrate their urine despite a rise in plasma osmolality after water deprivation, but they respond normally to exogenous vasopressin.

Nephrogenic DI is characterized by inability of the renal tubules to respond to endogenous or exogenous vasopressin. The high osmotic load per nephron which occurs in diabetes mellitus and chronic renal failure may also cause polyuria. In primary psychogenic polydipsia, polyuria is secondary to compulsive water drinking. This condition, far more common than central DI, is seen in patients with psychologic disturbances.

ETIOLOGY

Vasopressin Deficiency: Neurogenic Diabetes Insipidus (DI)

Idiopathic; posthypophysectomy, post-trauma; supra- or intrasellar tumors or cysts; histiocytosis or granuloma; intracranial aneurysm; Sheehan's syndrome; meningoencephalitis; Guillain-Barré syndrome; empty sella; familial (autosomal dominant)

Vasopressin Insensitivity (Nephrogenic DI)

Congenital: hereditary nephrogenic DI; polycystic or medullary cystic disease
Acquired tubulointerstitial renal disease: pyelonephritis, multiple myeloma, amyloidosis, after obstructive uropathy, sarcoidosis, hypercalcemia or hypokalemia nephropathy, sickle cell anemia, Sjögren's syndrome, analgesic nephropathy, renal transplantation; drugs or toxins

Osmotic Diuresis

Glycosuria, urea or mannitol infusion, radiographic contrast media, high-protein tube feedings; natriuretic syndromes (chronic renal failure; tubulointerstitial or medullary cystic disease; Bartter's syndrome; diuretic phase of acute tubular necrosis; diuretic agents)

Primary Polydipsia

Psychogenic; hypothalamic disease; drugs

Iatrogenic Causes of Polyuria

Excessive doses of corticosteroids; diuretics
Nephrogenic DI: vitamin D; lithium; demeclocycline; methoxyflurane; ethanol; phenytoin; propoxyphene; amphotericin
Primary polydipsia: thioridazine, chlorpromazine, anticholinergic agents

HISTORY TAKING*

Possible meaning of a positive response

1   **Mode of Onset**

1.1   How long have you been passing large quantities of urine?

Idiopathic diabetes insipidus (DI) is most often found in young adults, although it may occur at any age. Nephrogenic DI manifests itself early in life. The polyuria of DI is often well tolerated and not mentioned to a physician. Patients with primary psychogenic polydipsia usually do not complain of (thirst and) polyuria

1.2   Has the onset of polyuria been
  • *sudden?* in one or two days?
  • *gradual?* over weeks or months?

Most cases of pituitary DI
Suggests a disease other than pituitary DI. Acquired nephrogenic DI

2   **Character of the Polyuria**

2.1   What is the usual volume of urine passed per day?
  • less than 5 L?

Acquired nephrogenic DI: usually the urinary concentration defect is less severe than that in complete neurogenic DI, enabling patients to raise urine osmolality above plasma osmolality; recent onset of diabetes, pituitary or renal disease; hypokalemia; hypercalcemia; neurogenic DI with a partial deficiency of vasopressin

*In this section, items in *italics* are characteristic clinical features.

- *more than 5 to 6 L?*

- more than 20 L?

Idiopathic neurogenic DI; primary psychogenic polydipsia; osmotic diuresis
May be observed in psychogenic polydipsia

2.2 How many times a day do you urinate?

Urination typically occurs 5 to 6 times daily in adults. If urine volume rises to 3.5 L/day or greater, voiding increases in frequency to ten or more times daily

2.3 Do you pass at each urination
- *a large quantity of urine?*

- *a small quantity of urine?*

Polyuria (urine volume greater than 150 mL/hour)
Frequency (often with dysuria), not polyuria

2.4 Do you have to get up at night to urinate?

Nocturia: may occur in all the polyuric states; also in edema-forming states (congestive heart failure, nephrotic syndrome, hepatic cirrhosis with ascites); reduced bladder capacity; chronic partial bladder-outflow obstruction. Nocturia is usually absent in primary psychogenic polydipsia

2.5 Do you urinate more during the night than during the day?

May be an early complaint in chronic renal failure when urine is excreted at a uniform rate with loss of normal diurnal rhythm. (Normally, a much larger volume is excreted in the waking period)

2.6 Does your large urine flow
- *remain constant?*
- *vary from day to day?*

Idiopathic (spontaneous) DI
Episodic polyuria suggests compulsive water drinking (primary psychogenic DI)

3 Accompanying Symptoms

3.1 How much do you drink a day?
- Is your intake of fluid increased?

Polydipsia: an abnormally high intake of water or other fluids, commonly associated with polyuria. Polydipsia is secondary to the polyuria in: idiopathic DI, nephrogenic DI; osmotic diuresis; diabetes mellitus; chronic renal failure. Primary disorder in psychogenic polydipsia: patients with primary polydipsia drink enough water every day to produce polyuria. Polyuria due to primary polydipsia is often difficult to recognize because patients frequently deny excessive water ingestion

3.1a *Do you have a preference for very cold or iced drinks?*

Patients with spontaneous neurogenic DI characteristically prefer water rather than other beverages and desire ice cold water

• no preference?

Primary psychogenic polydipsia

3.1b Are there periods (from weeks to months) during which your intake of fluids is not increased?

Psychogenic polydipsia may be episodic

3.2 Do you have an excessive, insatiable thirst?

Thirst is secondary to loss of water in neurogenic DI; nephrogenic DI; osmotic diuresis. In primary polydipsia, thirst is often, but not necessarily, present

3.3 If you are deprived of water, do you urinate
• *less than usual?*
• *as much as usual?*

Psychogenic polydipsia
Spontaneous DI

3.4 Do you have
• headaches?

Increased intracranial pressure due to mass lesion

• a loss of vision?

Bilateral hemianopsia: compression of optic chiasma by a midline tumor: craniopharyngioma, pinealoma, glioma, metastases

• an increase of your appetite?
• a decrease of your appetite? nausea? vomiting?
• abdominal cramps? nausea? vomiting? diarrhea? headaches? irritability?
• muscular weakness?

Polyphagia of diabetes mellitus
Chronic renal failure; hypercalcemia; hypokalemia; intracranial tumor
Severe hypo-osmolality in primary psychogenic polydipsia

Potassium depletion; hypercalcemia

4 Iatrogenic Factors   See Etiology

5 Personal Antecedents Pertaining to the Polyuria

5.1 Have you ever had an examination of your urine? blood? an x-ray of your kidneys? your skull? When? With what results?

5.2 Do you have any of the following conditions: diabetes mellitus? a kidney disease? urinary tract infection? a prostate disease?
• an emotional problem? anxiety? depression?

A previous history of psychologic disturbances is nearly always present in patients with psychogenic polydipsia. Polyuria in patients being treated for manic-depressive illness is usually the result of lithium administration

| • a high blood pressure? | Chronic renal failure; aldosteronism (potassium depletion) |

5.3   Have you ever had
   • a severe head injury? a recent head trauma? intracranial surgery?

Point to pituitary DI as the cause of the polyuric state

6   Family Medical History Pertaining to the Polyuria

6.1   Is there someone in your family who also passes large amounts of urine?

Idiopathic neurogenic DI can be inherited as an autosomal dominant trait; rarely, nephrogenic DI is familial and congenital

PHYSICAL SIGNS PERTAINING TO POLYURIA

Possible significance

	Possible significance
Hypotension, tachycardia, decreased skin turgor, postural hypotension, (acute weight loss)	Depletion of intravascular fluid volume: in osmotic diuresis, recovery from acute tubular necrosis or bilateral obstruction
Acute weight gain, hypertension, edema	Solute administration with extracellular fluid excess
Abnormal neurologic examination	Intracranial space-occupying lesion
Exophthalmos; skin rash	Hand-Schüller-Christian disease: skull osteolytic lesions, exophthalmos, diabetes insipidus
Proximal muscular weakness; calcification in the cornea	Hypercalcemic states; hyperparathyroidism
Visual field defects	Intracranial tumor
Funduscopic examination: papilledema	Increased intracranial pressure
diabetic retinopathy	Diabetes mellitus with polyuria

LABORATORY TESTS PERTAINING TO POLYURIA[†]

Test	Finding	Diagnostic Possibilities
Urine		
24-h urine collection		To substantiate polyuria (and distinguish it from frequency)

[†]See the appendix on Laboratory Reference Values for the associated normal laboratory values.

Test	Finding	Diagnostic Possibilities
Specific gravity	1.005 or less	Hyposthenuria, the hallmark of DI, neurogenic or nephrogenic primary polydipsia
	>1.012	Polyuria due to solute administration, osmotic diuresis, use of diuretics, recovery from acute tubular necrosis or bilateral obstruction
Glucose	Positive	Diabetes mellitus: osmotic diuresis
Protein	Positive	Chronic parenchymal renal disease
Osmolality	Above serum osmolality: >700 mOsmol/kg	Osmotic diuresis; glycosuria
	Below serum osmolality: <200 mOsmol/kg	Hyposthenuria: neurogenic or nephrogenic DI; primary polydipsia
After fluid deprivation	Urine becomes concentrated	Primary polydipsia; partial DI
	Unchanged (hypotonic) osmolality	Vasopressin-sensitive or nephrogenic DI
After vasopressin test	Increase in urine osmolality	Vasopressin-sensitive neurogenic DI
	Unresponsive	Complete nephrogenic DI; psychogenic polydipsia

Blood

BUN, creatinine	Elevated	Chronic renal failure
Fasting glucose	Elevated	Diabetes mellitus
Electrolytes Calcium	Hypokalemia Elevated	Potassium depletion or hypercalcemia resulting in impaired ability to concentrate the urine maximally
CT of the head Visual field examination		To detect: mass lesion of the hypothalamic region; empty posterior sella

SELECTED BIBLIOGRAPHY

Hebert SC, Culpepper RM, Andreoli TE: The posterior pituitary and water metabolism, in Wilson JD, Foster DW (eds). *Williams Textbook of Endocrinology*, 7th ed., pp. 614–652, Philadelphia: Saunders, 1985.

26

Uremia and/or Proteinuria

INTRODUCTION

Uremia   The clinical syndrome associated with chronic renal failure.
Proteinuria   Presence of protein in the urine.

Many chronic renal diseases are inherently progressive and eventuate in uremia, a symptomatic state with disorders of various systems. With renal insufficiency, impaired urinary concentrating ability results in polydipsia, polyuria, and nocturia. The ability to reabsorb sodium from the tubular lumen is limited, resulting in a loss of sodium in the urine. In the later stages, sodium retention occurs, resulting in congestive heart failure, pulmonary edema, or hypertension. Metabolic acidosis is due to a decreased ability to excrete ammonium and to renal bicarbonate leak. Decreased renal function produces phosphate retention, secondary hypocalcemia, and secondary hyperparathyroidism. Decreased intestinal calcium absorption due to impaired hydroxylation of vitamin D also contributes to hypocalcemia. Decreased erythropoietin results in normochromic normocytic anemia. Some gastrointestinal, cardiovascular, neuromuscular manifestations of uremia are attributed to retention of by-products of protein and amino acid metabolism, "middle molecules", presumed polypeptides with molecular weight between 1,000 and 1,500, or to adaptive overproduction of polypeptide hormones.

Some protein is filtered by normal glomeruli (40 to 100 mg/24 h). Pathologic proteinuria is present when the protein in the urine is greater than 150 mg/24 h. Orthostatic proteinuria (protein present in the urine produced when the patient is in the upright position and absent when the patient is recumbent) occurs in about 3 percent of adolescents and is usually benign. Patients with transient (intermittent) proteinuria have various conditions and may show some renal histologic changes. Transient proteinuria (present on initial examination and absent on subsequent urinalysis) is a common type of proteinuria in young adults who have no evidence of renal disease. Persistent proteinuria is always pathologic. Massive proteinuria, in excess of 3.5 g daily (nephrotic syndrome), results from a gross increase in glomerular permeability; diseases of the glomeruli produce a proteinuria in which albumin predominates. Persistent proteinuria can be seen without glomerular disease. Overflow proteinuria occurs when increased production of filterable, low-molecular-weight proteins exceeds the tubular reabsorptive capacity, as in monoclonal gammopathies. Tubular proteinuria occurs when reabsorption of proteins from the tubular lumen is incomplete because of tubular damage.

ETIOLOGY

Chronic Renal Failure (Proteinuria Rarely Exceeding 1 to 2 g/24 h)

Glomerulonephritis* (progressive types): membranous; membranoproliferative; focal
   glomerulosclerosis
Tubulointerstitial renal disease
   Renal stone disease; nephrocalcinosis

Reflux nephropathy
Analgesic abuse; intoxication: lead, cadmium
Chronic pyelonephritis*
Vascular renal disease
    Hypertensive nephrosclerosis*
    Bilateral renal artery disease
Essential hypertension*
Diabetes mellitus*
Collagen-vascular disorders: systemic lupus erythematosus (SLE), polyarteritis
    nodosa, Wegener's granulomatosis, scleroderma, Henoch-Schönlein purpura
Gout; multiple myeloma; amyloidosis
Obstructive uropathy: stone; prostatic disease; congenital
Hereditary: polycystic kidney disease*; medullary cystic disease; chronic hereditary
    nephritis (Alport's syndrome)

Heavy Proteinuria: Nephrotic Syndrome

Idiopathic nephrotic syndrome[†] due to primary glomerular disease
    Primary glomerular disease: minimal change disease; focal glomerular sclerosis;
        membranoproliferative glomerulonephritis; membranous glomerulonephritis;
        IgA nephropathy; proliferative glomerulonephritis
Systemic: diabetes mellitus;[†] systemic lupus erythematosus;[†] Henoch-Schönlein pur-
    pura; amyloidosis[†]
Infections: poststreptococcal glomerulonephritis; infective endocarditis; "shunt
    nephritis;" hepatitis B; malaria; schistosomiasis
Neoplastic: solid tumors (lung, colon, stomach, breast); leukemia, lymphoma, Hodg-
    kin's disease; multiple myeloma
Toxins: drugs; heavy metals; allergens (bee sting, pollens, vaccines)
Miscellaneous: pregnancy-associated; chronic renal allograft rejection; hereditary dis-
    orders

Isolated Proteinuria (Usually Less Than 2 gm/daily, in Otherwise Healthy Individuals, With a Normal Urinary Sediment)

Transient (intermittent): strenuous exercise; congestive heart failure; emotional stress;
    exposure to cold; high fever
Orthostatic: postural
Constant: initial feature of idiopathic membranous glomerulonephritis, focal glomeru-
    losclerosis, IgA nephropathy; amyloidosis; asymptomatic essential hypertension;
    mild or latent diabetic nephropathy; overflow proteinuria (light chains); tubular
    proteinuria

Iatrogenic Causes of Uremia and/or Proteinuria (Partial List)

Nephropathies due to chronic analgesic abuse: phenacetin, salicylates(?)
Nephrotic syndrome: phenindione, probenecid, captopril, penicillamine, gold salts,
    fenopropen
Diuretics and antihypertensive drugs may induce sodium depletion and produce an
    elevation of BUN

*Common cause
†Common cause of nephrotic syndrome

HISTORY TAKING*

Possible meaning of a positive response

1 Mode of Onset and Duration

1.1 How long have you known that you have uremia and/or proteinuria?

The time of onset can provide useful information about how to proceed with the workup

1.1a How was it detected?
  • during a check-up examination?

Renal functional impairment may be asymptomatic. Proteinuria is usually detected on a urinalysis conducted during a routine physical examination or during a concurrent illness

  • because you were sick?

By the time patients present with general symptoms, at least 75 percent of renal function has been lost

1.2 Since when have you felt sick?

The onset of chronic renal failure is insidious

2 Character of the Urine

2.1 What is the appearance of your urine?
  • clear?
  • cloudy?

Chronic glomerulonephritis
Presence of phosphates, urates, pus, blood

  • reddish? bloody?

Acute glomerulonephritis, nephrolithiasis, tumor may cause hematuria

3 Precipitating or Aggravating Factors

All the extrarenal factors that can produce acute renal failure can worsen chronic renal failure and convert asymptomatic azotemia into uremia

3.1 Have you recently had
  • an infection? a urinary infection?

Infection, especially streptococcal, may seriously impair residual function

  • urinary tract obstruction?
  • an episode of vomiting? diarrhea? dehydration?

In symptom-free early stage of chronic renal failure: may compromise renal function still further, often leading to clinically overt uremia

  • black, tarry stools?

Bleeding into the intestine increases production rate of urea

*In this section, items in *italics* are characteristic clinical features.

3.2 What is your daily intake of fluid? salt? meat, fish?

Excessive ingestion of water may contribute to hyponatremia and weight gain. Excessive salt ingestion contributes to, or aggravates, congestive heart failure, hypertension, and edema formation. Excessive intake of protein may increase production rate of urea

4 Accompanying Symptoms

4.1 Do you feel weak? unwell? easily tired?

Almost universal in symptomatic uremia; anemia becomes a major cause of symptoms when hemoglobin falls below about 7 g/100 mL

4.2 Do you have
• a loss of appetite?

Common in early stage of chronic renal failure. Urea may account for anorexia

• nausea? *especially upon arising in the morning?* vomiting?

Glomerular filtration rate below 10 mL per minute

• a bad taste in the mouth?

Uremic fetor: a uriniferous odor to the breath: derives from the breakdown of urea in saliva to ammonia

• bloody diarrhea?

Uremic colitis: colonic ulcerations attributed to local irritation of the colonic mucosa by ammonia produced by the intestinal flora

• a dimmed, blurred vision?

Hypertension with lesions in the optic fundi

• a swelling of your eyelids? your face?

Nephrotic syndrome with hypoproteinemia. Parotitis in advanced uremia

• swollen legs?

Edema: hypertensive heart failure, one of the most common complications of uremia; hypoproteinemia: nephrotic syndrome; oliguric phase of terminal renal insufficiency with fluid overload

• trouble breathing?

Congestive heart failure; "uremic lung"; anemia

• fever?

Systemic lupus erythematosus; polyarteritis nodosa

• chest pain?

Pericarditis: now seen infrequently because of early initiation of dialysis

• abdominal pain?

Uremic colitis; pancreatitis occurs with increased frequency in chronic uremia

• epigastric pain?

Peptic ulcer disease occurs in as many as one-fourth of uremic patients

• drowsiness? insomnia? loss of memory?

Earliest symptoms of subtle disturbances of central nervous system function

• hiccups? cramps? twitchings of large muscle groups? nocturnal muscle cramps in the calves? thighs?

Signs of neuromuscular irritability and polyneuropathy: common in late chronic renal failure

- discomfort in your legs during rest and relieved by movement?

"Restless legs syndrome": peripheral neuropathy of advanced chronic renal failure

- numbness, tingling, burning of the toes? feet?

Peripheral demyelinating neuropathy; hypocalcemia

- easy bruising? abnormal bleeding?

Platelet defect of uremia: elevated plasma levels of guanidinosuccinic acid interfere with activation of platelet factor 3 by ADP, resulting in abnormal platelet aggregation and adhesiveness; thrombocytopenia

- itching?

Ascribed to calcium phosphate deposition in the skin; often associated with secondary hyperparathyroidism

- a skin rash?

Systemic lupus erythematosus

- bone pain?

Renal osteodystrophy: osteomalacia; secondary hyperparathyroidism (osteitis fibrosa cystica): evidence for chronicity because it develops over a period of months to years

- pain in your joints?

Lupus nephritis; gouty nephropathy (rare); Henoch-Schönlein purpura; renal osteodystrophy (calcium deposition in bursas)

- bloody expectorations?

Goodpasture's syndrome; Wegener's granulomatosis

4.3   During the day, do you urinate
- as much as usual?

Urine volume is usually normal or even mildly elevated in chronic renal failure because of lost concentrating ability

- less frequently than usual?

Oliguria: acute glomerulonephritis; end stage of renal failure; obstructive uropathy

- more frequently than usual?
  - without discomfort, and passing large amounts of urine?

Polyuria commonly accompanies isosthenuria: an early sign of chronic renal failure; hypercalcemia; hypokalemia; diuretic medication

4.3a   Do you have to get up at night to urinate? how many times?

Nocturia: loss of the urine concentrating ability in chronic renal failure

4.4   Do you drink more fluids than usual?

Polydipsia balancing the polyuria of chronic renal failure

5   Iatrogenic Factors   See Etiology

5.1   Have you regularly taken any drugs for headaches?

Phenacetin nephropathy; methysergide-induced retroperitoneal fibrosis. Denial of analgesic intake is common

| 5.2 | Are you taking any drugs for an elevated blood pressure? | Drug-induced hypotension and/or salt depletion tend to reduce renal function and may worsen renal insufficiency |

6 Personal and Social Profile

6.1 Are you exposed to any toxins?

| 6.1a | Do you use drugs? | "Street" heroin may cause nephrotic syndrome |

7 Personal Antecedents Pertaining to the Uremia and/or Proteinemia

7.1 Have you ever had blood, urine examinations? x-rays of the kidneys? When? With what results?

7.2 Have you ever had any of the following conditions: a renal disease? acute glomerulonephritis? stones? recurrent renal infections? elevated blood pressure? a recent febrile infection?

| | • gout? | Gouty nephropathy: uric acid stones and interstitial deposits of urate crystals in the kidney |
| | • diabetes? | The most common cause of secondary nephrotic syndrome in adults in the United States; proteinuria is usually the initial manifestation of renal disease in the diabetic patient |

8 Family Medical History Pertaining to the Uremia and/or Proteinemia

8.1 Does someone in your family have

| | • a renal disease? | Polycystic kidney disease |
| | • deafness? | Alport's syndrome (hereditary nephritis) |

PHYSICAL SIGNS PERTAINING TO UREMIA AND/OR PROTEINEMIA

Possible significance

Skin
  • pallor

Anemia: normochromic normocytic; due to diminished biosynthesis of erythropoietin by the diseased kidney; presence of erythropoietin inhibitors; hemolysis; gastrointestinal and chronic dialyzer blood loss. Absence of anemia suggests acute renal failure

• ecchymoses, hematomas	A bleeding tendency is common in late renal failure: disturbed ADP-mediated platelet aggregation and platelet adhesiveness
• calcium deposition	Secondary hyperparathyroidism
• scratch marks	Pruritus, particularly associated with secondary hyperparathyroidism
Hypertension	Present in more than 80 percent of patients with end-stage chronic renal failure; attributed to elevated renin production in the kidneys and sodium retention. Absence of hypertension suggests a salt-wasting form of renal disease (polycystic or medullary cystic disease, analgesic nephropathy); antihypertensive therapy; volume depletion (excessive gastrointestinal fluid losses, diuretic therapy)
Pulmonary edema; peripheral edema	Hypertensive heart failure: one of the most common complications of uremia; "uremic lung" (even in the absence of volume overload): due to increased permeability of the alveolar capillary membrane; impaired sodium and water excretion; nephrotic syndrome; acute glomerulonephritis; oliguric phase of terminal renal insufficiency with excessive fluid intake
Pericardial friction rub	Uremic pericarditis. Now infrequent because of early initiation of dialysis. Pericarditis in the well-dialyzed patient: viral infection or systemic disease
Diminished to absent deep tendon reflexes; muscle weakness	Peripheral neuropathy, a common complication of advanced chronic renal failure
Large kidneys	Obstructive uropathy; polycystic disease
Palpable liver or spleen	Amyloidosis with nephrotic syndrome
Arthritis; skin rash	Collagen-vascular disease
Metastatic calcification in the cornea	Band keratopathy: hypercalcemia with elevated serum phosphate
Funduscopic examination	May reveal: hypertensive retinopathy; diabetic retinopathy (patients with diabetic glomerulopathy almost invariably have retinal complications)

LABORATORY TESTS PERTAINING TO UREMIA AND/OR PROTEINURIA[†]

Test	Finding	Diagnostic Possibilities
Urine		
Protein quantitation		Nonalbumin proteins, such as immunoglobulin light chains (Bence-Jones proteins), may cause a false-negative dipstick test
	>150 mg/24 h; <50-mg excretion over 8 hours while recumbent	Orthostatic proteinuria
	<2 g/24 h	Interstitial or tubular disorder; chronic pyelonephritis; IgA nephropathy; overflow proteinuria; orthostatic proteinuria
	>3.5 g/24 h	Glomerular disease; nephrotic syndrome; overflow proteinuria: multiple myeloma
Sediment	Virtually normal	Obstructive uropathy; hypercalcemia
	Red blood cells and RBC casts	Glomerular cause of proteinuria
	Broad casts	Common in chronic renal failure (arise in dilated tubules)
	WBCs	Pyuria or tubulointerstitial disease
	Glycosuria	Diabetic nephropathy
Electrophoresis (if proteinuria above 150 mg/24 h)	Albumin more than 60 percent of urinary protein	Glomerular cause: nephritic or nephrotic disorder
	Low-molecular-weight protein; absence of albumin	Overflow or tubular proteinuria; Bence-Jones proteinuria; interstitial nephritis
Blood		
BUN:creatinine ratio	10 to 15:1	Renal parenchymal disease
	>10 to 15:1	Extrarenal disorder: dehydration, hypotension, hypovolemia, GI hemorrhage

[†]See the appendix on Laboratory Reference Values for the associated normal laboratory values.

Test	Finding	Diagnostic Possibilities
Hematocrit, hemoglobin	Decreased	Normocytic normochromic anemia in chronic renal failure
	Normal	Acute renal failure; early stage of urinary obstruction; renal artery stenosis; polycystic disease; erythropoietin-secreting tumor or cyst; polycythemia vera
Electrolyte	Metabolic acidosis	GFR below 20 mL/min
	Hyperkalemia	Terminal renal failure
Calcium	Decreased	Low serum albumin level; hyperphosphatemia; impaired GI absorption of calcium; formation of complexes with phosphate
Fasting glucose	Elevated	Diabetic nephropathy
Cholesterol, triglycerides	Elevated	Nephrotic syndrome
Serum electrophoresis	Hyperproteinemia; monoclonal peak	Multiple myeloma
	Hypoalbuminemia	Nephrotic syndrome
Antinuclear antibodies	Positive	Systemic lupus erythematosus
Serum complement	Decreased	Acute streptococcal nephritis; membranoproliferative glomerulonephritis; SLE

LABORATORY PROCEDURES PERTAINING TO UREMIA AND/OR PROTEINURIA

Procedure	To Detect
Ultrasound, abdominal scout film, pyelogram	Reduced kidney size: the hallmark of chronic renal failure; irregular renal outlines: chronic pyelonephritis. Normal renal size: acute renal failure. Large kidneys: obstruction; polycystic disease; amyloidosis
Renal biopsy*	Specific forms of parenchymal disease; causes of nephrotic syndrome; amyloidosis; polyarteritis nodosa; etc.

*When indicated

SELECTED BIBLIOGRAPHY

Abuello JG: Proteinuria: Diagnostic principles and procedures. *Ann Intern Med* 98:186–191, 1983.

Brenner BM, Lazarus JM: Chronic renal failure: Pathophysiologic and clinical considerations, in Wilson J, Braunwald E, Isselbacher KJ et al (eds). *Harrison's Principles of Internal Medicine*, 12th ed., Chap. 224, New York: McGraw-Hill, 1991.

Stone RA: Office evaluation of the patient with proteinuria. *Postgrad Med* 86(5):241–244, 1989.

Striegel J, Michael AF, Chavers BM: Asymptomatic proteinuria. *Postgrad Med* 83(8):287–294, 1988.

27

Abnormal Vaginal Bleeding

INTRODUCTION

Abnormal Vaginal Bleeding   Bleeding that occurs at an inappropriate time or in an excessive amount.

The menstrual cycle in normal women of reproductive age averages 28 ± 3 days. The average duration of menstrual bleeding is 4 ± 2 days and the average blood loss is 30 to 100 mL. For the first 10 to 14 days after the onset of menstrual bleeding, during the period of follicular maturation, a rising estrogen level results in proliferative changes of the endometrium (proliferative phase). During the latter part of the menstrual cycle (luteal phase), from ovulation to the onset of menstrual bleeding, the secretion of progesterone by the corpus luteum induces secretory activity of the glands of the endometrium. Uterine bleeding in ovulatory cycles results from a critical drop in the blood estrogen and progesterone levels. The interval between ovulation and menstruation is normally 14 days. In contrast, the preovulatory period (the interval from the first day of menstruation to the day of ovulation) may be variable. The variations in cycle length are thus related to changes in the duration of the follicular phase preceding ovulation.

Abnormal excessive bleeding may be due to anatomic lesions of the uterus, tubes, and ovaries. In general, ovulation continues in such cases. Systemic illnesses including various endocrinopathies may also present with abnormal bleeding. Dysfunctional uterine bleeding occurs in the absence of organic genital or extragenital cause. It is most frequently associated with anovulation and is usually due to either estrogen withdrawal or to estrogen breakthrough bleeding. In anovulatory women, estrogen stimulation of the endometrium is unopposed by progesterone. As a consequence, the endometrium proliferates, becomes thicker, and may shed irregularly, especially if estrogen levels drop. Anovulatory bleeding is a frequent cause of an irregular menstrual bleeding in adolescence and toward the end of the reproductive years.

ETIOLOGY

Anatomic Lesions

Cervical: malignancy; polyps; erosions; cervicitis; endometriosis
Uterine: malignancy; polyps; leiomyomas; endometritis; foreign body; endometriosis
Vaginal: malignancy; vaginitis; foreign body; trauma
Tubal and ovaries: malignancy
Complications of pregnancy: abortion; retained products of gestation; hydatidiform mole; chorioepithelioma
Ectopic pregnancy

Inflammation

Pelvic inflammatory disease

Extragenital Causes

Endocrinopathies; oral contraceptives; bleeding diathesis; drugs

Dysfunctional Uterine Bleeding

Iatrogenic Causes of Abnormal Vaginal Bleeding

Estrogens; progestogens; androgens; anticoagulants; nonsteroidal anti-inflammatory
agents

MENSTRUAL HISTORY TAKING*

Possible meaning of a positive response

1   Mode of Onset

1.1   How long have you had trouble
with your menstruations?

1.2   *On what date did your last period
occur?*

(Inaccurate in many cases) Indicates the
first day of the last normal menses.
When pregnancy is a possible diagnosis,
the identification of the last menstrual
period as truly normal becomes critical.
Every woman with abnormal vaginal
bleeding during the reproductive years
should be assumed to have a complication of pregnancy

1.3   Has your expected last menstruation been delayed?

Possible pregnancy

2   Onset of Menses

2.1   When did your menses begin?

The age at menarche is related to the
nutritional state of the woman and her
exposure to light. Normal menarche
(between 12 and 13 years) indicates a
normal maturation of the hypothalamic-pituitary ovarian axis

3   Frequency of Menses

3.1   How many days apart do your periods occur?
   • from 25 to 31 days?

Normal duration; longer menstrual cycles occur at menarche and prior to
menopause. A variation from the established pattern of normality for the
patient of greater than 5 days indicates a
disturbance in the feedback and control
mechanism of the hypothalamic-
pituitary-ovarian axis

*In this section, items in *italics* are characteristic clinical features.

• less than 21 days?

Polymenorrha: episodes of menstrual bleeding occurring at intervals of less than 21 days, with unaltered duration and character of menstrual flow; suggests disturbances in endocrine control; dysfunctional uterine bleeding (uterus likely to be normal); may be a normal variant

• more than 35 days?

Oligomenorrhea: a decrease in the frequency of menstrual flow with irregularity in the interval; dysfunctional uterine bleeding; disturbed endocrine control

3.2   *Are your periods still regular? predictable?*

Ovulatory cycles. Maintenance of cyclic regularity associated with excessive uterine bleeding suggests organic disease of the outflow tract

3.2a Do you have bleeding occurring
• irregularly between menstrual cycles?

Metrorrhagia (intermenstrual bleeding): organic disease: cervical or endometrial lesion (carcinoma, polyp); intrauterine device; vaginitis; oral contraceptives

• *after sexual intercourse? after douching?*

Contact bleeding; cervical carcinoma; cervical polyp; cervical erosion

• during the midintervals? with a dull aching pain?

Midcycle bleeding: associated with ovulation

• a few days before the onset of the normal cycle?

Premenstrual spotting, a variant of metrorrhagia

3.3   *Does the bleeding occur irregularly? Is it unpredictable as to amount and duration?*

Dysfunctional uterine bleeding (usually painless): due to failure of normal follicular maturation with consequent anovulation; transient disruption of the synchronous hypothalamic-pituitary-ovarian patterns necessary for regular ovulatory cycles: early menarche, perimenopausal period; temporary stresses, intercurrent illness; estrogen withdrawal bleeding; estrogen breakthrough bleeding (polycystic ovarian disease); progesterone breakthrough bleeding (with continuous low-dose oral contraceptives)

4   Duration of Menses

4.1   What is the duration of flow?
• from 2 to 7 days?

Normal duration: 4 ± 2 days. Considerable variation among women, but rather consistent over long periods of time for the individual woman

• more than 7 days?

Menorrhagia: prolongation of the menstrual flow often associated with an increase of flow: organic disease of the outflow tract: abnormalities of the ovaries, the uterus (submucous leiomyoma, adenomyosis, endometrial polyps)

• prolonged and with irregular intermenstrual bleeding?

Menometrorrhagia: totally disturbed menstrual cycle: chronic anovulation

5 Amount of Blood Loss

5.1 What is the amount of menstrual flow?

Most difficult to precisely determine. The average blood loss during a menstrual cycle is 30 to 100 mL

• increased? excessive?

Hypermenorrhea: increased quantity of menstrual flow during a regular cycle of normal duration; organic disease: conditions affecting the uterus rather than the ovary; bleeding diathesis. The complaint of abnormally heavy bleeding must be checked with a measurement of the patient's hemoglobin-hematocrit

• spotty? light bleeding? with regular, predictable menstruation?

Hypomenorrhea: decrease in the amount of menstrual flow, often with a decrease in duration; obstruction of the outflow tract: intrauterine synechiae, scarring of the cervix

5.2 How many tampons do you use per day? per period?

A rough (and inaccurate) estimate of blood loss. Normally: 4 per day, up to 12 per period. A fully saturated tampon contains between 15 and 25 mL of blood. Fastidious women may use a larger number of tampons, changing at a point well below blood saturation

5.2a Does the menstrual blood soak through a tampon and then onto your clothing?

Excessive amount of bleeding

5.2b Can you control bleeding with an intravaginal tampon?

A proprietary intravaginal tampon is never enough to contain abnormally heavy bleeding

6 Character of the Bleeding

6.1 Are there any clots in the menstrual flow?

The rate of normal menstrual flow permits prevention of clotting or lysis of existing clots (presence of fibrinolysin in the endometrial cavity). Clots may be observed during episodes of heavy bleeding

6.2 Is the blood
     • bright red, with clots?   Suggests a brisk nonmenstrual bleeding
     • dark?   Slower hemorrhage acted upon by cer-
                                                vical or vaginal secretions

7   Accompanying Symptoms

7.1 A few days before the onset of flow
     do you have
     • breast fullness? breast tender-   Premenstrual symptoms: may be pros-
       ness? abdominal distention? low   taglandin-mediated; ovulatory bleeding
       back pain? weight gain? mood   (absent in anovulatory bleeding)
       changes?

7.2 Do you have
     • abdominal cramping with, or just   Primary dysmenorrhea if no demon-
       prior to, your menstruations?   strable disorders of the pelvis; more
                                                common in ovulatory cycles
     • a dull aching pain at midcycle?   Pain associated with ovulation ("mit-
       (from a few minutes to hours)   telschmerz"): (?) peritoneal irritation
                                                by follicular fluid released at the time of
                                                ovulation
     • chronic pain in the lower abdo-   Secondary dysmenorrhea if associated
       men? increased during menstru-   with diseases of the pelvis; uterine ori-
       ation?   gin: leiomyoma, infection; adnexal
                                                pain: pelvic inflammatory disease; en-
                                                dometriosis
     • pain unrelated to the menses?   Pathology of nongenital organs

7.3 Is your abnormal bleeding pain-   Dysfunctional uterine bleeding; an-
     less?   ovulatory cycles

7.4 Do you have
     • fever?   Pelvic inflammatory disease (in young
                                                women); acute salpingo-oophoritis
     • a vaginal discharge? pruritus?   In women of childbearing age: acute
                                                salpingitis (gonorrheal, chlamydial);
                                                vaginitis (Candida, Trichomonas, Gard-
                                                nerella vaginalis)
     • a milky discharge from the nip-   Galactorrhea; with irregular menses:
       ples?   prolactinoma
     • easy bruising? a blood condition?   Thrombocytopenic purpura, von Wil-
                                                lebrand's disease, leukemia, may cause
                                                uterine bleeding

7.5 (In a perimenopausal woman): Do   Vasomotor instability; close temporal
     you have hot flashes? cold sweats?   relationship between the onset of the
                                                hot flash and pulses of LH secretion;
                                                alterations in catecholamines, prosta-
                                                glandins, endorphins may also play a
                                                role

8   Iatrogenic Factors   See Etiology

8.1	Do you use birth control pills? other contraceptive methods?	A common cause of abnormal bleeding
8.2	Do you take continuous low-dose oral contraceptives?	Progesterone breakthrough bleeding (abnormally high ratios of progesterone to estrogens)
8.3	Have you discontinued estrogen therapy?	In a postmenopausal woman: estrogen withdrawal bleeding (usually painless)

9   Personal and Social Profile

9.1	Age of the patient? • between 40 and 50 years old?	Perimenopausal and menopausal bleeding should be considered as caused by a malignancy until proved otherwise; dysfunctional uterine bleeding
	• fifth and sixth decade?	Bleeding in a postmenopausal woman: malignancy; estrogen therapy; atrophic vaginitis; foreign bodies (pessaries). Postmenopausal bleeding is typically uterine in origin. The appearance of bleeding in a woman more than 6 months beyond her last menstrual period requires appropriate diagnostic evaluation
9.2	Are you sexually active?	Abnormal vaginal bleeding may represent pregnancy complications
9.3	Do you think you are pregnant?	Implantation bleeding; threatened abortion; incomplete abortion; septic abortion; ectopic pregnancy

10   Personal Antecedents Pertaining to the Bleeding

10.1	Have you ever had a Pap test? a pelvic examination? an x-ray, an ultrasound of your uterus? When? With what results?	
10.2	Do you have any of the following conditions • diabetes? a thyroid condition? (hypothyroidism)	May cause dysfunctional uterine bleeding, anovulatory irregular menstrual bleeding
	• a recent pregnancy? abortion?	Retention of gestation products
	• a previous ectopic pregnancy? salpingitis? previous tubal procedure?	Major risk factors for ectopic pregnancy

- a liver disease?

May result in the failure of estrogen to be conjugated in the liver, with resulting increase of free estrogens and abnormal uterine bleeding

- a bleeding tendency?

Abnormal uterine bleeding may be the initial or principal manifestation of a generalized bleeding diathesis

11 Family Medical History Pertaining to the Bleeding

11.1 Does someone in your family have a uterine cancer?

A first-degree female relative of a patient with endometrial cancer has a fourfold greater risk of developing the disease

11.2 Did your mother take diethylstilbestrol (DES) as a fertility drug?

Daughter liable to clear cell adenocarcinoma of the vagina or cervix

PHYSICAL SIGNS PERTAINING TO ABNORMAL VAGINAL BLEEDING

Possible significance

Pelvic examination

May reveal or suggest: tumor, polyps, pelvic infection; threatened or incomplete abortion; ectopic pregnancy; endometriosis; atrophic vaginitis; foreign body in vagina

Rectal and urinary examination

To exclude extra-uterine bleeding. Bleeding from urethra or rectum may be interpreted by the patient as vaginal bleeding

Fever

Pelvic inflammatory disease

Ecchymoses, petechiae

Bleeding tendency

Pallor

Hypochromic anemia resulting from excessive blood loss; underlying malignancy

Abnormal abdominal examination

Tumor; ascites; intraabdominal inflammatory process

Ascites, hydrothorax

Meigs's syndrome (with ovarian tumors)

Dry coarse skin, periorbital puffiness; prolonged tendon reflex relaxation time

Hypothyroidism

Hirsutism (with or without obesity)

Stein-Leventhal syndrome (with polycystic ovaries)

LABORATORY TESTS PERTAINING TO ABNORMAL VAGINAL BLEEDING[†]

Test	To Detect
Complete blood count, platelet count, coagulation studies, thyroid function tests	
Urinary human chorionic gonadotropin	Uterine and ectopic pregnancies; hydatidiform mole; choriocarcinoma
Plasma estrogens, progesterone levels	Ovarian dysfunction; ovulation
Scraping, biopsy of cervix, vaginal canal	Tumor cells
Endometrial biopsy	Ovarian dysfunction; endometrial hyperplasia; endometrial neoplasm, polyps
Leukorrheal discharge: examination, culture	*Candida; Trichomonas; Gardnerella; Neisseria gonorrhoeae; Chlamydia*
Flat abdominal film	Tumors; fluid levels; distortion
Pelvic sonography	Uterine cavity content, volume; tumors; ectopic pregnancy
Hysterosalpingography	Submucosal myomas; polyps

[†]See the appendix on Laboratory Reference Values for the associated normal laboratory values.

SELECTED BIBLIOGRAPHY

Spellacy WN: Abnormal bleeding. *Clin Obstet Gynecol* 26(3):702–709, 1983.

Weingold AB: Abnormal bleeding, in Kase NG, Weingold AB, Lucas WE et al (eds). *Principles and Practice of Clinical Gynecology*, pp. 527–557, New York: John Wiley & Sons, 1983.

28
Amenorrhea

INTRODUCTION

Amenorrhea   Failure of menarche by age 16 (primary amenorrhea) or absence of menstruation for 3 or more months in a woman with past menses (secondary amenorrhea).

Normal menstrual cycles are regulated by gonadotropin secretion. During the period preceding ovulation, levels of blood follicle-stimulating hormone (FSH) and luteinizing hormone (LH) rise slowly. The FSH rise stimulates follicle growth, and the thecal cells of the developing follicle secrete increasing amounts of estradiol. At midcycle, as estrogen rises to a peak, it triggers the release of LH by the pituitary, through the LH-releasing hormone secreted by the hypothalamus. The LH surge results in ovulation, 18 to 36 h later, which in turn produces corpus luteum formation and function. During the period from ovulation to the onset of menstruation, a corpus luteum formed at the follicular site synthesizes and secretes estrogen and progesterone. The secretion of progesterone reaches a peak 5 to 8 days after the LH surge. As the estrogen and progesterone again decrease toward lower levels, the uterine endometrium sloughs and signals the onset of a new cycle. Gonadotropin secretion begins to rise between the ages of 8 and 9 years. This is followed by increasing amounts of estrogen, which are responsible for breast and genital development. At about age 13, puberty is signaled by the onset of periodic uterine bleeding.

A large proportion of women with primary amenorrhea have a 45,XO karyotype, resulting in the typical Turner syndrome. Secondary amenorrhea may result from primary defects of the gonad, primary or secondary aberrations of the hypothalamic-pituitary axis including various systemic illnesses, dysfunction of other endocrine glands, or drug-induced abnormalities. Amenorrhea may be an early sign of pituitary disease (tumor). Excess androgen production will suppress gonadotropin secretion and thereby induce amenorrhea. Amenorrhea following conception (the most common cause of secondary amenorrhea) is due to the rising titer of chorionic gonadotropin. The most common etiology of secondary amenorrhea, excluding pregnancy and menopause, is hypothalamic amenorrhea, a diagnosis of exclusion; it reflects a functional defect of the hypothalamic-pituitary axis with absent cyclic gonadotropin secretion.

ETIOLOGY

Anatomic Defects of the Outflow Tract

Congenital defect of the vagina; imperforate hymen; absence of vagina or uterus; cervical stenosis; intrauterine adhesions (Asherman's syndrome); hysterectomy; endometrial destruction (tuberculosis)

Ovarian Failure

Gonadal dysgenesis (Turner syndrome); abnormal chromosomes
Abnormal gonadal steroid synthesis: 17-alpha-hydroxylase deficiency; 17,20 desmo-
    lase deficiency
Resistant-ovary syndrome
Premature menopause
Ovarian failure after surgery, infection, irradiation; autoimmune oophoritis

Chronic Anovulation

With estrogen present
    Polycystic ovarian disease (Stein-Leventhal syndrome)
    Tumors of the ovary
    Adrenal dysfunction (production of excess androgen); thyroid disorders
With estrogen absent (hypogonadotropic hypogonadism)
    Hypothalamic lesion: craniopharyngioma; tuberculosis; sarcoidosis; Kallmann's
        syndrome
    Functional disorder of the hypothalamus or higher centers:[†] stress; weight loss;
        malnutrition; intense physical conditioning; depressive psychoses; anorexia ner-
        vosa; schizophrenia; chronic debilitating diseases, end-stage renal disease; drugs
    Pituitary disease
        Tumors: prolactinoma; chromophobe adenoma; craniopharyngioma; granu-
            lomas
        Simmonds' disease; postpartum necrosis (Sheehan's syndrome)
        Empty sella syndrome
        Panhypopituitarism

Pregnancy;[†] lactation

Menopause[†]

Iatrogenic Causes of Secondary Amenorrhea

Androgens; corticosteroids; oral contraceptives; cytotoxic drugs; ganglion-blocking
    agents; phenothiazines; tricyclic antidepressants; reserpine; spironolactone; dex-
    amphetamine; sulpiride; tranquilizers; methyldopa; drug addiction of various types

HISTORY TAKING*

	Possible meaning of a positive response
1 Duration of the Amenorrhea	
1.1 When have you ceased menstruat-ing?	Pregnancy should be excluded before initiating diagnostic studies

[†]Common cause
*In this section, items in *italics* are characteristic clinical features, and items in **boldface** are
potentially life-threatening or urgent conditions.

	• never menstruated?	Primary amenorrhea: anomalies of the genital tract; hypothalamic-pituitary disorders; ovarian insufficiency; gonadal dysgenesis, 17-alpha-hydroxylase deficiency
	• prior to age 40?	In a woman with no anatomic abnormalities of the hypothalamic-pituitary-ovarian axis and no other endocrine disturbances: hypothalamic chronic anovulation; premature ovarian failure (premature menopause): when due to ovarian antibodies, may be one component of polyglandular failure together with adrenal insufficiency, hypothyroidism, and other autoimmune disorders
1.2	How many menstrual periods have been missed?	If four to six: investigation is warranted
1.3	At what age did your first menstruation appear?	The normal menarche occurs between 12 and 13 years
1.4	What were your previous menstrual habits?	Oligomenorrhea frequently precedes amenorrhea

2 Precipitating Factors

2.1	Is there any possibility that you are pregnant?	All women with amenorrhea should be assumed to be pregnant until proved otherwise. During the reproductive years, pregnancy is the commonest cause of secondary amenorrhea
2.2	Have you recently had • an emotional stress? changes in family, school, employment, social relationships? • a severe weight loss?	A stressful event in a young woman can cause anovulation (functional disorder of the hypothalamus or higher centers) Weight loss, especially with vigorous exercise, is a common cause of amenorrhea

3 Accompanying Symptoms

3.1	Do you have • depression? anxiety?	Amenorrhea is common in depressive mental disorders
	• a loss of vision?	Visual field defects: pressure on the optic nerves due to a **pituitary tumor**
	• headaches? nausea? vomiting?	**Increased intracranial pressure:** pituitary tumor
	• cyclic, predictable episodes of abdominal pain?	May occur in amenorrhea due to anatomic defects with accumulation of menstrual blood behind the obstruction
	• episodes of irregular or profuse vaginal bleeding?	Menometrorrhagia: polycystic ovarian disease

- *a milky discharge from the nipples?* — Galactorrhea: indicates probable increased prolactin secretion in one third of women with amenorrhea; functional hyperprolactinemia without evidence of a pituitary tumor

- a heavy growth of hair on your face? arms? legs? back? — Virilism: overproduction of androgens: masculinizing tumors of the ovary; adrenal tumor; polycystic ovarian disease

- a loss of axillary and pubic hair? — Adrenal cortical failure; Sheehan's syndrome

- intolerance to heat? increased nervousness? — Hyperthyroidism

- intolerance to cold? — Hypothyroidism, primary or secondary to anterior pituitary disease

- purple striae on your skin? easy bruising? — Cushing's syndrome

- weakness? easy fatigability? — Cushing's syndrome; Addison's disease; panhypopituitarism; malignancy; chronic systemic illness; depressive state

- an impaired sense of smell? — Anosmia with primary amenorrhea: Kallmann's syndrome (rare): permanent LHRH deficiency

- a severe weight loss? — Addison's disease; hyperthyroidism; diabetes mellitus; chronic systemic illness; malignancy; in a young woman: anorexia nervosa with chronic anovulation (amenorrhea in anorexia nervosa can precede, follow, or appear coincidentally with the weight loss). Weight loss of 10–15 percent of total body weight often results in amenorrhea

- a gain in weight? — Cushing's syndrome; myxedema; acromegaly; polycystic ovarian disease

- hot flushes? profuse sweating? night sweats? — Menopause; premenopausal amenorrhea: the flush appears to coincide with a surge of LH

4 Iatrogenic Factors   See Etiology

4.1 Have you ever been treated for cancer? — Chemotherapy or radiation induce transient (months to a few years) or permanent ovarian dysfunction

4.2 Have you recently discontinued oral contraceptives? — Oral contraceptives can cause atrophy of the endometrium, leading to hypomenorrhea and amenorrhea (usually in women with prior menstrual abnormalities). Such patients should be evaluated in the same manner as any woman with amenorrhea

5   Personal and Social Profile

5.1   What is your usual diet?

May reveal nutritional deficiencies, food faddism, crash dieting (patients with anorexia nervosa often say that they are eating well). Undernutrition is a frequent cause of delayed menarche or amenorrhea in adolescents. A fat content of 17 percent of the total body weight is necessary for initiating menarche; 22 percent is the critical percentage required to maintain menstruation after the age of 16 years

5.2   What are your exercise habits? Do you practice jogging? (more than 30 miles per week)? running? dancing? ballet?

Excessive physical exercise that result in weight loss may cause loss of cyclic LH secretion and chronic anovulation (due to a decrease in the percentage of body fat and chronic stress)

6   Personal Antecedents Pertaining to the Amenorrhea

6.1   Have you ever had
- a meningitis? an encephalitis?
- a fracture (of the base) of the skull?

Disease or injury in the region of the midbrain causing disturbances in hypothalamic function

- a childbirth?

Possible ischemic necrosis of the anterior pituitary: Sheehan's syndrome

- (vigorous) curettage? endometritis?

May be followed by endometrial scarring or synechiae (Asherman's syndrome)

- radiation to your ovaries? When? Why?

Ovarian amenorrhea with underproduction of estrogen and progestogen

- your ovaries, your uterus removed? When? Why?

7   Familial Medical History Pertaining to the Amenorrhea

7.1   Did someone in your family have menstrual disorder?

Familial disorders: delayed menarche; premature menopause; polycystic ovarian disease; Kallmann's syndrome; pure gonadal dysgenesis

PHYSICAL SIGNS PERTAINING TO AMENORRHEA

Possible significance

Pelvic examination

May reveal or suggest: genital tract obstruction; pregnancy; ovarian tumor; agenesis of uterus and vagina

Absent secondary sexual characteristics | Gonadal dysgenesis (Turner syndrome); delayed puberty; hypopituitarism; psychogenic hypothalamic dysfunction; Kallmann's syndrome

Normal secondary sexual characteristics | Delayed menarche; pregnancy; hypothalamic dysfunction; stress; weight loss; pituitary tumor; ovarian tumor; polycystic ovarian disease; premature ovarian failure; müllerian dysgenesis; imperforate hymen

Female phenotype; sexual infantilism, absent secondary sexual characteristics; sparse hair growth; short stature; webbed neck; shield chest; short fourth metacarpals; coarctation of the aorta; multiple skin nevi | Gonadal dysgenesis (Turner syndrome, 45,X karyotype)

Nonpuerperal galactorrhea | Hypothalamo-pituitary dysfunction, usually with hyperprolactinemia: prolactinoma; pituitary tumor; sarcoidosis; eosinophilic granuloma; drugs (phenothiazines, methyldopa, reserpine)

Hirsutism; virilism | Virilizing ovarian tumor; adrenal tumor; polycystic ovarian disease; pure gonadal dysgenesis (46,XY karyotype)

Obesity | Polycystic ovarian disease

Signs of chronic illness | Renal or hepatic disease; hyperthyroidism; Cushing's syndrome; anemia; diabetes mellitus

Neurologic and ophthalmic abnormalities | Pituitary tumor; tumor of the third ventricle; glioma of the optic chiasma

LABORATORY TESTS PERTAINING TO AMENORRHEA[†]

Test	Finding	Diagnostic Possibilities
Pregnancy test	Serum or urine human chorionic gonadotropin elevated	Pregnancy; hydatidiform mole; chorioepithelioma

[†]See the appendix on Laboratory Reference Values for the associated normal laboratory values.

Test	Finding	Diagnostic Possibilities
Vaginal smear	Increased number of cornified cells; cervical mucus: arborization (ferning), increased elasticity	Estrogen stimulation
Serum prolactin level	Elevated	Prolactinoma; pituitary tumor (microadenoma); hypothalamic defect
Progesterone test	Positive: withdrawal bleeding	Chronic anovulation with adequate estrogen secretion and functional endometrium: polycystic ovarian disease; tumor of the ovary; hypothalamic amenorrhea
	Negative: no bleeding	Chronic anovulation with lack of estrogen production: ovarian failure; anatomic defect (müllerian agenesis); endometrial failure; hypogonadotropic hypogonadism due to organic or functional disorder of the pituitary or the CNS
Estrogen-progesterone test	Bleeding: withdrawal menses	Chronic anovulation (estrogen absent): functional hypothalamic amenorrhea; pituitary disease; ovarian failure
	No bleeding	Anatomic defect: müllerian agenesis; cervical obstruction; Asherman's syndrome
Serum gonadotropins	Elevated	Ovarian failure; gonadal dysgenesis; postmenopausal; polycystic ovarian disease (increased LH levels)
	Low or normal	Hypothalamic-pituitary disorder; anatomic defect of the outflow tract
Serum testosterone	Elevated	Androgen-producing tumor; polycystic ovarian disease
TSH level	Abnormal	Thyroid dysfunction

LABORATORY PROCEDURES PERTAINING TO AMENORRHEA

Procedure	To Detect
Endometrial biopsy	Ovarian dysfunction; endometrial responsiveness to hormonal stimulation
Chromosomal analysis	Ovarian dysgenesis
Pelvic ultrasonography	Uterine cavity; ovarian tumor; cyst; etc.
Hysterosalpingography	Uterine abnormalities (contraindicated if pregnancy or infection is suspected)
CT scan of the sella turcica; visual fields	Pituitary tumor
Culdoscopy; laparoscopy	Anatomic ovarian abnormalities

SELECTED BIBLIOGRAPHY

Kase NG: General evaluation of amenorrhea, in Kase NG, Weingold AB, Lucas WE et al (eds). *Principles and Practice of Clinical Gynecology,* pp. 271–277, New York: John Wiley & Sons, 1983.

Marut EL, Dawood Y: Amenorrhea (Excluding hyperprolactinemia). *Clin Obstet Gynecol* 26(3):749–761, 1983.

29
Impotence

INTRODUCTION

Impotence   Inability to obtain and maintain an erection that is suitable for sexual
intercourse.

The first phase of normal male sexual function, sexual desire or libido, is regulated by
psychic factors and by testicular androgens. The second phase, arousal, is primarily a
neurologic event controlled by both reflex and psychic stimuli that result in erection,
i.e., the penile engorgement with blood. The afferent sensory fibers originate in
pacinian corpuscles of the penis and pass via the pudendal nerve to the S2-S4 dorsal
root ganglia. The efferent limb begins with parasympathetic preganglionic fibers from
S2-S4 which synapse in the perivesicular, prostatic, and cavernous plexuses with
postganglionic fibers terminating on the blood vessels of the corpora cavernosa. The
central nervous system inhibits or stimulates erectile response via pathways descending in the lateral columns of the spinal cord. Erection is accomplished by increased
arterial inflow secondary to decreased arterial resistance with a subsequent decrease in
venous outflow. The vascular phenomenon results in enlargement and rigidity of the
penis.

The third phase, ejaculation, is controlled by the sympathetic nervous system and
consists of two processes. Contraction of the vas deferens, prostate, and seminal
vesicles causes seminal fluid to enter the urethra (seminal emission). Contraction of
the muscles of the pelvic floor including the bulbocavernous and ischiocavernous
muscles results in true ejaculation—expulsion of semen from the urethra. Partial
bladder neck closure mediated by the sympathetic nerves prevents retrograde ejaculation into the bladder. Orgasm, the fourth phase of normal sexual function, is a cortical
sensory phenomenon in which the rhythmic contraction of the bulbocavernous and
ischiocavernous muscles is perceived as pleasurable.

Erectile impotence may be due to organic causes (local, endocrine, neurologic,
vascular) or to psychological factors, such as anxiety or depression. Psychogenic
impotence should be a diagnosis of exclusion.

ETIOLOGY

Organic Causes of Impotence

Endocrine: primary testicular disorder; hypothalamic-pituitary disease; hyperprolac-
    tinemia; thyroid dysfunction
Vascular: large vessel atherosclerosis; arteritis
Neurological: temporal lobe lesions; spinal cord damage; multiple sclerosis; auto-
    nomic neuropathy; peripheral neuropathy: diabetic, tabes dorsalis; perineal prosta-
    tectomy; vascular surgery; sympathectomy; abdominoperineal resection
Systemic diseases: cirrhosis of liver; renal failure; congestive heart failure; angina
    pectoris; chronic debilitating diseases
Penile diseases: phimosis; Peyronie's disease; penile trauma; previous priapism

Psychogenic

Depression; anxiety; obsessional and affective disorders

Iatrogenic Causes of Impotence

Antihypertensive drugs (thiazides, guanadrel, clonidine, reserpine, methyldopa, propranolol); anticholinergics; antihistamines; cimetidine; ranitidine; antipsychotic drugs; tricyclic antidepressants; monoamine oxidase inhibitors; sedatives; levodopa; clofibrate; baclofen; amphetamines; aminocaproic acid; estrogens; antiandrogens; luteinizing-hormone-releasing hormone agonists; anticancer drugs

HISTORY TAKING*

	Possible meaning of a positive response
1 Character of the Impotence	
1.1 Are you unable to achieve and maintain an erection sufficient for penetration?	Impotence: impaired arousal phase of the sexual function
1.2 *Are you unable to adequately sustain and maintain an erection of any sort at any time?*	Organic impotence; incomplete suprasacral cord lesion; cerebral lesion; pudendal neuropathy
1.3 During coital activity • do you lose the erection?	Vascular impotence (pelvic steal syndrome): a partial blockage of the penile artery allows normal blood flow to the penis, except when exercise (intercourse) increases blood flow to the buttocks
• does the erection increase in rigidity?	Insufficient stimulation during foreplay prior to coitus
1.4 *Do you have nocturnal or morning erection?*	Generally present in psychogenic impotence; usually absent or reduced in frequency and intensity in organic impotence
1.5 Are you able to respond with an erection to erotic stimuli or fantasies? masturbation? an alternative partner?	Psychogenic impotence (patients with organic impotence are unable to obtain erection with these stimuli)

*In this section, items in *italics* are characteristic clinical features.

2   Mode of Onset and Evolution

2.1   How long have you had problems
      with impotence?
      • lifelong?   Primary impotence: the patient has
                                           never been able to achieve potency. Un-
                                           derlying organic etiology (in the pres-
                                           ence of abnormal nocturnal penile
                                           tumescence)
      • appearing at age 40 or less?   Psychological impotence
      • occurring in the sixth or seventh Vasculogenic impotence
        decade?

2.2   Has the decline in erectile function
      been
      • abrupt? sudden? (over several   Psychogenic impotence; situational
        days to weeks)   psychological etiology
      • insidious? gradual? (over months   Organic (usually vascular) impotence
        to years) with an initial decrease
        in erectile hardness followed by a
        decline in the frequency of erec-
        tions?

2.3   Is your impotence
      • constant? persistent? with pro-   Organic impotence
        gressive deterioration?
      • *selective? intermittent?* transient?
        with normal rigid erection in
        some circumstances but not in
        others?
                                           Episodic nature of psychogenic im-
                                           potence
2.3a Are you able to achieve erection
      with some but not all sexual part-
      ners?

2.4   How often do you have intercourse   Establishes a baseline coital frequency;
      at present and prior to onset of the helps the physician understand the
      problem?   patient's interpretation of his erectile
                                           problem

3   Precipitating or Aggravating Factors

3.1   Has there been any recent change   Psychogenic impotence temporally re-
      in your life? any stress? marital   lated to specific stress. Psychological
      difficulties? extramarital affairs? stress may occur secondarily or reac-
      loss of job? bereavement?   tively in patients with organic dysfunc-
                                           tion

4 Accompanying Symptoms

4.1 Have you lost any interest in sex?

Explores the desire phase of the sexual response. Loss of libido is usually situational and acquired: marital conflicts and disappointments, depression. Also in androgen deficiency; pituitary or testicular disease; hypogonadism; hyperprolactinemia; as a consequence of chronic illness. Patients with psychological impotence often have both libido and ejaculatory complaints. Sex drive is preserved in neurogenic or vascular impotence

4.2 Do you think you ejaculate
• normally when having sex?
• normally when masturbating?
• sometimes when asleep during dreams?

Orgasmic phase of the normal sexual response. Ejaculation is either unaffected or slightly premature in organic impotence

4.3 During ejaculation do you feel that
• ejaculation occurs too quickly? before there has been any penetration of the penis? very soon after penetration?

• there is no ejaculation?

Premature ejaculation: in psychogenic impotence. Usually the result of anxiety about sexual performance or the consequence of some other emotional state. Rarely organic in nature
Retrograde ejaculation: may occur following surgery on the bladder neck, sympathectomy (sympathetic denervation with absence of smooth muscle contraction at the time of emission and ejaculation); drugs; androgen deficiency. May occur spontaneously in diabetic men. In psychogenic ejaculatory failure the capacity to ejaculate is retained with masturbation. The inability to ejaculate intravaginally from organic cause is manifested uniformly despite the circumstances

4.4 Do you experience orgasm?

Failure to reach orgasm is almost always due to a psychologic disorder if libido and erectile function are normal

4.5 Do you have persistent painful erection unrelated to sexual activity?

Priapism: due to clotting within the penile vascular network; can be idiopathic or associated with sickle cell anemia, chronic granulocytic leukemia, spinal cord injury

4.6 Do you have any pain or curvature of the penis? (firm erection but the penis is bent when erect, making sexual intercourse impossible)

Peyronie's disease: fibrosed bands in the penis

4.7 Do you have
• pain in the calves when walking?

Intermittent claudication. With impotence: Leriche syndrome: atherosclerotic occlusion of the distal aorta and common iliac arteries: vascular impotence

• a decreased sensation in the penis? external genitalia?
  • in upper and lower extremity?
• decreased beard growth? increased size of breasts? visual disturbance?

Neuropathy: diabetes, alcoholism, uremic pudendal neuropathy
Multiple sclerosis; spinal cord trauma
Endocrine impotence: pituitary prolactin-secreting adenoma

• back pain? bowel or urinary dysfunction?
• an increased urinary volume? an increased intake of fluids?

Sacral cord disorder or cauda equina syndrome
Polyuria, polydipsia in diabetes mellitus

• excessive sweating? intolerance to heat? hand tremor?

Hyperthyroidism

• intolerance to cold? constipation?

Hypothyroidism

• feelings of anxiety? anger? depression? guilt? impaired worth?

Impotent men commonly have at least some psychological problems because self-esteem and ego are often closely allied to adequate sexual performance. Changes in mood and affect may be primary causes of impotence or secondary to an organic disorder

5   Iatrogenic Factors   See Etiology

6   Personal and Social Profile

6.1 What is your marital status? your sexual preference?

Conjugal difficulties or concealed homosexuality may cause psychogenic impotence

6.2 Do you smoke?

Tobacco has been linked to sexual dysfunction. Nicotine is a vasoconstrictor and is believed to interfere with penile blood flow

6.3 What is your alcohol consumption?

80 percent of chronic alcoholics may experience erectile failure, reduced libido, premature ejaculation. In chronic alcoholism: decreased testosterone level and frequently elevated prolactin levels

| 6.4 | Do you use (illicit) drugs? | Marijuana, methadone, heroin can diminish desire, impair erection, and delay or inhibit ejaculation |

6.5 Do you think that your problem is
• organic? — Psychogenic impotence
• psychological? — Organic impotence

7 Personal Antecedents Pertaining to the Impotence

7.1 Have you ever been investigated for impotence? When? With what results?

7.2 Have you ever had
• any neurologic injuries? back operations? a stroke?
• a blunt pelvic trauma? pelvic radiation therapy?
• prior episodes of priapism? other penile deformities? — Penile diseases causing organic impotence

7.3 Do you have
• diabetes? — Sexual dysfunction in diabetes mellitus includes retrograde ejaculation (damage to the pelvic parasympathetic nerves with relaxation of the internal vesical sphincter during orgasm) or impotence due to neuropathy or vascular disease. Impotence ultimately occurs in approximately half of diabetic men

• a neurologic disease? a thyroid disease?

PHYSICAL SIGNS PERTAINING TO IMPOTENCE

Possible significance

Examination of the pelvis and testes (size; abnormal masses) — Length of testes less than 3.5 cm: possible hypogonadism

Palpation of all pulses, including the penile pulse

Gynecomastia — Estrogen excess (testicular tumor); testosterone lack

Neurological evaluation

Anal sphincter tone; perineal sensation

Bulbocavernous reflex: the anal sphincter contracts around the examining finger upon squeezing the glans penis — A positive response indicates that sacral cord segments 2, 3, and 4 are intact

Distal muscle strength, tendon reflexes in the legs, tests for vibratory, position, tactile, pain sensation — Impaired in peripheral neuropathy

LABORATORY PROCEDURES PERTAINING TO IMPOTENCE[†]

Procedure	To Detect
Serum glucose level; thyroid function tests	
Serum testosterone; serum gonadotropins;* serum prolactin*	Hypogonadism with androgen deficiency causes impotence in 15 to 20 percent of men complaining of sexual dysfunction
Nocturnal penile tumescence (NPT) monitoring	Nocturnal erections occur during rapid eye movement sleep; average total time of NPT: 100 min per night. Normal number and duration of erectile episodes in psychogenic impotence. Erectile episodes are absent or decreased in number and duration in organic impotence
Penile brachial pressure index* (penile systolic pressure/brachial systolic pressure)	Low (< 0.6) in penile vascular disease; pelvic steal syndrome
Bulbocavernous reflex latency* (following electrical stimulation of the glans)	Normal: 13.5–35 msec: psychogenic impotence Prolonged (more than 40 msec): organic impotence

[†]See the appendix on Laboratory Reference Values for the associated normal laboratory values.
*When indicated

SELECTED BIBLIOGRAPHY

Krane RJ, Goldstein I, Saenz de Tejada I: Impotence. *N Engl J Med* 321:1648–1659, 1989.
Meyer JJ: Impotence. *Postgrad Med* 84(2):87–95, 1988.
Morley JE: Impotence in older men. *Hosp Pract* 23(4):139–158, 1988.
Sacks SA: Evaluation of impotence. *Postgrad Med* 74(4):182–197, 1983.

Neuromuscular System

30
Coma

INTRODUCTION

Coma   A state of total unresponsiveness to all external stimuli.

A normal level of consciousness (wakefulness) depends upon activation of the cerebral hemispheres by the reticular activating system (RAS), a diffuse system of upper brainstem and thalamic neurons. Both of the cerebral hemispheres, the RAS, and the connections between them must be preserved for normal consciousness. Coma may be produced by depression of either hemispheral or RAS activity.

Supratentorial mass lesions (tumor, abscess, hemorrhage) impair consciousness by compressing the diencephalic ascending reticular activating system.

Coma may result from infratentorial mass or destructive lesions, directly compressing or destroying the brainstem reticular formation structures (brainstem infarction, cerebellar hemorrhage). Toxic metabolic encephalopathy (anoxia, hypoglycemia, drug overdose) interfering with metabolism of both brainstem and cerebral cortical structures also produces coma. In psychogenic "coma" the patient is physiologically awake but appears comatose by not responding to his environment.

ETIOLOGY

Supratentorial Mass Lesions*

Intracranial hemorrhage: intracerebral, epidural, subdural
Tumor; abscess; infarction with surrounding edema

Infratentorial Structural Lesions*

Hemorrhage: pontine, cerebellar
Infarction: brainstem; cerebellar
Tumor; cerebellar abscess

*Common cause

Metabolic and Diffuse Lesions

Drugs;* alcohol; toxins

Endogenous metabolic disturbances: hypoglycemia;* hypoxia;* ischemia;* primary organ failure* (lung, kidney, liver); thyroid, adrenal, pituitary dysfunction; cardiovascular disturbances; acid-base, electrolyte disorders: hyponatremia, hypercalcemia, hypocalcemia, disturbances of osmolarity; systemic infection; hypothermia; heat stroke

Concussion-contusion; postictal states

Meningitis; encephalitis

Subarachnoid hemorrhage

Psychogenic

Catatonic states; hysteria; malingering

Iatrogenic Causes of Coma

Tricyclic antidepressants, sedatives, and tranquilizers; lithium; anticonvulsants; amphetamines; anticholinergic drugs; insulin; oral hypoglycemic agents; salicylates; cimetidine; vitamin D (hypercalcemia)

Stopping:
  corticosteroids: Addisonian coma
  insulin: diabetic acidosis
  thyroid hormone: myxedema coma
  alcohol, narcotics, sedatives, barbiturates: withdrawal syndrome

HISTORY TAKING*

	Possible meaning of a positive response
1 Mode of Onset, Duration, and Temporal Profile	
1.1 When was the patient found unconscious?	
1.2 Where was the patient found?	
• in a bar?	Acute alcoholism; head trauma
• in a locked room?	Exposure to toxic chemical agents: carbon monoxide
• in a locked garage? with automobile running?	Carbon monoxide poisoning
• at work?	Exposure to industrial toxic fumes

*In this section, items in *italics* are characteristic clinical features.

Note: Since the patient is inaccessible to questioning, contact should be made at once with whoever came with the patient, or with relatives and friends at home or elsewhere. Past physicians, pharmacists, employers should be contacted for questioning. Past medical records should be obtained. Patient should be interrogated during lucid intervals, if any.

1.2a If the patient was found in a room, were other persons found unconscious?

Carbon monoxide poisoning; common exposure to a toxic agent; narcotic abuse

1.3 Was the onset of the coma
• *sudden?*

Catastrophic brain lesion: cerebrovascular accident; subarachnoid hemorrhage; trauma; hypoxia; drug ingestion. In hemispheral lesions, the degree of decrease in alertness is often related to the acuteness of onset of the cortical dysfunction. Infarction in the territory of the middle cerebral artery, the commonest stroke, does not cause coma acutely

• acute but not instantaneous?

Basal ganglia and thalamic hemorrhage; drug ingestion

• gradual? subacute?

Preceding medical or neurologic problem: metabolic cause (e.g., renal insufficiency, ketoacidosis); subdural hemorrhage; drug intoxication; systemic infection. Most coma is metabolic or toxic in origin

1.4 Has the patient's unconsciousness fluctuated?

Chronic subdural hemorrhage

1.5 Has the patient had repeated episodes of unconsciousness?

Syncopal attacks; epilepsy; cerebrovascular accidents

2 Precipitating or Aggravating Factors

2.1 Is there any suggestion of
• head trauma? exposure to violence? riot?

Subdural or epidural hematoma (a negative history does not exclude the diagnosis of subdural hematoma); depressed skull fracture; concussion. Trauma may precipitate, or be secondary to, coma from other causes: Addisonian crisis, myxedema coma, stroke

2.2 Were any of the following items found in the vicinity of the patient or in a wallet or purse?
• physician appointment card? medications?

Depression: chronic or acute intoxication; suicide attempt; diabetes, kidney or liver disease

• syringes?

Narcotic abuse; insulin

• alcohol?

Alcoholic stupor

• household products?

Pesticide taken in error or for suicide attempt

3   Accompanying Symptoms

3.1   Has the patient recently had
 • severe headache?
   • for days or weeks before the onset of coma? — Increased intracranial pressure; meningitis; chronic subdural hematoma
   • *just before losing consciousness?* — (Without cranial trauma): subarachnoid hemorrhage; basal ganglia and thalamic hemorrhage; cerebellar hemorrhage
 • *(recurrent) vomiting?* — At the onset of coma: sudden increase in intracranial pressure: subarachnoid or intracerebral hemorrhage: basal ganglia and thalamic hemorrhage, cerebellar hemorrhage; basilar artery thrombosis
 • muscle weakness? speech difficulties? diplopia? dizziness? — Intracranial mass-expanding lesion; basilar artery thrombosis
 • fever? — Acute systemic infection; pneumonia; intracranial infection, bacterial meningitis; brain lesion disturbing the temperature-regulating centers
 • a change in mental status? behavior? — Evolving intracranial process; in the elderly, may be the presenting manifestation of gram-negative septicemia, pneumonia, other localized bacterial infections
   • just before losing consciousness? — Hypoglycemia

3.2   Has the patient had a convulsion? — Epilepsy; hypoglycemia; Stokes-Adams syndrome; sedative drug withdrawal; hyponatremia; hypocalcemia. Rare in cerebral infarction

3.3   Has any witness noticed
 • loss of urine? feces? — Convulsive seizure
 • blood froth around the mouth? bleeding from the ear or nose? — (Blood may have been swept away): epilepsy; trauma (may be secondary to a fall caused by a stroke)

4   Iatrogenic Factors   See Etiology

5   Personal and Social Profile

5.1   What is the patient's occupation? — Professional exposure to toxic products

5.2   Does the patient have a history of alcohol abuse? drug abuse?

6   Personal Antecedents Pertaining to the Coma

6.1   Does the patient have
  • any chronic disease? a hepatic
    condition? a heart disease? arte-
    rial hypertension? a chronic pul-
    monary disease? a neurologic
    disease? a bleeding tendency?
  • diabetes?

Coma in a diabetic patient: hypoglycemia; diabetic ketoacidosis; nonketotic
hyperosmolar coma; lactic acidosis

  • a renal disease?

Coma in a uremic patient: subdural
hematoma; seizures; Wernicke's encephalopathy; disequilibrium syndrome
(after rapid dialysis)

  • alcoholism?

Coma in an alcoholic patient: alcoholic
intoxication; subdural hematoma; hypoglycemia; delirium tremens; Wernicke's encephalopathy; ingestion of
toxic alcohol substitutes; drug intoxication; overwhelming infection

  • depression?   emotional   pro-
    blems? past attempted suicide?
    past psychiatric hospitalization?

Most cases of "coma of unknown
cause" are due to self-induced drug intoxication

  • convulsive disorders?

Coma in an epileptic patient: postictal
state; serious head injury with subdural
or epidural hematoma; overdose of
sedatives

PHYSICAL SIGNS PERTAINING TO COMA*

Possible significance

Vital signs: temperature, blood pressure,
pulse, respiratory pattern

Fever

Severe systemic infection; pneumonia,
bacterial meningitis; brain lesion disturbing   the   temperature-regulating
centers; heat stroke (42 to 44°C) with
dry skin

Hypothermia (30 to 36°C)

Bodily exposure to cold; drug poisoning
(alcohol, barbiturates, phenothiazines);
peripheral circulatory failure; extracellular fluid deficit; myxedema; hypoglycemia; severe lower brainstem injury

*In this section, items in *italics* are characteristic clinical features.

Hypotension	Low peripheral resistance: depressant drug poisoning, alcohol or barbiturate intoxication; internal hemorrhage; myocardial infarction; gram-negative bacillary septicemia; Addisonian crisis
Hypertension	Drug effect (amphetamines); cerebral hemorrhage; hypertensive encephalopathy; in a previously normotensive patient: may be a sign of subarachnoid hemorrhage (increased intracranial pressure)
Bradycardia	Heart block and Stokes-Adams syndrome; with hyperventilation and hypertension: increase in intracranial pressure
Tachycardia (> 160 beats per minute)	Ectopic arrhythmia with lowered cardiac output and impaired cerebral circulation
Respiratory patterns	Inconsistent localizing value of intracranial lesion
• shallow, slow, well-timed regular breathing	Metabolic or drug depression
• rapid, deep breathing	Kussmaul breathing: metabolic acidosis; pontomesencephalic lesion
• periodic (Cheyne-Stokes) respiration	Mild bihemispheral damage; metabolic suppression (commonly in light coma)
Hypertension, bradycardia, periodic breathing	Increased intracranial pressure
Skin	
• Ecchymosis behind the ear (Battle's sign); about the orbit (raccoon eyes)	Basal skull fracture
• cyanosis of lips and nail beds	Hypoxemia; methemoglobinemia
• cherry-red coloration	Carbon monoxide poisoning
• petechiae	Bleeding diathesis, thrombocytopenia causing intracranial hemorrhage; thrombotic thrombocytopenic purpura; meningococcemia; bacterial endocarditis; rickettsia
• track marks, other skin stigmata	Parenteral drug abuse
Breath odor	Alcohol intoxication; ketoacidosis; hepatic or renal failure

Stiff neck	Meningeal irritation: bacterial meningitis, subarachnoid hemorrhage; cerebellar tonsillar herniation
Multifocal myoclonus	Metabolic encephalopathy: drug ingestion
Symmetric or nonfocal neurologic signs	Metabolic origin
Focal or lateralizing neurologic abnormalities	Structural cause; supratentorial lesion causing upper brainstem dysfunction; subtentorial lesion destroying or compressing the reticular formation

Oculocephalic reflex (doll's head maneuver)

• intact: the patient's eyes deviate from the direction in which the head is rotated	Metabolic or bilateral hemispheric dysfunction
• decreased to absent	Brainstem damage

Pupillary light reactions

• absent	Structural brain lesion
• equal and reactive round pupils (2.5 to 5 mm in diameter)	Usually exclude midbrain damage as the cause of coma; metabolic coma; drug intoxication (exceptions: glutethimide and atropine intoxication; severe anoxia or asphyxia)
• unilaterally dilated and fixed pupil	Uncal herniation with pressure on the 3rd cranial nerve due to hemispheric (ipsilateral) mass effect
• bilaterally dilated and unreactive (fixed) pupils	Severe midbrain damage from secondary compression by transtentorial herniation or metabolic encephalopathy (anticholinergic drugs)
• reactive and bilaterally small pupils (1 to 2.5 mm)	Metabolic encephalopathy; profound barbiturate-induced coma; after deep bilateral hemispheral lesion
• pinpoint (less than 1 mm) and reactive pupils	Narcotic overdose; acute extensive bilateral pontine damage

Funduscopic examination

	May reveal lesions of diabetic retinopathy, bacterial endocarditis
• papilledema	Increased intracranial pressure; brain tumor, abscess, hemorrhage, or trauma
• exudates, hemorrhages, vessel-crossing changes	Hypertensive encephalopathy
• subhyaloid hemorrhages	Subarachnoid hemorrhage

LABORATORY TESTS PERTAINING TO COMA[†]

Test	Finding	Diagnostic Possibilities
Blood		
RBCs	Anemia	Acute blood loss
WBCs	Leukocytosis	Bacterial infection; cerebral hemorrhage
Glucose	Low	Hypoglycemia
	Elevated	Diabetic acidosis; diabetic hyperosmolar coma; massive cerebral lesion
BUN, creatinine	Elevated	Uremic coma
Electrolytes	Metabolic acidosis, anion gap	Diabetic ketoacidosis; uremic acidosis; intoxication (salicylates, methanol, ethylene glycol); lactic acidosis
Calcium	Abnormal	Hypercalcemic coma; hypocalcemia
Liver function tests, serum ammonia	Abnormal	Hepatic encephalopathy
PO_2, PCO_2, pH	Abnormal	Hypoxia; hypercapnia; acidosis; alkalosis
Thyroid function tests	Abnormal	Myxedema coma; thyroid storm
Blood culture	Positive	Septicemia
Toxicologic screen	Positive	Acute intoxication (other factors, particularly head trauma, may contribute to the clinical state)

[†]See the appendix on Laboratory Reference Values for the associated normal laboratory values.

LABORATORY PROCEDURES PERTAINING TO COMA

Procedure	To Detect
Computerized tomography (CT) scan	Tumor; hemorrhage, intracerebral, subarachnoid; hydrocephalus. A normal CT scan does not exclude anatomic lesions as the cause of coma

Procedure	To Detect
EEG	Diffuse metabolic encephalopathy; postictal state; focal or epileptic disturbance
Lumbar puncture (to be avoided in any patient suspected of having an intracranial mass lesion)	In suspected cases of meningitis; encephalitis; occasional cases of subarachnoid hemorrhage; in cases with obscure origin of coma and normal CT
• bloody	Subarachnoid hemorrhage; brain hemorrhage; cerebral contusion
• pleiocytosis, elevated protein, low glucose	Bacterial meningitis (tuberculous meningitis: lymphocytosis in CSF)

SELECTED BIBLIOGRAPHY

Bleck TP, Klawans HL: Neurologic emergencies. *Med Clin North Am* 70:1167–1184, 1986.
Plum F, Posner JB: *The diagnosis of stupor and coma*, 3rd ed., Philadelphia: Davis, 1980.

31
Confusional State

INTRODUCTION

Confusional state A state characterized by abnormal orientation, attention, arousal, thought, and memory.

Delirium A state of gross disorientation in the presence of heightened alertness and psychomotor overactivity.

Dementia Deterioration of all intellectual or cognitive functions without disturbances of consciousness, awareness, or perception.

Confusion alone generally indicates a metabolic derangement. Direct interference with the metabolic activities of the nerve cells in the cerebral cortex and central thalamic nuclei of the brain appears responsible. Sedatives (barbiturates, phenothiazines) impair consciousness by their direct suppressive effect on the neurons of the cerebrum and diencephalon.

The most common cause of delirium is the withdrawal of alcohol, barbiturates, or other sedative drugs following a period of chronic intoxication. These drugs have a depressant effect on the high brainstem reticular activating system. Withdrawal of these drugs is followed by the release and overactivity of this area, which are the basis of delirium. The delirious state observed in bacterial infections and drug intoxication probably results from the direct action of the toxin or chemical agent on the same areas of the brain. The function of these neuronal formations may be disturbed by destructive neurologic diseases, with resulting delirium.

Dementia is usually associated with structural diseases of the cerebrum and the diencephalon.

ETIOLOGY

Acute Confusional States Associated with Delirium

Neurologic diseases: vascular or neoplastic; cerebral contusion; bacterial meningitis; tuberculous meningitis; encephalitis; subarachnoid hemorrhage; postconvulsive delirium

Infections: septicemia; pneumonia; rheumatic fever; malaria; typhoid fever

Endocrine condition: thyrotoxicosis; ACTH intoxication

Postoperative and posttraumatic states; after cardiac surgery

Abstinence states:* withdrawal of alcohol, sedatives following chronic intoxication

Drug-induced states:* drugs of abuse (hallucinogens, cocaine, amphetamines)

Acute Confusional States Associated with Reduced Mental Alertness and Responsiveness

Neurologic disease: cerebral vascular disease; tumor; abscess; subdural hematoma; meningitis; encephalitis

Metabolic disturbances: hepatic stupor; uremia; hypoglycemia; hypoxia;

hypercapnia; porphyria; electrolyte imbalance; congestive heart failure with hypoxia; obesity-hypoventilation syndrome
Infections: typhoid fever
Postoperative, posttraumatic, and puerperal psychoses

Dementia

Diffuse degenerative diseases: Alzheimer's disease;* Pick's disease; Creutzfeldt-Jakob disease; Huntington's disease; Parkinson's disease; leukodystrophies; Wilson's disease
Vascular: multi-infarct dementia*
Intrarenal neoplasm: primary; metastatic
Trauma: brain trauma; chronic subdural hematoma; posttraumatic state
Normal pressure hydrocephalus
Chronic CNS infections: cryptococcosis, toxoplasmosis, AIDS-associated dementia; neurosyphilis; brain abscess
Metabolic and endocrine disorders: hypothyroidism; hypoparathyroidism; Cushing's disease; hypoglycemia; uremia; hepatic failure; pulmonary failure; cerebral hypoxia; Wernicke-Korsakoff syndrome; pellagra; vitamin B_{12} deficiency; folic acid deficiency; lipid storage diseases
Collagen-vascular diseases; SLE
Intoxications: alcohol dementia;* heavy metals (lead, mercury, manganese); chronic drug toxicity*

Iatrogenic Causes of Confusional or Delirious States

Anticholinergics; barbiturates; bromides; digitalis; salicylates; lithium; cimetidine; levodopa; anti-parkinsonian drugs; beta-adrenergic blocking agents; bromocriptine; clonidine; methyldopa; metrizamide; aminophylline; sedatives and hypnotics; phenothiazines; antidepressants; corticosteroids; isoniazid; amantadine; penicillins

HISTORY TAKING†

Possible meaning of a positive response

1   Mode of Onset and Evolution

1.1   Where has the patient been found?
       From where has he been brought?
       • his home? the street?
       • a locked room?   Exposure to toxic chemical agents; carbon monoxide poisoning
       • a bar?   Acute alcoholism

*Common cause
†In this section, items in *italics* are characteristic clinical features.
Note: The history should always be supplemented by information obtained from a person other than the patient.

1.2 Were any of the following items found in the vicinity of the patient:
- medications? prescriptions?   Chronic or acute intoxication
- syringes?   Suggest use of medications or illicit drugs

1.3 How long has the patient been confused?   If recent onset of disordered state of consciousness: metabolic encephalopathy (interference with brain metabolism by extracerebral disease). If the onset of delirium occurs 48 to 72 h after hospital admission: withdrawal from drug dependency or addiction

1.4 Have similar episodes previously occurred?   Hypoglycemia; porphyria

1.5 Has the onset of confusion been
- acute? (hours to days)   Toxic state; acute brain injury; delirium
- subacute? (weeks)   Extracerebral disease with toxic or metabolic encephalopathy; confusional psychosis or delirium (onset can be acute)

- gradual? insidious? (months to years)   Dementia, degenerative or symptomatic; chronic use of sedatives

1.5a In case of gradual onset, has the mental impairment
- *fluctuated?*   Metabolic encephalopathy; chronic subdural hematoma; chronic sedative intoxication

- progressively worsened?   Alzheimer's disease

1.6 In the elderly patient: *Has the mental deterioration been "stepwise"?*   Episodes of strokelike events suggest arteriosclerosis with multi-infarct dementia

2 Character of the Mental Impairment

2.1 What is the patient's mental status?   See Chapter 35 "Mental Status Examination"

2.2 Does the patient have
- lack of initiative? irritability? loss of interest? forgetfulness? inability to perform up to the usual standards?   Earliest signs of dementia

- inability to think with customary clarity? defective memory, especially for recent events? apathy? excessive lability of mood?   More advanced stage of dementia

- impaired judgment? lapses in social conduct? speech and language disturbances? paranoid ideas? delusions?

Loss of almost all intellectual faculties in dementia. The demented patient has little or no realization of these changes in behavior and lacks insight into their meaning

2.3 Does the patient have reduced responsiveness? slow, undecisive reactions? difficulty in sustaining a conversation? apathy? disorientation?

Confusional state with psychomotor underactivity

2.4 Does the patient repeat the same questions? make the same remarks over and over again?

In acute confusional state with reduced alertness and decreased psychomotor activity

2.5 Does the patient answer with a single word or a short phrase? no longer notice or respond to much of what is occurring?

More advanced stage of confusion: failure to recognize the surroundings and loss of all sense of time

2.6 Is the patient irritable? restless?

Delirium or confusional state

2.7 Does the patient manifest excessive activity? tremulousness? insomnia? poor appetite? terrifying dreams?

Approaching attack of delirium

2.8 Does the patient talk incessantly? incoherently? look distressed? perplexed?

Delirium

2.8a Is the patient inattentive? unable to think coherently? incapable of self-orientation?

"Clouded" sensorium in delirium

2.9 Does the patient
- misinterpret the meaning of ordinary objects? ambient sounds?
- have hallucinations?

In delirium: visual, auditory, tactile hallucinations, often of a most unpleasant type; metabolic encephalopathy (in schizophrenia: usually auditory hallucinations only)

2.10 In an elderly patient: Does the patient have
- loss of memory for recent events? depression? anxiety? an inappropriate behavior?

Dementia; Alzheimer's disease

- urine, fecal incontinence? reduced responsivity? mutism?

Late stage of dementia

3   Precipitating or Aggravating Factors

3.1   Has the patient recently had

• a trauma, an operation? cardiac surgery?

Postoperative or posttraumatic confusional state; an operation or any hospitalization may induce a withdrawal syndrome in a chronic abuser of alcohol or sedatives

• a head trauma?

Subdural hematoma (a negative history does not exclude the diagnosis); posttraumatic confusional state

• an emotional, personal problem? a change of environment?

In the elderly patient: may be causal factors of altered mental status

• pneumonia? other infections? cardiac arrhythmias? anemia? fever?

Increase clinical expression of dementia dysfunctions

• (female): a pregnancy?

Puerperal psychosis

3.2   *Has the patient abruptly stopped*

• *a chronic alcohol habit?*

Withdrawal syndrome; alcoholic hallucinosis appears within 24 to 36 h, delirium tremens within 72 h of withdrawal

• *a chronic benzodiazepine, other sedatives habit?*

Adrenergic hyperarousal state with tremor, tachycardia, delirium. Withdrawal syndrome appears between second and fourth days of abstinence

4   Accompanying Symptoms

4.1   Does the patient have

• fever? chills?

Acute infectious disease (intra- or extracranial)

• headache?

Intracranial evolving process

• abdominal pain?

Acute intermittent porphyria

• a seizure?

Postconvulsive delirium; hypoglycemia; Stokes-Adams episode with cerebral hypoxia

• involuntary abnormal (choreoathetotic) movements? odd postures?

In a young or middle-aged adult with progressive dementia: Huntington's disease

• arthralgias?

Systemic lupus erythematosus

5   Iatrogenic Factors   See Etiology

6   Personal and Social Profile

6.1   Age of the patient?

Huntington's disease appears between 35 and 50 years. All mental illnesses beginning in middle or late adult life are due either to structural disease of the brain or to a depressive psychosis

6.2	What is the patient's occupation?	Acute psychosis or behavioral changes due to lead (organic), mercury, carbon disulfide, manganese, solvents in: handling gasoline, seed handling, fungicide, wood preserving, viscose rayon industry, battery makers, smelting, degreasing, dental amalgam workers, manufacturing/repair of scientific instruments
6.3	What is the patient's intake of	
	• alcohol?	Intoxication due to acute alcoholism, particularly in the elderly; chronic alcoholism: Wernicke-Korsakoff syndrome
	• drugs?	Consumption of opiates, sedatives, hallucinogens, or other recreational drugs should be considered in confused patients: chronic drug intoxication; delirium due to psychoactive drugs [phencyclidine ("Angel dust", PCP), MDMA ("ecstasy"), cocaine, "crack"]
6.4	What is the patient's sexual orientation?	Mental impairment in a homosexual man: CNS toxoplasmosis, cryptococcal meningitis, progressive multifocal leukoencephalitis, CNS lymphoma; AIDS-associated dementia

7 Personal Antecedents Pertaining to the Confusional State

7.1	Has the patient ever had an x-ray of the skull? an EEG? a CT scan? a lumbar puncture? When? With what results?	Commonest reversible causes of dementia: drugs, depression, metabolic
7.2	Did the patient have an abnormal mental status prior to the present episode?	Preexisting dementing brain disease, possibly complicated by a medical disease
7.3	Does the patient have	
	• depression?	The distinction between depression and dementia with mental deterioration may be difficult
	• a previous psychiatric hospitalization? previous suicide attempts?	Preexisting dementia; depression
	• a cardiac disease? chronic bronchitis? emphysema?	Cerebral hypoxia

- a liver disease?   Hepatic encephalopathy
- a renal disease?   Confusional state of uremia
- a thyroid, an adrenal condition? Medication may have become irregular
                                     or abandoned
- hypertension?   In the elderly patient: antihypertensive
                                     drugs may cause mental impairment by
                                     reducing the blood pressure below an
                                     optimal level
- Parkinson's disease?   Anticholinergic drugs may cause con-
                                     fusional states

8 Family History Pertaining to the Confusional State

8.1 Are there similar cases in the pa-   Huntington's disease; lipid storage dis-
     tient's family?   eases of the nervous system; Pick's dis-
                                            ease; Alzheimer's disease

PHYSICAL SIGNS PERTAINING TO THE CONFUSIONAL STATE

Possible significance

Flushed countenance; rapid pulse; raised temperature; sweating — Delirium: signs of overactivity of the autonomic nervous system distinguish delirium from all other confusional states

Fever
- with profuse perspiration — Most delirium states; delirium tremens; salicylate intoxication; acute infectious disease; gram-negative sepsis
- without perspiration — Anticholinergic drug ingestion

Hypothermia — Myxedema; hypoglycemia; barbiturate intoxication

Hyperventilating delirious patient — Diabetic ketosis; uremia; lactic acidosis; methyl alcohol poisoning; pulmonary or cardiac disease; hepatic encephalopathy

Hypoventilating patient — Chronic pulmonary disease with CO_2 retention; depressant drug poisoning

Hypoventilation; obesity — Obesity-hypoventilation syndrome

Fluctuations of mental status — Metabolic encephalopathy (also in chronic subdural hematoma)

Flapping tremor — Asterixis: in hepatic encephalopathy; uremia; ventilatory failure

Myoclonus — Metabolic brain disease; drug ingestion; Creutzfeldt-Jakob disease

Asterixis	Metabolic encephalopathy; drugs
Increased psychomotor activity	Delirium tremens; drug withdrawal states
Focal neurologic abnormalities	Multi-infarct dementia; cerebrovascular disease; brain tumor
Jaundice; asterixis; fetor hepaticus	Hepatic encephalopathy
Sixth nerve palsy; nystagmus (horizontal and vertical); paralysis of conjugate gaze; ataxia of stance and gait; polyneuropathy; retrograde and anterograde amnesia; confabulation	Wernicke-Korsakoff syndrome
Choreoathetotic movements	Huntington's disease
Funduscopic examination: papilledema	Increased intracranial pressure: brain tumor, chronic subdural hematoma; hypercarbic encephalopathy

LABORATORY TESTS PERTAINING TO THE CONFUSIONAL STATE[†]

Most useful diagnostic studies: CBC, blood glucose, blood PO_2, PCO_2, pH, ammonia, electrolytes, BUN, liver function tests, vitamin B_{12} and folate levels, sedative drug screen, lumbar puncture, blood and CSF cultures

Procedure	To Detect
Computerized tomography (CT) scan; magnetic resonance imaging (MRI)	Tumor; subdural hematoma; normal pressure hydrocephalus; multi-infarct dementia
EEG	Diffuse generalized slowing: diffuse metabolic brain disease Seizure activity; focal depression of activity; structural brain disorder
Lumbar puncture	Subarachnoid hemorrhage; cerebral contusion; bacterial meningitis; neurosyphilis; encephalitis

[†]See the appendix on Laboratory Reference Values for the associated normal laboratory values.

SELECTED BIBLIOGRAPHY

Adams RD, Victor M: Delirium and other acute confusional states, in *Principles of Neurology*, 4th ed., pp. 323–333, New York: McGraw-Hill, 1989.

Cadieux RJ: Early differentiation of senile dementia. *Hosp Pract* 24(12):77–94, 1989.
Consensus Conference: Differential diagnosis of dementing diseases. *JAMA* 258:3411–3416, 1987.
Furlan AJ: Unexplained acute changes in behavior. *Postgrad Med* 84(2):173–178, 1988.
Martin RA, Guthrie R: Office evaluation of dementia. *Postgrad Med* 84(3):176–187, 1988.

32
Epilepsy

INTRODUCTION

Epilepsy   Recurrent episodes of brain dysfunction (seizures) present over months or years, often with a stereotyped clinical pattern.

The epileptic seizure is characterized by a rhythmic and repetitive hypersynchronous discharge of many neurons in a localized area of the brain. If the neuronal hypersynchrony is large, a focal, simple seizure follows. The earliest symptomatology (aura) generated by this focal discharge allows localization of the epileptic focus. A focal seizure can spread locally or generalize throughout the brain, resulting in a generalized seizure. Widely ramifying thalamocortical pathways are likely to be responsible for the rapid generalization of some forms of epilepsy. Epileptic hyperactivity may be due to local alterations of cerebral cortex structures resulting in a tendency to abnormal synchronization, local and systemic biochemical and metabolic factors altering a neuron's firing characteristics, and variations of the interconnections between cortical and subcortical regions that integrate normal cerebral function.

The disturbances of cerebral function caused by a seizure must be distinguished from syncope, transient ischemic attacks, migraine, and hysteria.

Classification of Epileptic Seizures

Partial seizures (beginning locally)
  Simple: consciousness not impaired (with motor, sensory, autonomic, or psychic symptoms)
  Complex: consciousness impaired
  Partial seizures, secondarily generalized
Primary generalized (bilaterally symmetrical, without focal onset): tonic-clonic; absence; myoclonic; atonic

ETIOLOGY

Idiopathic*
Structural lesions
  Severe birth trauma
  Intracranial infections:* meningitis; encephalitis (herpes simplex); cerebral abscess; parasitic brain disease
  Cerebral traumatism;* concussion of the brain
  Cerebrovascular diseases:* stroke; subdural hematoma; intracranial hemorrhage; rupture of an aneurysm; cortical thrombophlebitis; SLE; polyarteritis nodosa
  Intracranial neoplastic disease:* primary and metastatic tumors
  Cerebral degenerative and developmental diseases: Alzheimer's disease; tuberous sclerosis; Sturge-Weber disease; hydrocephalus

*Common cause

Metabolic disorders: hypoglycemia; hypoxia; marked hyperglycemia (nonketotic hyperosmolar states); hypocalcemia; hyponatremia; acid-base disturbances; uremia; hepatic encephalopathy; porphyria; thyrotoxic storm; pyridoxine deficiency; alcohol;* hypertensive encephalopathy; eclampsia; phenylketonuria
Drug intoxication;* drug withdrawal

Iatrogenic Causes of Seizures

Tricyclic antidepressants; amphetamines; dopamine antagonists (neuroleptics, metoclopramide); insulin; isoniazid; lidocaine; lithium; penicillins; phenothiazines; theophylline; vincristine
Withdrawal from barbiturates, hypnosedatives, ethanol

HISTORY TAKING*

Possible meaning of a positive response

1 Mode of Onset and Duration

1.1 When did your seizures appear for the first time? | The likely etiology depends on the age of the patient and the type of seizure
• in childhood? (2 to 12 years) | Birth injury; trauma; infections; idiopathic; febrile illness
• in adolescence? (age 12 to 18) | Idiopathic; head trauma; arteriovenous malformations
• in early adulthood? (18 to 35) | Trauma; idiopathic; alcohol withdrawal; brain tumor
• in middle age? (35 to 60) | Trauma; brain tumor; cerebrovascular disease; metabolic disorder; alcohol or drug withdrawal
• in late life? (over 60) | Cerebrovascular disease; brain tumor; degenerative disease; trauma

1.2 What is the frequency of the seizures? | Important for treatment program; generalized seizures may occur once or twice yearly to many times daily; in women, the seizures may appear with or immediately before the menstrual periods
• several spells of unconsciousness per day or month? | In a young person: more suggestive of epilepsy than of syncope

1.2a Has there been any recent change in frequency?

1.3 Do the seizures occur day or night? regardless of your position? | Frequent in seizures, rare in syncope (exception: the Stokes-Adams attack)

*In this section, items in *italics* are characteristic clinical features, and items in **boldface** are potentially life-threatening or urgent conditions.
Note: If the patient has amnesia for portions of the attack and is unable to report what has occurred, careful questioning of the family and/or witnesses to the attack is mandatory.

2 Location, Spread, and Character of the Seizures

2.1 Does the seizure consist of sudden twitching in the thumb and index fingers? the great toe? the corner of the mouth? without loss of consiousness?

Simple partial ("Jacksonian") seizure with motor signs: origin in contralateral frontal lobe, precentral gyrus

2.2 Does the seizure consist of forced conscious turning of the head and eyes?

Simple partial motor adversive seizure; onset in opposite lateral frontal or supplementary motor region

2.3 Does the seizure consist of masticatory movements?

Simple partial motor attack; localization in amygdaloid nuclei

2.4 Does the seizure consist of a tingling, numbness of the fingers? lips? toes? without loss of consciousness?

Simple partial somatosensory seizure; epileptiform discharges in the contralateral parietal, post-central gyrus

2.5 Does the twitching or the tingling sensation spread to adjacent ipsilateral body parts? (thumb to hand to arm to face?) with preserved consciousness?

"March" of epileptic discharge into adjacent parts of the cortex; the partial seizure may remain limited to the extremity

2.6 Does the seizure consist of paroxysmal nausea, vomiting? abdominal discomfort? excessive salivation? sweating? trouble breathing? palpitation?

Simple partial autonomic seizures: insular cortex

2.7 Does the seizure consist of
   • forced thinking? overwhelming fear? déjà vu? without altered consciousness?

Simple partial psychic seizure; discharges in temporal and frontal lobe

   • olfactory hallucinations?
   • visual hallucinations? unformed images?

Onset: medial temporal lobe (uncus)
Onset: in the occipital lobe

   • auditory (unformed), vertiginous hallucinations?

Superior temporal gyrus

   • peculiar sensations of taste?

Gustatory hallucinations: insular cortex

2.8 Does the seizure consist of activities being carried out in a state of impaired consciousness? out of contact with other people?

Complex partial seizure: involvement of the temporal lobe and limbic system. May begin as simple partial seizure and progress to impairment of consciousness or with impaired consciousness at onset

2.9 Does the onset of impaired consciousness consist of
   • altered perception (déjà vu, feeling of strangeness or unreality)?

Complex partial seizure: medial temporal (amygdala)

- altered affect? intense emotional feeling? fear? elation? depression?
- formed sensory hallucinations? illusion of objects growing smaller (micropsia)? illusion of objects growing larger (macropsia)?
- chewing, swallowing? lip smacking? walking aimlessly? mumbling? picking at your clothes?

2.10 Does the seizure (2.1 to 2.9) terminate in a general convulsion with loss of consciousness?

2.11 Do you have a sudden loss of consciousness and generalized convulsions? without warning?

2.11a *What do other people observe when you have a seizure?* Have you been told that the seizure begins with
- a forceful fall to the ground?
- a cry?

- *biting of the tongue?* inside of the cheeks?
- *loss of urine? feces?*

2.11b How long does your convulsive attack last?

2.11c How long does your period of unconsciousness last?

2.12 Does the seizure consist of brief episodes (10 to 45 seconds) of loss of awareness of the environment? sudden cessation of ongoing conscious behavior?
- with or without chewing? blinking movements (3 per second)? a stare?
- without warning, convulsions, or fall?

Complex partial seizure: medial temporal

Complex partial seizure: temporal neocortex or amygdaloid-hippocampal complex

Automatisms: complex partial seizure; localization: temporal and frontal regions. Some minor motor activity may occur in complex partial seizure

A simple partial seizure (with preserved consciousness) may exist alone, or progress to a complex partial seizure (with altered consciousness) and/or to a generalized tonic-clonic seizure (with altered consciousness). A complex partial seizure (with altered consciousness) may progress to a generalized tonic-clonic seizure

Tonic-clonic seizure: may occur alone as a primary generalized seizure or as the result of secondary generalization from partial seizure

Loss of postural control
"Tonic stage": contraction of the respiratory muscles with forced expiration
The tongue is frequently caught between the teeth during the tonic stage
Bladder and bowel may be emptied during the tonic stage (rare in syncope)

Habitual duration of convulsions ("clonic stage") less than 5 min

The coma may last for many minutes to ½ hour

Absence seizure (childhood and adolescence); localization in frontal cortex, amygdaloid-hippocampal complex, reticular-cortical system

3 Precipitating or Aggravating Factors

3.1 Are your seizures precipitated by
- flickering lights? driving through trees in the sunshine? sounds? music? reading? tactile stimulation?
- an intercurrent infection? alcohol? cessation of therapy?
- sleep deprivation?

- (in women) menstrual periods?
- oral contraceptives? pregnancy?

Focal or generalized seizures can be evoked in certain epileptic patients by a physiologic or psychologic stimulus ("reflex" epilepsy)

Common causes of exacerbation of a chronic seizure disorder

May induce generalized tonic-clonic seizures in neurologically normal individuals

Catamenial epilepsy

Estrogens tend to exacerbate seizures

4 Relieving Factors

4.1 Do you take any drug for your seizures?

4.1a How does medication influence your seizures?

With adequate therapy, most patients with occasional generalized and complex partial seizures achieve complete or nearly complete reduction of seizures

5 Accompanying Symptoms

5.1 Have you been told that the loss of consciousness is
- *associated with cyanosis?*
- *preceded by pallor?*

Seizure
Syncope

5.2 Do you have any warning, minutes to hours before a seizure? apathy? depression? irritability? headache?

A prodromal phase of altered emotional reactivity may precede generalized seizures

5.3 *What is the first thing that happens in a (typical) seizure a few seconds before consciousness is lost?*

"Aura": a simple partial seizure produced by the onset of the epileptic discharge; perceived (and remembered) by the patient before consciousness is lost. Some patients with generalized seizures have no warning but become unconscious at once. An aura provides the most reliable clue to the location of the seizure focus. In case of generalized seizures: indicates a partial seizure with secondary generalization

5.4 After the attack, do you have
- mental confusion? drowsiness? headache? muscular pain? tiredness? fatigue?
- a transitory (minutes to hours) weakness of an extremity?

Postictal symptoms in generalized seizures

Todd's postictal paralysis: an important clue to a focal origin to the seizure; onset in a motor strip

• a transitory disorder of speech?

Postical aphasia: attack occurring in the dominant hemisphere

5.5 When you awaken, are you aware of the eventual aura? your attack?

Postical amnesia for events which took place during the complex partial seizure and for generalized seizure. Patient may remember prodromal phase or aura

5.6 Do you regain full consciousness
• *slowly?* (minutes to hours)
• *promptly?*

Usual duration in epilepsy
Syncope rather than epilepsy

5.7 Do you have
• headaches? vomiting? disorders of speech? of gait? weakness of an extremity?

Increased intracranial pressure; underlying mass lesion (tumor, abscess), chronic subdural hematoma; meningitis

• fever?

Brain abscess; meningitis; encephalitis

• blurred vision?

Hypertensive encephalopathy with altered fundi

• cough? bloody expectorations?

Bronchogenic carcinoma with cerebral metastases

5.8 (Question for observers): Is the patient's mental function impaired?

Recurrent subclinical seizures not controlled by medication; drug intoxication; postseizure psychosis; subdural hematoma; brain disease causing both dementia and seizures

6 Iatrogenic Factors See Etiology

7 Personal and Social Profile

7.1 What is your occupation?

Occupational exposure to toxic products; patient's disease may require job alteration

7.2 Do you have any problems due to your seizures with your family? at school? professionally?

Patients with convulsive seizures often have emotional problems, usually in response to environmental restrictions

7.3 What is your consumption of alcohol?

Seizures in an alcoholic may be due to: alcohol withdrawal: seizures ("rum fits") usually occur between 12 and 36 h after cessation of drinking; old cerebral contusion (from falls or fights); chronic subdural hematoma; metabolic disorder; liver disease

8 Personal Antecedents Pertaining to the Seizures

8.1 Have you ever had an x-ray of your skull? an EEG? a CT scan? a lumbar puncture? When? With what results?

8.2 Did you ever hurt yourself from the fall during a seizure?	Injury may be sustained during the fall (protective reflexes are abolished instantaneously) or may result from violent muscular contraction (crushed vertebra). Injury is rare in syncope
8.3 Have you had any of the following conditions: a birth trauma? a head trauma? meningitis? encephalitis? a cerebral vascular accident (stroke)?	
• febrile seizures during childhood?	Significant risk of subsequent epilepsy if the febrile convulsion is prolonged or focal
8.4 Do you have any of the following conditions: arterial hypertension? a renal disease? a hepatic disease ? drug abuse?	
• diabetes?	Hypoglycemia: overdose of insulin
• a recent febrile illness, with headaches? a change in mental status?	Acute CNS infection: meningitis, encephalitis

9 Family Medical History Pertaining to the Seizures

9.1 Are there other members of your family who have epilepsy? other neurologic disorders?	The relatives of patients with idiopathic epilepsy have a prevalence rate of seizures 3 times that of the overall population (incidence in the ordinary population: 0.5 to 2 percent)

PHYSICAL SIGNS PERTAINING TO EPILEPSY

	Possible significance
Focal neurologic deficit(s)	Localizing value; intracranial mass lesion: tumor, abscess, cerebral vascular lesion
Fever	Brain abscess; meningitis; encephalitis
Stiff neck; fever	Bacterial meningitis
Ear infection	Brain abscess
Heart murmur; valvular or septal lesions; fever	Subacute bacterial endocarditis with cerebral embolism
Clubbing; abnormal lung examination	Bronchogenic carcinoma or lung abscess with metastatic tumor or abscess
Café au lait spots; subcutaneous nodules, pedunculated tumors	Neurofibromatosis with intracranial glioma or neurofibroma

Sebaceous adenomas of the face; shagreen patches; white spots over the trunk and limbs	Tuberous sclerosis
Portwine facial stain	Sturge-Weber disease (with venous hemangioma of the leptomeninges and cerebral calcifications)
Body or limbs asymmetries	Congenital or infantile cerebral lesion
Funduscopic examination: papilledema	Increased intracranial pressure: tumor; abscess; hypertensive encephalopathy

LABORATORY TESTS PERTAINING TO EPILEPSY[†]

Test	To Detect
Blood	
Glucose; BUN, creatinine; electrolytes; liver function tests; drug screen	Metabolic disturbances; hypoglycemia; uremia; hypo- or hypernatremia; hypo- or hypercalcemia
EEG	Focal or generalized abnormalities of cortical activity; absence seizure (a normal EEG does not exclude the diagnosis of epilepsy)
CT scan; magnetic resonance imaging	Anatomic lesion: hemispheric mass; ventricular size and position; cerebral atrophy
Lumbar puncture*	Suspected acute or chronic CNS infection; subarachnoid hemorrhage

[†]See the appendix on Laboratory Reference Values for the associated normal laboratory values.
*When indicated

SELECTED BIBLIOGRAPHY

Adams RD, Victor M: Epilepsy and other seizure disorders, in *Principles of Neurology*, 4th ed., pp. 249–272, New York: McGraw-Hill, 1989.
Bleck TP: Epilepsy. *DM* 33(11):601–679, 1987.
Porter RJ, Theodore WH (eds): Epilepsy. *Neurol Clin* 4(3):495–700, 1986.

33
Fatigue

INTRODUCTION

Fatigue (tiredness, lassitude)   Loss of that sense of well-being typically found in persons who are healthy in body and mind; it is a subjective feeling of lack of energy, not necessarily associated with physical activity.

Fatigue is a normal physiologic reaction when associated with or occurring after sustained muscular exertion. Under these circumstances a rest period rapidly restores the subject's feeling of well-being and capacity for work. In a normal subject continuous muscular work results in depletion of muscular glycogen and an accumulation of lactic acid and other metabolites which reduce the power of muscular contraction. Fatigue may result from overwork. It also occurs in various infectious, metabolic, endocrine, and nutritional diseases. Fatigue may be associated with true muscular weakness in thyroid dysfunction, adrenal insufficiency, or neurologic disorders. Even when fatigue is associated with an organic lesion, it may not be attributable to it, but rather to independent or related psychogenic disturbances. The role of Epstein-Barr virus in chronic fatigue is debated. Psychiatric disorders account for approximately two thirds of cases of chronic fatigue.

Fatigue must be distinguished from weakness of neural or muscular origin.

ETIOLOGY

Physiological: increased physical exertion; inadequate rest; environmental stress (noise, vibration, heat)

New physical disability, recent illness, surgery, or trauma

Sleep pattern disruption

Acute infection: virtually any; influenza; acute viral hepatitis; acquired immunodeficiency syndrome

Chronic infections: tuberculosis; infectious mononucleosis; brucellosis; subacute bacterial endocarditis; Lyme disease; asymptomatic urinary tract infection; hookworm, parasitic infection

Inflammatory: rheumatic fever; glomerulonephritis; collagen-vascular diseases: systemic lupus erythematosus; rheumatoid arthritis; chronic hepatitis; inflammatory bowel disease

Neurologic disorders: Parkinson's disease; multiple sclerosis; posttraumatic syndrome; encephalitis; narcolepsy; dementia

Endocrine and metabolic diseases: adrenal insufficiency; aldosterone deficiency; panhypopituitarism; Cushing's disease; hypothyroidism; hyperthyroidism; hypogonadism; hypercalcemic and hypocalcemic states; hyponatremia; hyperaldosteronism; hypokalemia; uncontrolled diabetes mellitus; hypoglycemic states; chronic renal failure

Nutritional deficiencies

Cardiovascular disorders: "silent" myocardial infarction; congestive heart failure; low cardiac output syndromes; mitral valve prolapse; cardiomyopathy

Pulmonary insufficiency: emphysema; chronic bronchitis
Neoplastic disorders: lymphomas; carcinomas; occult malignancy
Persistent chronic pain causing lack of sleep
Miscellaneous: anemia; pregnancy; medications; chronic drug intoxication; alcohol
Psychogenic: chronic anxiety; tension states; depression; stress reaction
Controversial: chronic fatigue syndrome; chronic infectious mononucleosis

Iatrogenic Causes of Fatigue

Large doses of corticosteroids (causing depression); sedatives; tranquilizers; antihistamines; analgesics; anticonvulsants; anti-inflammatory agents; antihypertensive medications (beta-blockers, methyldopa, reserpine, clonidine); progestational agents; cimetidine

HISTORY TAKING*

Possible meaning of a positive response

1 Character of the Fatigue

1.1	Are you able to perform tasks of daily living? drive a car? run to catch a bus? climb stairs? carry an object?	The patient with fatigue is able to do a task at least once and perform normal activities, but lacks the ability to perform a task repetitively
1.2	Do you experience trouble on exercise? when you begin to move?	True weakness of muscular or neural origin
1.3	Do you feel tired before you begin activities? before a physical effort?	Fatigue: psychological or systemic disorder
1.4	Do you feel tired while lying in bed?	Fatigue, lassitude
1.5	Is the fatigue	
	• constant?	Fatigue due to an organic disease; depression; also: muscular weakness
	• intermittent?	Psychogenic fatigue; weakness: in periodic paralysis
1.6	When do you feel at your worst?	
	• on awakening? *in the morning?*	Psychogenic fatigue (frequently worse in the morning): possible depression
	• at the end of the day?	Organic cause of fatigue; psychogenic fatigue
	• all day?	Chronic anxiety
1.6a	*Do you feel just as tired when you awaken as you do later on in the day?*	Psychogenic fatigue
1.7	When do you feel at your best?	
	• in the morning?	Fatigue due to an organic factor
	• *in the evening?*	Psychogenic fatigue; depression

*In this section, items in *italics* are characteristic clinical features.

2 Mode of Onset and Duration

2.1	How long have you been feeling tired?	If the patient has "always" felt tired: psychogenic fatigue. More than 4 months: probably psychological; the patient with organic fatigue is usually seen within 4 months of onset
2.2	Has the onset of the fatigue been	
	• sudden? (days)	Acute infection; disturbance of fluid balance, extracellular deficit; rapidly developing circulatory failure (outspoken objective phenomena present)
	• gradual? (weeks to months)	Psychogenic fatigue or fatigue due to an organic disease
2.3	Is your lassitude	
	• fluctuating?	Psychological fatigue
	• progressive?	Organic fatigue: underlying deteriorating condition, anemia, malignancy

3 Precipitating or Aggravating Factors

3.1	Does your fatigue appear	
	• during exertion?	Weakness; organic fatigue
	• only after a strenuous physical effort?	Physiological fatigue
	• *without any relation to physical effort?*	Psychogenic fatigue
3.2	Is the fatigue related	
	• more to some activities than to others? to unpleasant emotional experiences?	Psychogenic fatigue
3.3	What is your sleep pattern?	Insufficient or poor-quality sleep may produce fatigue or may be due to depression, chronic pain, alcohol, or drugs

4 Relieving Factors

4.1	Is the fatigue relieved by	
	• rest? additional sleep? weekends and vacations?	Fatigue due to an organic disease; weakness; chronic stress related to employment (if not relieved: psychogenic fatigue likely)
	• physical activity?	Psychological fatigue

5 Accompanying Symptoms

5.1	Do you feel anxious? depressed? irritable? unable to concentrate?	Depression; anxiety neurosis; tension states
5.2	Do you have	
	• headache? poor sleep? a lack of interest in sex?	Frequently observed in depression with psychogenic fatigue

• a loss of weight?

Thyrotoxicosis; chronic infection; tuberculosis; diabetes mellitus; Addison's disease. (Neoplasms are seldom manifested primarily by fatigue; however, carcinoma of the lung, pancreas, or right colon may be introduced by fatigue). May occur in depressive reaction

• a weight gain?

Fatigue associated with weight gain suggests a depressive syndrome; hypothyroidism

• constipation? cold intolerance?

Hypothyroidism

• a decreased appetite?

Chronic infection; uremia; Addison's disease; panhypopituitarism; depression

• fever?

Chronic infection; tuberculosis; inflammatory disease; subacute bacterial endocarditis; lymphoma

• shortness of breath?

Cardiorespiratory disease

• cough? night sweats?

Pulmonary tuberculosis

• inappropriate sweating?

Psychological fatigue

• palpitations?

Fever; thyrotoxicosis (arrhythmias); psychogenic fatigue; mitral valve prolapse

• changes in your bowel habits?

Carcinoma of colon or pancreas; depression; inflammatory bowel disease

• double vision? difficulty in speaking? in chewing?

Weakness in myasthenia gravis with involvement of cranial nerves (diplopia, dysarthria); never present in psychogenic fatigue

6   Iatrogenic Factors   See Etiology

7   Personal and Social Profile

7.1   Have you been under much pressure lately?
  • a recent death in your family? financial loss? job stress? childbirth?

Stress-related psychogenic fatigue (discussion of life stresses can make the patient feel better). Patients with organic disease may erroneously attribute their fatigue to a psychological problem

7.2   Do you have any job problems?

Possible overwork with fatigue; possible psychogenic cause of fatigue

7.2a   Do you take any vacation? How many weeks a year?

May reveal an overworked patient with no time for diversion and sleep. Fatigue is frequently ascribed to overwork when it actually reflects a psychological problem or depression

7.3 Do you feel more tired at home
     than on your job?   } Familial psychogenic factor

7.3a Do you have any family problem?

7.4 What is your daily diet? your alco-   A nutritional deficiency and/or alcohol-
     hol intake?   ism may cause fatigue due to psy-
                                                 chosocial problems, nutritional de-
                                                 ficiencies and/or organic diseases (liver
                                                 cirrhosis)

7.5 Do you use illicit drugs?   Fatigue in a drug addict may be due to a
                                                 psychiatric problem, acute or chronic
                                                 hepatitis

7.6 What is your sexual orientation?   Fatigue in a homosexual man: AIDS-
                                                 related condition; amebiasis; hepatitis

8   Personal Antecedents Pertaining to the Fatigue

8.1 Do you have any of the following
     conditions: anemia? any chronic
     disease? malignancy? alcoholism?
     a psychiatric condition?
     • a cardiac condition?   Fatigue due to congestive heart failure:
                                                 related to the reduction of cardiac out-
                                                 put

8.2 Have you recently had
     • a systemic or prolonged illness? a   Convalescing, postinfectious, and post-
       stroke? an operation? childbirth?   operative states responsible for fatigue
       influenza? infectious hepatitis?
     • infectious mononucleosis?   Alleged cause of chronic fatigue (con-
                                                 troversial)

9   Family History Pertaining to the Fatigue

9.1 Are there any psychiatric disorders   Major depression is a familial disorder.
     in your family? depression? alco-   Familial stress can contribute to the
     holism? psychosis?   patient's fatigue

PHYSICAL SIGNS PERTAINING TO FATIGUE

                                                 Possible significance

Reduced muscular power; neurologic   Primary myopathic or neurologic dis-
abnormalities; muscle wasting   order

Cranial muscle weakness; nasal voice   Myasthenia gravis (exclude emotional
                                                 fatigue states)

Lack of facial expression; paucity of   Depression
movements; inertia; slow speech; paucity
of ideas

Pallor; tachycardia	Moderate to severe anemia (mild anemias are usually asymptomatic and any associated fatigue is probably attributable to some other condition)
Fever; cardiac murmur	Subacute bacterial endocarditis
Dry skin; bradycardia; delayed relaxation phase of the tendon reflexes	Hypothyroidism
Thyroid enlargement; tremor; sweating palms	Thyrotoxicosis
Hyperpigmentation of skin and mucosae; hypotension; postural hypotension; muscular weakness	Adrenal insufficiency
Cardiomegaly; gallop rhythm; bilateral basal crackles; distended jugular veins; hepatomegaly; edema	Congestive heart failure; decrease in cardiac output and inadequate tissue perfusion and oxygenation
Prolonged expiration; rhonchi; wheezes; cyanosis	Chronic pulmonary disease with chronic dyspnea and fatigue
Hepatosplenomegaly; lymphadenopathy	Chronic active hepatitis; lymphoma; leukemia; chronic infection

LABORATORY TESTS PERTAINING TO FATIGUE[†]

Test	To Detect
Blood	
Hematocrit	Anemia: a possible cause for fatigue if hematocrit less than 30 percent
WBCs	Leukemia; infection
Erythrocyte sedimentation rate	Infection; collagen-vascular disorders; etc.
Liver function tests	Liver disease
BUN, creatinine	Chronic renal failure
Fasting glucose	Uncontrolled diabetes mellitus
Electrolytes	Endocrinopathies: Addison's disease, hyperaldosteronism; renal tubular acidosis; diuretic intake
Calcium	Hyperparathyroidism; other hypercalcemic states

[†]See the appendix on Laboratory Reference Values for the associated normal laboratory values.

Test	To Detect
Iron	Iron-deficiency anemia
Thyroid function tests	Thyrotoxicosis; myxedema
Cortisol*	Addison's disease
Epstein-Barr virus serologic testing	Infectious mononucleosis
Stool	
Occult blood tests	Gastrointestinal tumor
Chest x-ray	Pulmonary tuberculosis; lung tumor; chronic pulmonary disease
ECG	Silent myocardial infarction
Psychologic evaluation*	Depression or anxiety states

*When indicated

SELECTED BIBLIOGRAPHY

Holmes GP, Kaplan JE, Gantz NM et al: Chronic fatigue syndrome: A working case definition. *Ann Intern Med* 108:387–389, 1988.
Jarvis RG: The "tired person" syndrome. *Postgrad Med* 81(8):321–324, 1987.
Solberg LI: Lassitude. A primary care evaluation. *JAMA* 251:3272–3276, 1984.
Swartz MN: The chronic fatigue syndrome—One entity or many? *N Engl J Med* 319:1726–1728, 1988.

34
Headache

INTRODUCTION

Headache   Painful or unpleasant sensations in the region of the cranial vault.

Structures sensitive to pain in the region of the head and face include all extracranial tissues, especially the arteries, the basal dura mater, the venous sinuses and their tributary veins, the arteries within the dura mater and piarachnoid, and nerves with sensory afferents (fifth, ninth, tenth cranial nerves, first three cervical nerves).

Headache may originate from extracranial or intracranial structures. Vascular headaches involve vasoconstriction followed by painful dilatation and distention of extracranial branches of the external carotid artery. Most of the pain of migraine is attributed to dilatation of the extracranial, temporal, and intracranial arteries, with stretching of surrounding sensitive structures. Abnormalities of platelet aggregation, blood serotonin concentration, and other metabolites have been observed in classic migraine. Cluster headache is believed to be a vascular headache related to migraine. The headache associated with febrile states or some cases of hypertension is probably due to dilatation and distention of intracranial arteries. Some tension headaches are due in part to painful neck or scalp muscle spasm; in others, no sustained contraction is found. Tension headache usually coincides with anxiety and depression. Pain of infection or blockage of paranasal sinuses is due to changes in pressure and irritation of pain-sensitive sinus walls. Headache of ocular origin is believed to be caused by ocular muscle imbalance. Intracranial mass lesions may cause headache by deforming, displacing, or exerting traction on vessels and dural structures at the base of the brain. Headache of meningeal irritation is ascribed to increased intracranial pressure, and dilatation and congestion of inflamed meningeal vessels. The pain of trigeminal neuralgia (over the distribution of one or more branches of the fifth cranial nerve) can occur spontaneously or may be brought on by stimulating a trigger zone, which may exist in any part of the face.

CLASSIFICATION OF HEADACHE (ABBREVIATED FROM THE INTERNATIONAL HEADACHE SOCIETY)

Migraine:* without aura; with aura: hemiplegic, basilar; ophthalmoplegic
Tension-type headache:* with or without disorder of pericranial muscles
Cluster headache and chronic paroxysmal hemicrania
Miscellaneous headaches unassociated with structural lesion: benign cough headache; benign exertional headache; headache associated with sexual activity
Headache associated with head trauma
Headache associated with vascular disorders: acute ischemic cerebrovascular disease; intracranial hematoma; subarachnoid hemorrhage; vascular malformation; giant cell (temporal) arteritis; venous thrombosis; arterial hypertension
Headache associated with non-vascular intracranial disorder: high cerebrospinal fluid

*Common cause

284

(CSF) pressure; low CSF pressure (postlumbar puncture headache); intracranial infection; intracranial sarcoidosis; intrathecal injections; intracranial neoplasm

Headache associated with substances or their withdrawal: carbon monoxide; alcohol; monosodium glutamate; drugs

Headache associated with non-cephalic infection: viral; bacterial; other infection

Headache associated with metabolic disorder: hypoxia; sleep-apnea; hypercapnia; hypoglycemia

Headache or facial pain associated with disorder of: cranium; neck; eyes; ears; nose; sinuses; teeth; mouth; jaws; temporomandibular joint disease

Cranial neuralgias, nerve trunk pain, and deafferentiation pain

Headache not classifiable

Iatrogenic Causes of Headache

Nitrates, nitrites, nitroglycerin; hydralazine; reserpine; oral contraceptives; analgesics abuse; withdrawal of caffeine, ergotamine, corticosteroids, narcotics

HISTORY TAKING*

	Possible meaning of a positive response
1 Location of Headache	
1.1 Where do you have pain?	If the source of the headache is in extracranial structures, the correspondence with the site of the pain is fairly precise. Involvement of deeper structures leads to less precise localization
1.1a Can you point to the painful area?	Local disorder: frontal sinus; ear; temporal arteritis
1.2 Is the pain	
• *unilateral?*	Migraine; cluster headache (male preponderance); one-sided intracranial lesion; trigeminal neuralgia
• *recurrent and always on the same side of the head?*	Intracranial vascular malformation, tumor, or other organic lesion of the head and neck; cluster headache; migraine uncommonly involves the same side of the head in every attack
• on one side of the head in one attack and on the other in the next?	May occur in common migraine
• occipital?	Temporal arteritis; arterial hypertension (diastolic pressure $\geqslant$120 mmHg)
• *temporal?*	Temporal arteritis; cluster headache

*In this section, items in *italics* are characteristic clinical features, and items in **boldface** are potentially life-threatening or urgent conditions.

• *orbital or supraorbital?*	Cluster headache; glaucoma
• frontotemporal?	Migraine; intracranial supratentorial lesion
• over the antrum? in the forehead?	Infection or blockage of paranasal sinuses
• around the eye(s)?	Blockage of the ethmoid and sphenoid sinuses
• in the orbit, forehead, temple?	Pain of ocular origin; cluster headache
• around the ear?	Disease in the ear; referred pain from the neck
• spreading from one to both sides of the head?	May occur in migraine
• bilateral?	Tension headache; it is common for migraine to be bilateral
• bitemporal? bifrontal?	Tension headache; posterior fossa lesion may cause bifrontal headache
• occipitonuchal?	Tension headache; arterial hypertension; cervical spondylosis; referred eye pain; intracranial lesion in posterior fossa
• generalized?	Tension headache; **meningeal irritation** (meningitis, subarachnoid hemorrhage)

1.3   Does the pain spread to the
• face?   Trigeminal neuralgia
• face, neck, shoulder?   May occur in cluster headache and in pain referred from lesions of the upper cervical portion of the spinal column; subarachnoid hemorrhage

1.4   Does your pain seem
• deep-seated?   Pain arising from structures deep to the skin: extracranial, subdermal, intracranial; meningeal irritation; cluster headache
• superficial?   Localized to the skin

2   Mode of Onset and Chronology

2.1   How long have you had headaches?   If many years: benign, tends to eliminate intracranial or inflammatory lesion; probably vascular or tension headache. Migraine usually begins in adolescence; its commencement after age 50 is uncommon

2.2   Was the onset
• *sudden (over a period of minutes) and violent?*   Subarachnoid hemorrhage
• acute? (over several minutes to an hour)   Meningitis; epidural hematoma; glaucoma; purulent sinusitis
• more gradual?   Tension headache

2.3 Is your headache
- continuous?

  Tension headache, functional problem;
  temporal arteritis (intermittent at onset)

  - lasting days to a week?
    Meningeal irritation
  - continuous for weeks or months?
    Temporal arteritis
  - continuous for months to years? often waxing and waning from hour to hour or day to day?
    Tension headache
  - recurrent?
    Organic: migraine, cluster headache; trigeminal neuralgia

2.4 In case of recurrent headache: What is the frequency of the episodes?
  - a single attack every few weeks?
    Migraine: a greater frequency is exceptional
  - several attacks per week?
    Usually combination of migraine and tension headaches
  - once to four daily, for several weeks?
    Cluster headache

2.4a Are the headaches becoming more frequent and severe over a period of months?
  Expanding intracranial lesion; brain tumor; subdural hematoma; aneurysm

2.4b At what time in the day does your headache appear?
  - *upon awakening in the morning?*
    Hypertensive headache (occipital); cerebral tumor; infection or blockage of paranasal sinuses (filling at night); sleep apnea-hypersomnia syndrome
  - on awakening, with gradual disappearance on erect position and coming again in the late morning hours?
    Sinus headache
  - in early afternoon or evening?
    Tension headache
  - at night? *2 to 3 h after onset of sleep?*
    Cluster headache (over a period of several weeks to months); chronic pulmonary disease with hypercapnia. Tension headaches seldom awaken the patient from sleep
  - at any time of day or night?
    Intracranial tumor

2.4c What is the duration of your headaches?
  - 1 to 2 s?
    Iceprick-like headaches: uninterpretable; no serious underlying disease
  - minutes to hours?
    Brain tumor
  - dissipates within an hour?
    Cluster headache
  - several hours up to 1 to 2 days?
    Migraine
  - days or weeks?
    Temporal arteritis; sinusitis
  - weeks or months with fluctuations?
    Tension headache

2.4d How quickly does your headache reach a maximum?

- abruptly, rapidly peaking? (5 to 10 min)   Cluster headache

- gradually? in a half hour or so?   Migraine

3   Character and Intensity of the Pain

3.1   Is the pain

- dull, aching? burning?   Cranial or temporal arteritis (giant cell arteritis); headache of ocular origin

- sharp? stabbing?   Trigeminal neuralgia

- throbbing? pulsatile?   Vascular, migraine headaches; hypertensive headache; in some cases of tension headache; temporal arteritis; blockage or infection of paranasal sinuses; febrile illness

- like a head soreness rather than headache?   Temporal arteritis

- persistent? steady? nonthrobbing?   Subarachnoid hemorrhage; brain tumor; cluster headache; febrile illness

- tight? *bandlike? pressing?* nonthrobbing? bursting? dull?   Tension headache (psychogenic); muscular tension; psychologic state

3.2   Is the pain severe? intense?   Subarachnoid hemorrhage; meningitis; migraine; cluster headache (paroxysmal nocturnal). Discomfort is minimized by stoical persons and dramatized by depressed patients

3.3   Does your headache

- allow performance of your day's work?   Rare with a severe migraine attack. Degree of incapacity is a good index of the intensity of the pain

- *awaken you from sleep at night?* prevent sleep?   Headache with demonstrable organic basis; intracranial tumor

4   Precipitating or Aggravating Factors

4.1   Is your headache caused or worsened by

- stooping? straining? coughing? sneezing? lifting? exertion?   Intracranial mass lesion; subarachnoid hemorrhage; infection of nasal sinuses

- sudden head movement?   Cervical disease; sinus headache

- active and passive motion of the spine?   Cervical disease (ligaments, muscles, apophyseal joints)

- touching the scalp?   Scalp sensitivity in migraine, temporal arteritis

- bright light? noise? stress? too much sleep?   Migraine

- head-low position?   Migraine (vascular origin of the headache); brain tumor

- dietary factors? (red wine, chocolate, nuts, coffee, tea, fermented cheeses)

  Migraine

- alcohol?

  Migraine; cluster headache

- prolonged reading? watching movies, TV?

  Eyestrain headache

- anxiety? fatigue? emotional upset? excitement? nervous strain?

  Psychogenic (tension) headache; common migraine; hypertensive headache; cluster headache

- sudden temperature changes?

  Sinusitis

- exposure to cold?

  Arthritic or neuralgic condition; temporal arteritis

- *touching a trigger point around the lips?*

  Trigeminal neuralgia

- exertion?

  Leaking berry aneurysm; brain tumor; arterial dissection; benign exertional headache

4.2 Does your headache occur
- during weekends?

  Migraine may occur at the time of relaxation following a stressful situation

- before the time of your menstrual periods?
  - disappearing after the first day of vaginal bleeding?

  Migraine; tension headache (as part of the premenstrual syndrome)

5 Relieving Factors

5.1 Is your headache relieved by
- dark room and sleep? pressure? ergot preparations?

  Migraine

- recumbency?

  Brain tumor

- neck massage?

  Cervical disease

- heat? local massage of muscles? removal of stress?

  Tension headache

5.2 Do you have periods with complete freedom from pain?

  Organic headache: migraine; cluster headache. Patients with psychogenic headache are reluctant to admit symptomless periods

6 Accompanying Symptoms

6.1 Do you have
- hours before your headache: thirst? a craving for sweet foods? drowsiness? depression?

  Prodromal stage: may occur in common migraine; suggests a hypothalamic involvement in the pathogenesis of migraine

- 10 to 30 min before your headache: *scintillating scotomas?* depression? fatigue? photophobia? nausea? vomiting?

  Prodrome of classic migraine: due to arteriolar constriction and decreased cerebral blood flow

6.1a Is your headache accompanied by nausea? vomiting? intolerance to noise and light? — Often observed in migraine

6.2 Do you have
• fever? malaise? — **Meningitis; subarachnoid hemorrhage;** headache of febrile illness; temporal arteritis

• nausea? vomiting? — Migraine; brain tumor; meningoencephalitis; subarachnoid hemorrhage; vomiting is rare in cluster headache and tension headache

• *watering of an eye? running of the ipsilateral nostril? ipsilateral conjunctival injection?* — Ipsilateral lacrimation, nasal congestion, and rhinorrhea in cluster headache

• blurred or decreased vision? — **Malignant hypertension; temporal arteritis**

• muscle aches? pain in the joints? — Temporal arteritis (with polymyalgia rheumatica); febrile illness

• weakness, numbness in (a) limb(s)? — Organic intracranial involvement; basilar or carotid artery insufficiency (after age 50). May precede or accompany complicated migraine

• depression? anxiety? insomnia? nervousness? — Tension headache

• pain on mastication? impairment of vision? muscular aches? pain in peripheral joints? fever? weight loss? — (In older persons): temporal arteritis associated with polymyalgia rheumatica

• jaw pain? — Temporomandibular joint dysfunction

• attacks of severe headache with palpitations, sweating, pallor? — Pheochromocytoma

7   Iatrogenic Factors   See Etiology

8   Personal and Social Profile

8.1 Age of the patient? — In a man after the third to fourth decade of life: cluster headache
In middle and late adult life: cervical spondylosis
In a patient over 50: temporal arteritis

8.2 What is your profession? — Headache due to carbon monoxide, solvents in: firefighting, automobile exhaust, foundry, wood finishing, dry cleaning

8.3 Do you have a personal, familial, professional problem? — Tension headache

8.4 What is your consumption of beer? alcohol? wine? — Alcohol-induced headache; alcohol withdrawal headache (hangover). Alcoholics are prone to subdural hematoma

| 8.5 | What is your sexual orientation? | Persistent headache in a homosexual man: CNS toxoplasmosis; cryptococcal meningitis; herpetic meningoencephalitis, CNS lymphoma |

9 Personal Antecedents Pertaining to the Headache

9.1	Have there been similar episodes in the past? When? Diagnosis?	
9.2	Have you ever had a skull x-ray? a CT scan? an EEG? When? With what results?	
9.3	Do you have a sinus disease? glaucoma?	
9.4	Have you had during the preceding weeks or months	
	• a head injury? an injury to the neck?	Posttraumatic dysautonomic cephalalgia; chronic subdural hematoma
	• an infection? an ear infection?	Brain abscess

10 Family Medical History Pertaining to the Headache

| 10.1 | Are there other members of your family who have headaches? | 70 percent of patients with migraine give a family history |

PHYSICAL SIGNS PERTAINING TO HEADACHE*

	Possible significance
Fever	Headache accompanying febrile illnesses; meningitis; temporal arteritis
Fever; pallor (anemia); *tender thickened temporal artery*	Temporal arteritis
Homolateral lacrimation, rhinorrhea, nasal congestion, conjunctival injection, flush and edema of the cheek, myosis, ptosis	Cluster headache
Severe diastolic hypertension (>120 mmHg)	May produce headache (hypertension is an infrequent cause of headache)
Stiffness of neck on bending forward	Meningeal irritation: infection, hemorrhage
Painful active and passive movements of the cervical spine	Disease of ligaments, muscles, and apophyseal joints of the cervical spine
Tender contracted muscles of head, neck, upper part of back; localized tender areas or nodules	Muscle contraction headache

*In this section, items in *italics* are characteristic clinical features, and items in **boldface** are potentially life-threatening or urgent conditions.

Sinus tenderness	Infection or blockage of nasal and para-nasal sinuses
Neurologic abnormalities; slow mentation	Intracranial space-occupying lesion: brain tumor, chronic subdural hematoma

Funduscopic examination
- papilledema

Brain tumor with increased intracranial pressure

- hypertensive retinopathy   Arterial hypertension
- subhyaloid hemorrhages   Subarachnoid hemorrhage

LABORATORY TESTS PERTAINING TO HEADACHE†

Test	Finding	Diagnostic Possibilities
Blood		
Hemoglobin	Anemia ⎫	Temporal arteritis (in elderly patients)
Erythrocyte sedimentation rate	Elevated ⎭	

†See the appendix on Laboratory Reference Values for the associated normal laboratory values.

LABORATORY PROCEDURES PERTAINING TO HEADACHE

Procedure	To Detect
Sinuses: x-rays, transillumination	Purulent sinusitis
Eye examination	Increased intraocular pressure in glaucoma; refraction errors
Computerized tomography (CT) scan*	Space-occupying lesion; primary or metastatic neoplasm; abscess; subdural hematoma
Biopsy of temporal artery*	Temporal arteritis
Lumbar puncture*	Subarachnoid hemorrhage; meningitis; encephalitis
Psychologic evaluation*	Underlying anxiety or tension state (even positive evidence of neurosis does not rule out brain tumor or other organic disease)

*When indicated

SELECTED BIBLIOGRAPHY

Diamond S, Freitag FG, Solomon GD et al: Migraine headache. *Postgrad Med* 81(8):174–183, 1987.

Edmeads J: The worst headache ever. 1. Ominous causes. 2. Innocuous causes. *Postgrad Med* 86(1):93–104; 107–110, 1989.

Elkind AH: Muscle contraction headache. *Postgrad Med* 81(8):203–217, 1987.

Headache Classification Committee of the International Headache Society: Classification and diagnostic criteria for headache disorders, cranial neuralgia and facial pain. *Cephalalgia* 8(Suppl 7):1–96, 1988.

35
Mental Status Examination

The patient must be prepared for the questions about the mental status to enlist his or her full cooperation. He or she must be reassured that these are not tests of intelligence or of sanity.

Give simple introductory explanations, be tactful and flexible in your approach.

HISTORY TAKING

Possible meaning of response

1 Insight

Insight, the state of being fully aware of the nature and degree of one's deficits, is impaired in all types of cerebral disease that cause complex disorders of behavior

1.1 What are your complaints? Are you ill?

Through lack of insight, patients are often unaware of their illness

1.2 When did your illness begin?

1.3 Do you recognize the need for treatment?

The patient's understanding of the illness may guide the physician's therapeutic planning

2 Orientation

Depends on both memory and attention. Tests the patient's knowledge of personal identity and present situation

Note: Questions of the Mini-Mental Status Examination are *italicized*. Normal scores: 27 to 30; dementia: less than 20; depression: intermediate scores

2.1 What is your name?

2.2 What is your occupation?

2.3 Where do you live?

2.4 Are you married?

2.4a Do you have children?

2.5 What are you doing now?

2.6 How long have you been in your present home?

2.7 Orientation to time

The passage of time is the most sensitive of all components involved in orientation; disorientation in time usually appears first, followed in more severe disturbances by disorientation for place and persons in that order

2.7a *What is the date today? (day of week, day of month, month, year, season)* (score: 5)

2.7b What time of day is it?

2.7c When was the last holiday?

2.8 Orientation to place

2.8a *Where are we? (hospital, state, county, town, floor)* (score: 5)

2.8b Where is the nurse's or secretary's desk?

2.8c Where is the bathroom?

3 Memory

Amnesia (disorders of past memory) indicates cortical disturbance of a permanent nature (brain atrophy or other gross destructive lesion), or of a transient nature (delirium, marked disorders of thinking of the affective and schizophrenic type). Memory defects appear early in organic diseases of the brain which cause dementia; memory for distant events may remain relatively unaffected until the dementia becomes gross. Major depression alone does not directly impair memory

3.1 Memory for remote past events

3.1a Tell me your birth date

3.1b When were you married?

3.1c What was your mother's maiden name?

3.1d What are the names of your children? their birth dates?

3.1e What was the name of your first school teacher?

3.1f When did you graduate from school?

3.1g What jobs have you held?

3.2   Memory for recent past experiences (in the past 24 h)

In dementia, recent memory is most affected, with faulty recall of day-to-day happenings

3.2a What did you have for breakfast today?

3.2b What were the headlines in the newspaper today?

3.2c What is my name?

3.2d When did you see me for the first time?

3.2e What tests were done yesterday?

3.3   Present, short-term, immediate memory

Recall of immediate impressions. Registration is the ability to repeat phrases or numbers to be learned. Inability to recall a list of items or a story is commonly associated with dementia, chronic alcohol abuse, and drug abuse

3.3a Please repeat these numbers after me
      • series of 3, 4, 5, 6, 7, 8 digits (at the speed of one per second)

A normal person can repeat seven to eight digits without errors

3.3b *Please listen to, and repeat the names of the three following objects* (score: 3).
      Try to remember them because I will ask for them in a little while

3.3c *(After 5 min): Please name the three objects* (score: 3)

4   General Intellectual Evaluation

The intellectual functions are invariably impaired when there is brain damage, whether focal or generalized, e.g., cerebrovascular disease, cerebral tumor, damage from head injury, generalized cortical atrophy; similar disturbances occur transiently in association with toxic or inflammatory disease of the brain

4.1   General information

4.1a Please give the names of five large cities in the United States

4.1b Please give the names of five large rivers in the United States

4.1c Please give the names of 10 fruits, 10 flowers, 10 vegetables as quickly as possible

4.1d What is the name of the capital of: this state? the United States? England? France? Italy?

4.1e What is the name of the last four presidents? their political parties?

4.2 Attention and calculation

Attention: refers to the ability to focus or concentrate over time on one task or activity

4.2a Test ability to add, subtract, multiply, divide

Capacity for sustained mental activity

4.2b *Starting from a hundred, subtract 7, and keep subtracting 7* (five steps) (score: 5)

A good test of attention, concentration, and ability to calculate; normal average time: 90 s with fewer than 4 errors. Poor performance in delirium, dementia, mental retardation, lack of education, anxiety, depression

4.2c If 5 times X equals 20, how much is X?

5   Language and Praxis

5.1 *(Point to a pencil and a watch) Please name these objects* (score: 2)

5.2 *Please repeat: "No ifs, ands, or buts"* (score: 1)

5.3 Three-stage command: *"Take a paper in your hand, fold it in half, and put it on the floor* (score: 3)

5.4 *Read the following sentence: "Close your eyes". Do what it says* (score: 1)

5.5 *Please write a sentence*

The sentence should contain a subject and a verb and should make sense (score: 1)

5.6 *Copy exactly as it is two intersecting pentagons*

All 10 angles must be present and 2 must intersect (score: 1)

5.7 Please draw a clock face complete with numbers and hands

Constructional ability: impaired in dementia; parietal lobe damage, mental retardation

6   Discrimination and Judgment

6.1   Can you state the difference or similarity between:
   • a dwarf and a child? a lie and a mistake? a tree and a bush?

Abstract reasoning: commonly disturbed in organic mental disease

6.2   Please explain the meaning of the following proverbs:
   "A stitch in time saves nine."
   "People who live in glass houses should not throw stones."

Patients with organic brain disease often treat such proverbs entirely literally and seem unaware of their underlying meaning

7   Depression

Note: Major depressive episode if at least five of the following symptoms have been present nearly every day for a period of at least 2 weeks

7.1   Do you feel depressed? (sad, blue, moody, down?)

7.1a Do you often cry?

7.2   Have you lost interest in or get less pleasure from things that you used to enjoy? Job, friends, family, sex, hobbies?

7.2a Have you had decreased contact with people? being less active in church, club, bowling, etc.?

7.2b Do you prefer to be by yourself?

7.3   Do you have to force yourself to eat?

7.3a Are you eating less than usual?

7.3b Have you had an increase in appetite?

7.3c Have you lost/gained any weight since . . .?

7.4   Do you have trouble sleeping?

7.4a Are you sleeping longer or more than usual?

7.5   Are you unable to sit still? (psychomotor agitation)

7.5a Do you have to keep moving?

7.6   Do you feel slowed down? (psychomotor retardation)

7.6a Do you have trouble moving as quickly as usual?

7.6b Is your speech slowed down?

7.7   Do you have less energy than usual to do things?

7.7a Do you get tired more easily?

7.8   Do you have feelings of guilt? which you cannot explain?

7.8a Do you have feelings of worthlessness? inadequacy? failure?

7.9   Do you have any difficulty making everyday decisions? (indecisiveness)

7.9a Do you have trouble concentrating?

7.10 Have you thought about dying or killing yourself?

Depressed patients do not resent this question and are often relieved to be able to admit their feelings

8   Generalized Anxiety

8.1   Do you feel anxious? frightened? tense? nervous?

8.2   Are you bothered by
      • difficulty falling asleep? palpitations? shortness of breath? sweating? dizziness? muscular tension? worrying much of the time about things that might happen?

8.3   Anxiety attacks

8.3a Do you have attacks when you suddenly feel very frightened? with sudden intense anxiety? shortness of breath? palpitations? chest pains? choking? dizziness? tingling? sweating? faintness? fear of dying?

9   Special Preoccupations and Experiences

9.1   Are there any thoughts that come to your mind over and over again and which you feel are abnormal?

Obsessions: persistent intrusive thoughts

9.2   Do you have to repeat some act over and over which you cannot resist repeating? like constantly washing your hands? checking on things? assuring yourself that the light has been turned off? the door has been locked?

Compulsions: intrusive behaviors: in obsessive-compulsive neurosis; minor variations of this neurosis are extremely common

9.3   Do you have irrational fears of animals? heights? elevators? closed places? crowds? certain animals (reptiles, insects, rodents)? being closed in? going out alone?

Phobia: irrational fear of a specific object, activity, or situation which the patient tends to avoid; the irrational nature of the uncontrollable thoughts, acts, or phobias is recognized by the patient (mild phobias are frequent)

9.4   Do you hear voices or things that are not there or that other people cannot hear?

9.4a Do you see things that are invisible to other people?

9.4b Do you notice strange or unusual smells that other people do not notice?

Hallucinations: perceptions of auditory, visual, olfactory, or tactile sensations in the absence of identifiable external stimulation. In metabolic encephalopathy; delirium; certain psychotic states (hallucinations in schizophrenia are usually auditory only)

9.5   Do you believe that people are trying to harm you?

9.5a   Do you believe that you have a great mission in life?

9.5b   Do you believe that your thoughts and actions are being controlled or broadcast to others?

Delusions: false belief in which the patient persists in spite of demonstrations of its falseness. Common in many psychiatric illnesses, particularly manic-depressive and schizophrenia states; in dementing illnesses; in chronic infections of the CNS

SELECTED BIBLIOGRAPHY

Frazier SH (ed): Anxiety and depression. *Med Clin North Am* 72:743–977, 1988.

MacKinnon RA, Yudofsky SC: *The psychiatric evaluation in clinical practice.* Philadelphia: Lippincott, 1986.

Rovner BW, Folstein MF: Mini-mental state exam in clinical practice. *Hosp Pract* 22(1A):99–110, 1987.

36
Sleep Disorders

INTRODUCTION

Insomnia   Persistent difficulty falling or staying asleep that compromises daytime functioning.
Hypersomnia   Excessive daytime sleepiness.
Parasomnias   Dysfunctions associated with sleep or specific sleep stages.

There are two kinds of sleep: the REM sleep and the NREM (non-REM) sleep. The REM sleep is characterized by tumultuous brain activity, rapid eye movements (REM), and simultaneous muscular paralysis (paradoxical sleep). The NREM sleep lacks rapid eye movements; it is divided into four separate stages on the basis of the EEG record; during NREM sleep the brain is resting. REM sleep alternates with NREM sleep approximately every 90 to 100 min, the first REM period usually occurring about 90 to 100 min after the onset of sleep. In a normal individual NREM sleep always comes first. Five sleep cycles represent an average night's sleep. About three-fourths of the night are spent in NREM sleep. Cerebral oxygen metabolism, which is always depressed with coma or anesthesia, remains equivalent to waking levels during natural sleep.

The majority of cases of insomnia are secondary to psychologic disturbances or are associated with another disease, including any condition in which pain and physical discomfort are important symptoms. Most insomniacs have normal-appearing polysomnograms. Narcoleptic patients are subject to either complete or partial sleep attacks which begin with REM sleep rather than with the usual NREM sleep observed in normal subjects. In contrast to narcolepsy, the excessive sleep of hypersomnia is not irresistible but is usually much longer (hours to days). The sleep-stage pattern of hypersomniac patients resembles normal sleep except in terms of duration. Hypersomnia may be primary or, more often, secondary to organic neurologic or metabolic diseases.

ETIOLOGY

Insomnia

Psychophysiologic:* situational or persistent
Psychiatric disorders
Drug dependency or withdrawal;* chronic alcoholism*
Sleep-induced respiratory impairment: sleep apnea syndrome; alveolar hypoventilation syndrome
Sleep-related (nocturnal) myoclonus and "restless legs" syndromes
Medical, toxic, or environmental conditions: fever, pain, cardiopulmonary disease

*Common cause

Hypersomnia

Psychophysiologic: situational or persistent
Psychiatric disorders
Drugs and alcohol
Sleep-induced respiratory impairment: sleep apnea syndrome; alveolar hypoventilation syndrome (with obesity: Pickwickian syndrome)
Sleep-related (nocturnal) myoclonus and "restless legs" syndromes
Narcolepsy-cataplexy
Medical, toxic, environmental conditions: uremia, liver failure, severe hypothyroidism, chronic pulmonary disease with hypercapnia, diabetes mellitus with incipient coma or with severe hypoglycemia; central nervous system disorders; encephalitis
Idiopathic CNS hypersomnolence; Kleine-Levin syndrome

Disorders of the Sleep-Wake Schedule

Transient: jet lag; work shift
Persistent: delayed or advanced sleep phase syndrome

Parasomnias

Sleep walking; sleep terror; enuresis; others

Iatrogenic Causes of Sleep Disorders

Sleep disturbances: anorexiants; levodopa; monoamine oxidase inhibitors; sympathomimetics; caffeine; analeptics, amphetamine
Withdrawal insomnia: from chronic high-dose use of hypnotics
Drowsiness: anxiolytic drugs: major tranquilizers, tricyclic antidepressants; antihistamines; methyldopa; clonidine, reserpine

HISTORY TAKING*

Note: Observations by the bed partner of snoring, partial arousing, or kicking may suggest a more specific diagnosis

Possible meaning of a positive response

Insomnia

1   Duration of the Insomnia

1.1   How long have you been unable to sleep at night?
• acute insomnia? (up to several days)   Jet lag; anxiety before a highly stressful event
• short-term insomnia? (lasting less than 3 weeks)   Situational stress and anxiety; severe personal loss; acute illness

*In this section, items in *italics* are characteristic clinical features.

• persistent? (for months or years)	Underlying medical or psychologic cause (depression)

2 Character and Severity of the Insomnia

2.1 How many hours do you sleep at night?	Many patients who complain of insomnia far overestimate their actual time awake
2.2 *Do you have difficulty falling asleep?*	In patients with anxiety and obsessive disorders
2.2a Do you awake 2 to 3 hours after sleep onset?	Situational insomnia: anxiety; emotional cause (sick individuals may show no evidence of anxiety or depressive disorder); use of drugs or alcohol; painful or debilitating medical illness; periodic movements of legs; nonobstructive sleep apnea. The pattern of insomnia helps relatively little in estimating its seriousness as a symptom
2.3 *Do you fall asleep easily but wake up too early in the morning?*	Depression (or anxiety); abuse of CNS depressants; situational insomnia; also in the elderly: frequently reflects a declining need for sleep

(Note: The patterns 2.2 and 2.3 may appear singly or in combination)

2.4 Do you have daytime drowsiness?	Clinically significant sleep deprivation with impaired performance; periodic leg movements of sleep. May be a symptom of hypersomnia with sleep apnea or narcolepsy. Excessive daytime sleepiness may result from inappropriate dosage or scheduling of hypnotics

3 Precipitating or Aggravating Factors

3.1 Have you recently had an acute work-shift change? a rapid time-zone change?	Jet lag: due to both sleep deprivation and the circadian phase-shift change
3.2 Do you engage in strenuous physical activity during the day?	Excessive fatigue may give rise to abnormal muscular sensations which delay the onset of sleep
3.3 Do you engage in vigorous mental activity late at night?	May contribute to difficulty falling asleep
3.4 Do you drink much coffee, tea in the afternoon? before retiring?	Caffeine and stimulant xanthines producing insomnia
3.5 At night, do you have • pain?	The pain may keep the patient awake

• in the spine?	Vertebral lesion
• in the abdomen?	Gastroesophageal reflux; duodenal ulcer
• in the chest?	Nocturnal angina pectoris; gastroesophageal reflux
• shortness of breath?	Unrecognized orthopnea due to heart disease; asthmatic attack
• frequent disturbing dreams? excessive night-time noise or heat? cough? pruritus? diarrhea? tinnitus? nocturia?	Any of these conditions may disturb sleep and awaken the patient

3.6	*Are you awakened about 2 to 3 h after falling asleep by headaches?* (unilateral? orbital?)	Cluster headache
3.7	Do you take afternoon naps?	Elderly patients often complain of insomnia as a consequence of taking several naps during the day

4   Accompanying Symptoms

4.1	During sleep, do you have (or has your bedpartner observed) • repetitive dorsiflexion of the foot and big toe? • jerking movements of your legs? (flexion of the knee and hip) recurring every 20 to 30 s? (lasting about 2 s each)	Periodic movements of sleep (nocturnal myoclonus), usually during NREM sleep: in middle-aged persons with drug-dependency insomnia, sleep apnea, narcolepsy-cataplexy
4.2	Do you feel • an irresistible urge to move the legs, when sitting or lying down, especially prior to sleep? • a discomfort deep inside the calves? alleviated by moving, exercising, or walking about?	Restless legs syndrome: interferes with sleep onset and may recur during the night
4.3	Do you feel anxious? depressed?	Insomnia secondary to psychologic disorder
4.4	Do you have • headache? lethargy? unsatisfactory daytime performance?	May be due to sleep pathology
	• chronic fatigue? irritability?	May become persistent or worsened by worry about sleep loss. The complaints may be due to underlying depression

4.5   Do you have
         • sleepwalking?

Somnambulism: occurs normally in children and adolescents: in stage III or IV of NREM sleep. Psychopathology may be found if the episodes begin or persist into adulthood

         • frightening or "bad" dreams?
             • with detailed dream recall?

Nightmares: occur during REM sleep; in adolescence and adulthood: recurrent nightmares are suggestive of psychopathologic causes

             • without recall of the episode?

Night terrors: psychopathology suspected if onset is in adulthood

5   Iatrogenic Factors   See Etiology

5.1   Do you use hypnotics? sedatives? tranquilizers?
         • regularly and chronically?

As tolerance develops with continuous use, the sleep promoting properties of such drugs are lost

5.1a Have you recently stopped using hypnotics?

Withdrawal from hypnotic agents may cause both insomnia and nightmares

6   Personal and Social Profile

6.1   What is your consumption of alcohol?

Heavy and sustained ingestion of alcohol severely disrupts sleep-stage organization: REM sleep periods are shortened and nightly awakenings occur. In the abstaining alcoholic, abnormal sleep patterns may persist for many weeks

6.2   Has your sleep difficulty affected your work or social life?

Insomniacs may avoid family and social interactions by insisting they are too tired

7   Personal Antecedents Pertaining to the Insomnia

7.1   Do you have
         • personal, familial, professional problems?
         • a psychiatric condition?

Psychoneuroses and psychoses commonly produce sleeplessness

         • paroxysmal nocturnal dyspnea? nocturnal asthma? a rheumatic illness? a gastrointestinal illness?

Hypersomnla

1   Duration of the Hypersomnia

1.1   How long have you felt sleepy all
       day?
       • since adolescence?   The narcolepsy-cataplexy syndrome
                                               may begin in childhood and persist
                                               throughout life
       • of recent onset?   Structural nervous system disease

2   Character of the Hypersomnia

2.1   Do you have
       • an irresistible urge to sleep dur-
         ing the day?   Hypersomnia (excess daytime sleepi-
       • excessive yawning?   ness is sometimes confused with a lack
       • increased total sleep time over a   of energy, weariness, or depression)
         24-hour period?

2.1a   Do you have difficulty fully waking   Sleep drunkenness in hypersomnia
       in the morning?

2.2   How many hours do you sleep at   Inadequate sleep is a common cause of
       night?   excess daytime sleepiness

2.3   Do you have recurrent attacks of
       irresistible sleepiness   Narcolepsy-cataplexy syndrome with
       • at any time of the day? lasting   sleep-onset REM attacks. Attacks often
         about 15 min? since adoles-   precipitated by boredom, but also occur
         cence?   inappropriately during athletics, while
                                               driving an automobile, or during coitus
2.3a   Do you awake refreshed after the
       attack of sleep?

2.3b   Between attacks, are you sleepy?
       inattentive?
                                               Narcolepsy-cataplexy syndrome
2.3c   Is nocturnal sleep usually disturbed
       by frequent awakening?

2.4   Has your bed partner observed   Sleep-induced respiratory impairment
       • intermittent inspiratory snoring?   (sleep apnea-hypersomnia syndrome).
         alternating with periods of ap-   Stages III and IV of NREM sleep are
         nea?   decreased. Periods of apnea lasting from
       • talking while asleep? (somnilo-   10 to 60 s or more may result in oxygen
         quy)   desaturation and cardiac arrhythmias.
                                               Patients with obstructive sleep apnea
                                               often are unaware of their many sleep-
                                               time obstructive arousals

2.4a Do you awake unrefreshed? still sleepy? with a generalized headache?	In sleep apnea-hypersomnia syndrome

3 Accompanying Symptoms

3.1 Do you sometimes experience • a sudden loss of muscle power provoked by strong emotion? anger? laughter? fear? surprise?	Cataplexy: total flaccid paralysis without loss of consciousness; in about 70 percent of narcoleptic patients
• when falling asleep (or at awakening): • an inability to move or speak? • visual or auditory hallucinations?	Sleep paralysis in narcolepsy Hypnagogic (at sleep onset) or hypnosomnic (on awakening) hallucinations in narcolepsy
3.2 Do you have • attacks of excessive sleepiness lasting for a few days to several weeks? • with excessive eating? disturbances in mood? disorientation? sexual hyperactivity?	Kleine-Levin syndrome (rare): in adolescent males
• headaches? vomiting? loss of muscular strength in a limb?	Brain tumor (a central nervous system lesion may produce chronic hypersomnia)
• intolerance to cold?	Hypothyroidism, if severe, may cause hypersomnia

4 Personal and Social Profile

4.1 Has your excessive sleepiness provoked poor school performances? accidents? job disruptions? depression?	Narcolepsy-cataplexy has severe psychosocial consequences and may lead to social withdrawal. The patient is often accused of malingering or of being lazy

5 Personal Antecedents Pertaining to the Hypersomnia

5.1 Have you ever had a head injury? a brain inflammation? encephalitis?	CNS lesion producing hypersomnia
5.2 Do you have a renal illness? a liver illness? a chronic pulmonary disease?	May cause excessive somnolence

6 Family Medical History Pertaining to the Hypersomnia

6.1 Are there similar cases in your family?	A family history of disorders of excessive sleep is often present in narcolepsy and hypersomnia

PHYSICAL SIGNS PERTAINING TO SLEEP DISORDERS

	Possible significance
Periorbital puffiness; cold coarse skin, delayed relaxation phase of the tendon reflexes	Hypothyroidism with sleepiness; hypothyroid myxedema with sleep apnea-hypersomnia syndrome
Obesity; cyanosis; periodic respiration; drowsiness	Approximately two-thirds of the patients with the sleep apnea-hypoventilation syndrome are obese
Enlarged tonsils or adenoids; mandibular abnormalities; pharyngeal soft tissue alterations	May cause narrowing of the upper airway with obstructive apnea in the sleep apnea-hypersomnia syndrome; in acromegaly; hypothyroid myxedema

LABORATORY PROCEDURES PERTAINING TO SLEEP DISORDERS

Procedure	To Detect
Polysomnography	Sleep apnea; idiopathic insomnia; narcolepsy
EEG	Structural brain lesion producing hypersomnia
Psychologic evaluation*	Anxiety state; depression

*When indicated

SELECTED BIBLIOGRAPHY

Gillin JC, Byerley WF: The diagnosis and management of insomnia. *N Engl J Med* 322:239–248, 1990.
Gross PT: Evaluation of sleep disorders. *Med Clin North Am* 70:1349–1360, 1986.
Kales A, Soldatos CR, Kales JD: Taking a sleep history. *Am Fam Physician* 22(2): 101–107, 1980.
Kales A, Soldatos CR, Kales JD: Sleep disorders: Insomnia, sleepwalking, night terrors, nightmares, and enuresis. *Ann Intern Med* 106:582–592, 1987.

37
Syncope

INTRODUCTION

Syncope (Faint)   Generalized weakness of muscles with loss of postural tone, inability to stand upright, and temporary loss of consciousness.

Syncope results from a transient impairment in cerebral metabolism as a consequence of essential energy substrates deprivation. This deprivation may be due to a decrease in cerebral blood flow or to insufficient concentration of oxygen or glucose in the blood perfusing the brain. Decreased cerebral blood flow may be caused by arterial hypotension, diminished cardiac output, or obstruction to cerebral blood flow. A decrease in blood pressure may result from a decrease in peripheral vascular resistance or failure of vasoconstrictive reflexes. The ordinary vasovagal (vasodepressor) syncope appears to be due to a decrease in splanchnic and extremity vascular resistance with sudden excess of vagal activity; the loss of consciousness usually occurs when the systolic pressure falls to 70 mmHg or below. Cardiac output may be reduced as a consequence of decreased stroke volume (diminished cardiac contractility, decreased cardiac filling), arrhythmias, or anatomic obstructive lesions (aortic stenosis, pulmonary hypertension). Cerebral arterial obstruction generally due to arteriosclerosis is one of the less common causes of syncope. An inadequate oxygen or glucose concentration in the blood delivered to the brain may cause loss of consciousness which generally persists longer than in the other types of syncope. More than one mechanism may be involved in syncope. Hyperventilation with resulting hypocapnia simultaneously produces cerebral vasoconstriction and peripheral vasodilatation. Carotid sinus hypersensitivity may occur in a cardioinhibitory (bradycardia) type, a vasodepressor (hypotension without bradycardia) type, and a possible rare central (without bradycardia) type.

ETIOLOGY

Neurogenic (Defective Vasoconstrictor Mechanisms)

Vasovagal (vasodepressor) syncope*
Postural (orthostatic) hypotension:* peripheral neuropathies; primary autonomic insufficiency; prolonged bed rest; physical deconditioning; varicose veins; pregnancy; postsympathectomy; drugs*
Hypovolemia: bleeding, external or internal; sodium loss
Reflex: cough; micturition; acute painful states; carotid sinus hypersensitivity

Cardiac Dysfunction

Disturbances of rate and rhythm: bradyarrhythmias; tachyarrhythmias; conduction abnormalities

*Common causes

Reduced cardiac output
  Obstructive lesions: aortic stenosis; hypertrophic cardiomyopathy; pulmonic valve
    stenosis; primary pulmonary hypertension; pulmonary embolism; tetralogy of
    Fallot; atrial myxoma or thrombus; cardiac tamponade
  Massive myocardial infarction; cardiomyopathy

Defective Quality of Blood to the Brain

Hypoxia; anemia; hyperventilation with hypocapnia; hypoglycemia

Cerebral Disorders

Cerebrovascular disturbances: vertebrobasilar transient ischemic attacks; hypertensive
  encephalopathy
Seizures
Hysterical seizures

Iatrogenic Causes of Syncope

Orthostatic hypotension: vasodilators; antihypertensives, diuretics; nitrates; calcium
  channel blockers; levodopa; phenothiazines, tricyclic antidepressants
Drug-induced ventricular tachycardia (with prolonged Q-T interval and torsades de
  pointes): quinine, disopyramide, procainamide; phenothiazines, tricyclic anti-
  depressants
Digitalis: heart block, drug-induced tachyarrhythmias
Insulin, oral hypoglycemic agents: hypoglycemia
Anticoagulants: acute internal hemorrhage

HISTORY TAKING*

Possible meaning of a positive response

1   Mode of Onset and Duration

1.1   When did your syncope occur?

1.1a What was your body position or posture?	Most syncope occurs when the patient is in the upright position, sitting or standing (exception: Stokes-Adams attacks)
1.2 Do you have recurrent episodes of syncope?	In a young adult: vasovagal syncope (the most usual form of syncope); epilepsy; hypoglycemia; postural hypotension; hysteria

*In this section, items in *italics* are characteristic clinical features, and items in **boldface** are
potentially life-threatening or urgent conditions.

In a middle-aged or elderly patient: complete heart block; aortic stenosis; myocardial dysfunction; cardiac arrhythmia; pulmonary emboli; postural hypotension; chronic postganglionic autonomic insufficiency; carotid sinus syncope; cerebrovascular arterial disease; cough and micturition syncope (If single episode in elderly, consider silent myocardial infarction)

In a young woman (showing little concern about her fainting episodes): hysteria

1.2a In case of recurrent episodes of unconsciousness: How long and how frequently have you had syncopes?

Several per day, per month: epilepsy, Stokes-Adams attacks, other cardiac arrhythmias

1.3 Is the onset of the syncope
   • sudden? abrupt? (over 1 or 2 seconds)

Arrhythmia: sudden **atrio-ventricular block, ventricular tachycardia or fibrillation;** carotid sinus syncope; epilepsy

   • rapid? (a few seconds)

Vasovagal syncope; postural hypotension

   • gradual? (over several minutes)

Hyperventilation; **hypoglycemia**

1.4 Do you feel weak? without loss of consciousness?

Faintness (incomplete faint): anxiety; hyperventilation; hypoglycemia; cerebral ischemic attacks; drop attack

1.5 Do you lose consciousness? Do you slump on the floor?

Full syncope: alteration of consciousness progressing to complete syncope

1.6 What is the duration of the unconsciousness?
   • a few seconds to a few minutes?

Vasovagal syncope; carotid sinus syncope; postural hypotension

   • more than a few minutes? (but less than 1 h)

Aortic stenosis; hysteria; hypoglycemia; hyperventilation

2 Precipitating or Aggravating Factors

2.1 *What were you doing during the hours or minutes preceding the faint?*

Vasovagal syncope occurs in conditions which favor peripheral vasodilatation: sight of an accident, blood; hot, crowded rooms; emotional stress

2.2 Does the loss of consciousness occur
   • *only in a standing, sitting position?*

Faintness associated with a decline in blood pressure; orthostatic hypotension; vasovagal syncope; ectopic tachycardia; carotid sinus attack

• *upon suddenly arising from a recumbent to a standing position?*	Orthostatic hypotension; hypertrophic obstructive cardiomyopathy
• *after prolonged standing?*	Pooling of blood in the lower extremities and viscera without compensatory reflex peripheral vasoconstriction; vasovagal hypotension; orthostatic hypotension; hypertrophic obstructive cardiomyopathy
• *in any body position? while recumbent?*	Most probably not vasovagal syncope; Stokes-Adams syncope; hypoglycemia; hyperventilation; epilepsy; partial complex seizure
• upon bending, leaning? *when leaning over?* (as to tie a shoe lace)	Left atrial myxoma; ball-valve thrombus: with movements of the tumor or clot into, and obstruction of, the left ventricular inflow tract and sudden reduction of cardiac output
• *during or immediately after exertion?*	Any form of obstruction to left ventricular outflow; aortic stenosis; hypertrophic obstructive cardiomyopathy; arrhythmia; cyanotic congenital heart disease; primary pulmonary hypertension; in elderly subjects: postural hypotension
• after upper extremity exertion?	Subclavian steal syndrome: decreased vascular resistance in the arm during exercise with redirection of flow away from the brain
• *during or following an emotional stress?* (fright, anxiety, pain, surgical instrumentation, sight of blood)	Vasovagal syncope; hyperventilation
• after severe coughing paroxysms?	"Tussive syncope": in overweight middle-aged or elderly men with chronic obstructive pulmonary disease or a history of heavy alcohol abuse: prolonged Valsalva maneuver: increased intrathoracic pressure interfering with the venous return to the heart; hypertrophic obstructive cardiomyopathy
• during or after micturition? defecation?	A form of reflex syncope; usually in the elderly after arising from bed at night: rapid release of intravesical pressure causes sudden, reflex vasodilatation of the peripheral vasculature, augmented by standing and orthostatic hypotension
• on sudden movements of the head? when wearing a tight collar? shaving the neck?	Carotid sinus hypersensitivity

3   Relieving Factors

3.1   Can you avert an impending faint
       by
       • *promptly lying down?*   Vasovagal syncope; postural syncope;
                                         most types of syncope, except anxiety
                                         attacks, hyperventilation
       • eating?   Hypoglycemia

4   Prodromal and Accompanying Symptoms

4.1   Is the syncope preceded by
       • lightheadedness?   giddiness?   Faintness: usually precedes full syn-
       weakness? nausea? sweating?   cope: presyncopal symptoms of de-
       yawning? visual spots? dim vi-   creased cerebral blood flow and au-
       sion? ringing in the ears? a sensa- tonomic hyperactivity in vasovagal
       tion of impending loss of con-   syncope. Absence of prodromal symp-
       sciousness?   toms suggests a sudden fall in cardiac
                                           output
       • palpitations?   Ectopic tachycardia; hypoglycemia; hy-
                                         perventilation; anxiety
       • chest pain?   Cardiac origin of syncope; myocardial
                                         ischemia associated with arrhythmias;
                                         aortic stenosis; hypertrophic obstructive
                                         cardiomyopathy
       • deep sighing? numbness, tingling Hyperventilation
       in the hands? face?
       • a sensation of hunger? weak-   Hypoglycemia (faintness rather than
       ness? mental confusion? sweat-   true syncope)
       ing?
       • unilateral weakness? unilateral Cerebral ischemic attack
       numbness?   dizziness?   thick
       speech? aphasia? confusion?

4.2   *Do you have no warning of any sort*   Stokes-Adams syndrome; arrhythmia;
       before the fainting spell?   carotid sinus syncope; epileptic attack

4.3   After the loss of consciousness:
       • do (did) you lie motionless?   Usually in syncope
       • do (did) you have
         • convulsive movements?   Epilepsy; clonic muscle contractions
                                          can also occur in syncope, if uncon-
                                          sciousness persists for 15 to 20 s
         • loss of urine? feces? biting of Frequent in epilepsy, rare in syncope
         the tongue?

4.4   Do (did) you regain full conscious-
       ness
       • *promptly?*   Syncope
       • slowly?   Seizure disorder

4.5   Did you hurt yourself when falling to the ground during a fainting spell?

Common in epilepsy; occasionally syncope of cardiac origin; rare in emotional disturbances; absent in hysteria. In elderly patients, fracture or other trauma due to the fall is the chief hazard of a faint

4.6   Following a syncopal attack, do you have
• headache? drowsiness? mental confusion?

Do not follow a syncopal attack. Common in seizure disorders with postictal confusional state. The patient with syncope awakens feeling weak but mentally clear, without headache or drowsiness (slight confusion in Stokes-Adams attacks)

• a slurred speech? transitory paralysis?

Epilepsy; may occur in Stokes-Adams syndrome; cerebral arterial occlusive disease

4.7   Prior to, or after the faint, did you notice the passage of black, tarry stools?

Acute gastrointestinal hemorrhage with syncope

4.8   Do you have impotence? sphincter disturbances? absence of sweating?

Chronic autonomic insufficiency with orthostatic hypotension; autonomic neuropathy (diabetic, others)

4.9   Questions for witnesses of the syncope: Did the patient have any turning of the eyes or head? any twitching of the face or extremities?

Epileptic seizure

4.9a Was the patient's skin *sweaty? pale?* or blue?

Pallor is usual with disorders of the peripheral circulation; cyanosis suggests epilepsy

5   Iatrogenic Factors   See Etiology

6   Personal and Social Profile

6.1   What is your alcohol consumption? Do you use (illicit) drugs?

Severe alcohol or drug intoxication may be accompanied by "passing out," a state of deep, barely arousable sleep

7   Personal Antecedents Pertaining to the Syncope

7.1   Do you have any of the following conditions: epilepsy? any neurologic disease? hypertension? prior sympathectomy?
• anemia? fever? a cardiac disease?

Factors which increase the possibility of vasovagal syncope in susceptible individuals

- (Prior to the blackout): poor physical condition? excessive fatigue?
- diabetes?

- Parkinson's disease?

Factors which increase the possibility of vasovagal syncope in susceptible individuals
Iatrogenic hypoglycemia; diabetic neuropathy may cause postural hypotension
Shy-Drager syndrome (idiopathic autonomic failure) with chronic orthostatic hypotension

8   Family Medical History Pertaining to the Syncope

8.1   Are there members of your family who have fainting spells?

Chronic autonomic insufficiency with orthostatic hypotension may be familial; hypertrophic obstructive cardiomyopathy; ventricular tachyarrhythmias associated with Q-T prolongation. A family history of epilepsy is positive in approximately 4 percent of patients with convulsive disorders

PHYSICAL SIGNS PERTAINING TO SYNCOPE

Possible significance

Pallor without cyanosis

Disorder of the peripheral circulation. Pallor is an early finding in all types of syncope, except: chronic postganglionic autonomic insufficiency, anxiety attacks, hyperventilation syndrome

Pallor, cyanosis, dyspnea, distended jugular veins

Disorder of cardiac function with reduced cerebral blood flow

Bradycardia (<40 beats per minute)

Complete atrioventricular block with Stokes-Adams attacks; sick-sinus syndrome; vasovagal syncope

Tachycardia (>160 beats per minute)

Ectopic cardiac rhythm; paroxysmal tachycardia

Significant differences in blood pressures and pulses of the patient's arms

Subclavian steal syndrome

Lack of change in pulse and blood pressure or color of the skin

Hysterical fainting

Attempts to reproduce the attacks:
   Valsalva maneuver

Tussive syncope

   Having the patient breathe rapidly and deeply for 2 to 3 min

Hyperventilation

   Carotid sinus massage (with caution)

May reveal carotid sinus hypersensitivity

Response of blood pressure, pulse rate, and symptoms to standing:

Replication of symptoms with hypotension (systolic blood pressure <100 mmHg) and:

Bradycardia	Carotid sinus syndrome; vasovagal syncope; sick-sinus syndrome
Increased pulse rate	Hypovolemia: diuretics, salt and water deprivation, adrenal insufficiency
Unchanged pulse rate	Chronic autonomic insufficiency
Heart murmurs	Aortic stenosis; hypertrophic obstructive cardiomyopathy; tetralogy of Fallot; primary pulmonary hypertension; left atrial myxoma; ball-valve thrombus
Muscle weakness; depressed or absent deep-tendon reflexes	Neuropathy with chronic orthostatic hypotension
Focal neurologic deficits, dysarthria, carotid bruits	Cerebral arterial occlusive disease with ischemic attacks
Tremor, extrapyramidal rigidity, pupillary paralysis, anhydrosis	Shy-Drager syndrome with chronic preganglionic autonomic insufficiency and orthostatic hypotension
Tachycardia, sweating, tremulousness	Hypoglycemia
Rectal examination	May reveal gastrointestinal hemorrhage

LABORATORY PROCEDURES PERTAINING TO SYNCOPE

Procedure	To Detect
ECG	Arrhythmia, ischemia, preexcitation syndrome, heart block
Ambulatory ECG monitoring	Rhythm disorders and conduction disturbances responsible for the syncopal episodes
Intracardiac electrophysiologic studies*	Rapid ventricular tachycardia; His bundle conduction delays; sick-sinus syndrome; atrial flutter
Echocardiography*	Hypertrophic obstructive cardiomyopathy; left atrial myxoma; ball-valve thrombus
EEG, head CT scan*	For patients with focal neurologic findings or a history compatible with seizure disorder

*When indicated

SELECTED BIBLIOGRAPHY

Adams RD, Victor M: Faintness and syncope, in *Principles of Neurology*, 4th ed., pp. 291–301, New York: McGraw-Hill, 1989.

Dohrmann ML, Cheitlin MD: Cardiogenic syncope. Seizure versus syncope. *Neurol Clin* 4(3):549–562, 1986.

Mader SL: Orthostatic hypotension. *Med Clin North Am* 73(6):1337–1349, 1989.

von Dohlen TW, Frank MJ: Presyncope and syncope. *Postgrad Med* 86(2):85–96, 1989.

INTRODUCTION

Vertigo   An illusion of self- or environmental movement, most commonly a rotation.

Impulses from the retinas, the labyrinths, the proprioceptors of joints and muscles maintain balanced posture and awareness of the body's position in relation to its surroundings. The cerebellum, the vestibular nuclei, the oculomotor nucleus and the red nucleus in the brainstem, and certain ganglionic centers in the basal ganglia integrate these sensory data and provide for postural adjustment and locomotion.

Generally the problem of vertigo resolves itself into deciding whether it has its origin in the labyrinth, in the vestibular division of the eighth cranial nerve, or in the vestibular nuclei and their immediate connections with other structures in the brainstem. Labyrinthine lesions are the usual causes of paroxysmal vertigo (Ménière's disease, vestibular neuronitis). Vertigo of acoustic nerve origin (acoustic neuroma) is usually mild and intermittent. The association of vertigo with auditory signs and symptoms indicates an aural or eighth nerve lesion. In vertigo of brainstem origin, auditory function is nearly always spared, since the vestibular and cochlear fibers separate upon entering the medulla and pons. Central causes of vertigo are associated with signs of involvement of other structures within the brain.

Giddiness (pseudovertigo) is a sensation of uncertainty or lightheadedness, without a feeling of rotation or impulsion. It is frequently of circulatory or psychologic origin.

ETIOLOGY

Physiologic Vertigo

Motion sickness; height vertigo; space sickness

Peripheral Causes Ear or Eighth Cranial Nerve)

Ménière's disease*; benign paroxysmal positional vertigo; vestibular neuronitis*
Cerebellopontine-angle tumors; acoustic neuroma
Tumors of middle ear and inner ear, cholesteatoma
Middle ear trauma
Ototoxic drugs*
Otitis media; chronic otomastoiditis; otosclerosis; impacted cerumen
Head injury:* temporal bone fracture
Perilymphatic fistula (following head trauma)

Central Causes (Brainstem or Cerebellum)

Brainstem tumors; cerebellar tumors
Demyelinating diseases; multiple sclerosis

*Common cause

Vascular: vertebrobasilar insufficiency*
Drugs
Infections: brain abscess; meningoencephalitis; herpes zoster (Ramsay-Hunt syndrome)
Temporal lobe epilepsy
Cervical origin: neck trauma; upper cervical sensory root irritation
Ocular disturbances; ocular muscle paralysis

Pseudovertigo (Without Sensation of Motion)

Psychogenic: depression; anxiety; hyperventilation syndrome; introspective persons
Cardiovascular disorders: cardiac diseases; arrhythmias; hypertension; postural dizziness (unstable vasomotor reflexes); hyperactive carotid reflex
Anemia; emphysema; posttraumatic; hypoglycemia

Iatrogenic Causes of Vertigo or Giddiness

Antihypertensive drugs (particularly guanethidine); neomycin; dilantin (toxic doses); quinine; salicylates (large doses); aminoglycosides; ristocetin; viomycin; polymyxins; tobramycin; vancomycin; minocycline; diuretics: ethacrynic acid, furosemide; sedatives; anticonvulsants (large doses)

HISTORY TAKING*

Possible meaning of a positive response

1   Character of the Dizziness

1.1   During your dizzy spell, do you feel
• *a rotating sensation? a rotation of your surroundings? "spinning"?*
• *a sensation of lateral pulsion when walking?*

True vertigo; a rotational sensation and a feeling of impulsion are particularly characteristic of vertigo. Usually: disturbance in the vestibular system

1.2   Does the spell consist of
• "lightheadedness"? giddiness? without rotatory sensation, sense of motion?

Pseudovertigo

• staggering? a sensation of imbalance? "dizziness in the feet"?

Disequilibrium (to be distinguished from vertigo): suggests cerebellar, proprioceptive, or motor abnormalities

2   Mode of Onset and Chronology

2.1   How long have you had dizzy spells?

Acute process: lesion of middle ear; basilar insufficiency
Chronic process: Ménière's disease

*In this section, items in *italics* are characteristic clinical features.

2.2   Do you have
      • repeated episodes of vertigo?   Acute and recurrent peripheral vestibu-
                                               lopathy; chronicity: Ménière's disease;
                                               benign positional vertigo. If single at-
                                               tack: acute etiology, inflammation or
                                               infection of middle ear; vestibular neu-
                                               ronitis

      • persistent dizziness?   Chronic suppurative otitis with labyrin-
                                               thine fistula; acoustic neuroma

2.3   How long does an episode of dizzi-
      ness last?
      • a few seconds? less than 1 min?   Benign positional vertigo; almost al-
                                               ways precipitated by movements of the
                                               head into a certain position
      • from minutes to hours?   Labyrinthine disease; Ménière's disease
      • from hours to days?   Vestibular neuronitis; Ménière's disease
      • for days to weeks?   Chronic suppurative otitis with labyrin-
                                               thine fistula; acoustic neuroma; toxic
                                               labyrinthitis; brainstem origin

2.4   Was the onset of vertigo
      • *abrupt?*   Usually in true vertigo: Ménière's dis-
                                               ease; vestibular neuronitis
      • gradual? insidious?   Central pathology: multiple sclerosis;
                                               brainstem or cerebellar neoplasm;
                                               acoustic neuroma; benign positional
                                               vertigo; pseudovertigo

3   Intensity of the Vertigo

3.1   Is your attack of vertigo
      • usually mild?   Acoustic neuroma; central vertigo is
                                               generally less severe than peripheral
                                               vertigo
      • intense? severe enough to con-   Ménière's disease; vestibular neuronitis
        fine you to bed or resting posi-   (the nearer the pathology is to the pe-
        tion?   ripheral labyrinthine system, the more
                                               severe the vertigo)

3.2   Does your dizziness progress grad-   Acoustic neuroma
      ually in intensity?

3.2a Do the attacks
      • become more frequent? more
        disabling?   } Natural course of Ménière's disease
      • have less warning?

4   Precipitating or Aggravating Factors

4.1   Do you have dizziness
      • only on change of position? on   Vertigo originating from pathology in
        rolling over in bed?   the vestibular system of the dependent
                                               ear: Ménière's disease; vestibular neu-
                                               ronitis; benign positional vertigo

- when the head is positioned to one side? tilting the head back to look up?
- when coughing? sneezing? straining? (Valsalva maneuvers)
- *on abrupt arising from a recumbent or sitting position?*

Vertigo originating from pathology in the vestibular system of the dependent ear

Perilymphatic fistula: may occur following trauma

Postural dizziness (without a feeling of rotation or impulse): may occur in normal persons or in individuals in poor physical condition, in many elderly persons, in persons convalescing from debilitating illness

- on standing?

Postural dizziness with orthostatic hypotension

- on sudden head movement? on stooping over?

Benign positional vertigo; other vestibular disorders in which vertigo is present at other times; vascular insufficiency, vertebrobasilar involvement

5 Accompanying Symptoms

5.1 Is your dizzy spell accompanied by
- nausea? vomiting? profuse sweating?

Autonomic symptoms frequently accompany severe vertigo of peripheral origin: Ménière's disease, vestibular neuronitis; vertebrobasilar insufficiency

- *a need to keep the head immobile?*

Vertigo increases with quick head movements

- *a state of imbalance?*

Usually in true vertigo of labyrinthine origin (vestibular end-organs): Ménière's disease; also in vertigo of acoustic neuroma

- a feeling of unsteadiness? lightheadedness?

Giddiness: pseudovertigo

- choking? tingling around the mouth, in the fingers? sweating? anxiety?

Pseudovertigo with hyperventilation: in depressed or anxious patients

- *a hearing loss? tinnitus?*

Peripheral vestibular pathology: Ménière's disease; acoustic neuroma; drug ototoxicity

- a fluctuant hearing loss, improving as the attack subsides?
- tinnitus? worse during attacks of vertigo? subsiding between attacks?

Ménière's disease

- unilateral tinnitus?

Acoustic neuroma

- a normal hearing? no tinnitus?

Absence of auditory symptoms in: vestibular neuronitis; benign positional vertigo; central lesions; vertebrobasilar insufficiency; demyelinating lesion

5.2 Do you sometimes fall to the ground, without loss of consciousness?

May occur in abrupt and severe attack of vertigo

5.3 Following the acute attack, do you have
   • a period of imbalance or unsteadiness? (for several days?)

Ménière's disease

5.4 Do you have
   • blurring of vision? double vision?

Central vestibular disease; multiple sclerosis

   • difficulty swallowing? a loss of strength? numbness?

Brainstem origin of vertigo: involvement of other cerebral structures

   • a decreased hearing? tinnitus? present for months before the vertigo?

Ménière's disease; acoustic neuroma

   • disturbances of gait?

Acoustic nerve origin; labyrinthine origin

   • an aural discharge?

Otorrhea: in chronic otitis media

   • ear pain? fullness in the ear?

Peripheral vestibular pathology; otalgia in herpes zoster (with seventh nerve paralysis): Ramsay-Hunt syndrome

   • vomiting? a slurred speech?

Vertebrobasilar insufficiency (hearing loss and tinnitus: rare)

6   Iatrogenic Factors   See Etiology

7   Personal and Social Profile

7.1 What is your sexual orientation?

Loss of balance in a homosexual man: CNS toxoplasmosis; CNS lymphoma

8   Personal Antecedents Pertaining to the Vertigo

8.1 Do you have any of the following conditions:
   • a neurologic disease? an ear condition? hypertension? anemia?
   • a past cranial trauma?

May be followed by persistent or positional vertigo (traumatic labyrinthine vertigo); temporal bone fracture

   • epilepsy?

Patients with temporal lobe epilepsy occasionally experience vertigo as an early symptom

   • a recent neck trauma?

Cervicogenic vertigo: the articulations and musculature of the cervical region provide extensive proprioceptive signals to the brainstem vestibular system

   • a recent infectious illness?

Vestibular neuronitis: appears 2 weeks or so following a viral illness

9   Family Medical History Pertaining to the Vertigo

9.1   Does someone in your family have vertigo?

A family history is often present in Ménière's disease and otosclerosis. Vestibular neuronitis may affect several members of the same family

PHYSICAL SIGNS PERTAINING TO VERTIGO

	Possible significance
Otalgic examination	May reveal otitis media; perforated tympanic membrane; cholesteatoma
Nystagmus	
Unidirectional	Central and peripheral causes of vertigo
Bidirectional and vertical	Vertigo of central origin
Unidirectional nystagmus; hearing loss; disturbed balance; unsteadiness of gait; no other neurologic findings	Labyrinthine vertigo (hearing is normal in benign positional vertigo, vestibular neuronitis)
Hearing loss; facial weakness (fifth, sixth, seventh cranial nerves); disturbed balance; ipsilateral ataxia of the limbs; nystagmus	Acoustic neuroma (cerebellopontine-angle tumor) (with tinnitus)
Café au lait spots; neurofibromas	Unilateral or bilateral acoustic neuromas are common in neurofibromatosis
Nystagmus; involvement of cranial nerves, motor and sensory tracts; disequilibrium; hearing spared	Central cause of vertigo, brainstem origin (no tinnitus); cerebrovascular disease; multiple sclerosis
Nystagmus; bilateral internuclear ophthalmoplegia	Multiple sclerosis

LABORATORY TESTS PERTAINING TO VERTIGO

Test	Finding	Diagnostic Possibilities
Caloric and rotational testing	Abnormal	Vestibular dysfunction: lesion of labyrinth, vestibular nerve, central vestibular connections
Pure-tone and speech audiometry	Normal	Vestibular neuronitis; benign positional vertigo; vertigo of central origin
	Abnormal	Lesion of the middle ear, labyrinth, cochlear nerve: Ménière's disease; cerebellopontine-angle tumor

LABORATORY PROCEDURES PERTAINING TO VERTIGO

Procedure	To Detect
Skull x-rays and tomograms	Erosion of internal auditory meatus: acoustic neuroma
Cervical spine x-rays	Cervical spondylosis with possible cervicogenic vertigo
Computerized tomography*, magnetic resonance imaging* of the head	Intracranial lesions; cerebellopontine-angle tumor; temporal lobe mass lesions; posterior fossa lesions
Brainstem auditory-evoked response*	To differentiate cochlear or sensory-hearing losses from retrocochlear or neural hearing losses
Electronystagmography*	To identify a lesion of the labyrinth or eighth nerve

*When indicated

SELECTED BIBLIOGRAPHY

Adams RD, Victor M: Deafness, dizziness, and disorders of equilibrium, in *Principles of Neurology*, 4th ed., pp. 226–246, New York: McGraw-Hill, 1989.

Hanson MR: The dizzy patient. *Postgrad Med* 85(2):99–108, 1989.

Harner SG: Peripheral labyrinthine causes of dizziness. *Postgrad Med* 81(4):251–258, 1987.

Slater R: Vertigo. *Postgrad Med* 84(5):58–67, 1988.

39
Weakness

INTRODUCTION

Weakness Reduction in the maximum force of muscular contraction and in muscular force on repeated contraction.

The stimulus for voluntary movement originates in the cerebral cortex. The motor impulse passes from the motor cortex down the corticospinal tract to the anterior horn cell of the spinal cord and thence down the motor nerves to the neuromuscular junction and to the muscle. Muscle tone and movement are also influenced by the effect of the extrapyramidal, cerebellar, and proprioceptive pathways on the anterior horn cells. Motor dysfunction may result from involvement of the upper motor neuron (motor cortex and corticospinal tract), the lower motor neuron (anterior horn cell and motor nerve), the neuromuscular junction, and the muscle fibers. A lesion of the upper motor neuron affects muscle groups diffusely and is associated with spasticity, increased tendon reflexes, clonus, extensor plantar reflex, and no or slight atrophy due to disuse. Lesions of the lower motor neuron may affect individual muscles and are accompanied by marked atrophy, flaccidity, loss of tendon reflexes, and normal plantar reflex, if present; muscular twitchings may be present. Sensory changes are generally absent when the lesion is localized to the anterior horn cell (progressive muscular atrophies) or anterior roots, and are usually present when the lesion is in the peripheral nerves (neuropathies). Weakness may be due to disorders of the neuromuscular junction (myasthenia gravis). Myasthenia gravis is associated with acetylcholine receptor (AChR) deficiency at the motor end plate and usually with circulating AChR antibodies. Diseases affecting muscle fibers without interfering with their nerve supply (myopathies) also result in weakness with atrophy, flaccidity, and decreased tendon reflexes; sensory loss and fasciculations are absent. In contrast to neuropathies, myopathies are associated with normal nerve conductions; serum enzymes [creatine kinase (CK), lactic dehydrogenase (LDH), serum aspartate and alanine aminotransferases (AST, ALT), aldolase] are usually elevated.

Weakness must be distinguished from fatigue, a subjective sense of loss of energy. The loss of strength of true weakness can generally be demonstrated objectively.

ETIOLOGY

Central Nervous System Lesions

Vascular; tumor; infection; trauma; demyelinating; hereditary

Anterior Horn Cells

Poliomyelitis; syringomyelitis; amyotrophic lateral sclerosis; tumor; myelitis; trauma

Neuropathies

Nutritional: alcoholism; malnutrition; pellagra; pernicious anemia; chronic gastrointestinal disease; postgastrectomy conditions

Malignancy: carcinoma; lymphoma; multiple myeloma

Collagen-vascular disease: polyarteritis nodosa; systemic lupus erythematosus; rheumatoid arthritis

Metabolic and endocrine disorders: diabetes mellitus; uremia; porphyria; amyloidosis; macroglobulinemia; acromegaly; myxedema

Toxins: heavy metals (lead, arsenic, thallium, mercury); organophosphate compounds; industrial poisons; drugs

Inflammatory states: serum sickness; acute inflammatory polyneuropathy (Guillain-Barré syndrome); sarcoidosis

Infections: diphtheria; leprosy; infectious mononucleosis; herpes zoster

Hereditary disorders: progressive hypertrophic polyneuropathy; peroneal muscular atrophy; Refsum's disease; metachromatic leukodystrophy

Entrapment neuropathies

Nerve Roots

Herniated intervertebral disk; spondylosis

Muscle Diseases

Hereditary

Muscular dystrophy: Duchenne, Becker, myotonic, fascioscapulohumeral, limb-girdle, oculopharyngeal, distal

Congenital myopathies: glycogen storage diseases, lipid storage diseases

Mitochondrial diseases: central core disease, nemaline myopathy, others

Myotonia; periodic paralysis

Endocrine and metabolic disorders

Hyper- and hypothyroidism; hyperparathyroidism; Cushing's syndrome; Addison's disease; electrolyte abnormalities: potassium, sodium, calcium, magnesium, phosphate

Inflammatory myopathies

Polymyositis, dermatomyositis

Collagen-vascular diseases: SLE; rheumatoid arthritis; scleroderma

Polymyalgia rheumatica; sarcoidosis

Infections: influenza B; toxoplasmosis; leptospirosis; trichinosis

Tumors: primary and metastatic neoplasms

Toxic: alcohol; drugs

Disorders of Neuromuscular Transmission

Myasthenia gravis

Carcinomatous myopathy (Eaton-Lambert syndrome)

Toxins and chemicals: botulism; organophosphate poisoning; snake venoms; drugs

Iatrogenic Causes of Weakness (Partial List)

Drug-induced polyneuropathies: clofibrate; amiodarone; perhexilene; chloroquine; procarbazine; ethambutol; ethionamide; glutethimide; chlorpropamide; polymyxins; tricyclic antidepressants; metronidazole; disopyramide; clioquinol; dimercaprol (BAL); phenytoin; disulfiram; gold salts; hydralazine; isoniazid; nitrofurantoin; vincristine; cis-platinum; excessive pyridoxine administration

Exacerbation of myasthenia: aminoglycosides; polymyxins; quinidine; β-adrenergic blockers

Drug-induced myopathy: chloroquine; corticosteroids; clofibrate; pentazocine; vincristine

Drug-induced intracerebral bleeding and stroke: anticoagulants; oral contraceptives; monoamine oxidase inhibitors associated with sympathomimetic amines or tricyclic antidepressants

Hyperkalemic weakness: injudicious administration of oral potassium preparations, alone or in combination with potassium-sparing diuretics

Diuretic-induced hypokalemia

HISTORY TAKING*

Possible meaning of a positive response

1   Mode of Onset and Evolution

The patient with weakness, particularly of gradual onset, may not recognize it: "signs of muscle weakness precede symptoms of weakness"

1.1   When was the weakness first noted?
- by age 5?   Duchenne's muscular dystrophy
- before age 20?   Becker's dystrophy; fascioscapulohumeral dystrophy; limb-girdle type
- age 20+?   Distal dystrophy
- after age 35?   In case of muscle diseases: polymyositis; myotonic dystrophy appears early or late

1.2   Has the onset of the weakness been
- sudden? (developing over a period of minutes to hours)   Vascular disorder of spinal cord or brain; upper motor neuron lesion; myelitis; metabolic or toxic disorder of the neuromuscular junction or the muscle (sudden alteration in electrolytes, botulism)
- acute? (over the course of 24 h)   Electrolyte, metabolic, or toxic disorder; periodic paralysis; acute inflammatory myopathy; acute polyneuropathy
- subacute? (over days)   Peripheral nerve or neuromuscular junction disease; myasthenia gravis; Guillain-Barré syndrome; acute intermittent porphyria; diphtheric, toxic neuropathies; severe polymyositis and dermatomyositis; weakness from endocrine disorders; poliomyelitis

*In this section, items in *italics* are characteristic clinical features.

- slowly progressive? (over weeks to months)

Polymyositis or dermatomyositis; endocrinopathy; muscular dystrophy, neuromuscular junction defect (myasthenia gravis); spinal muscular atrophy; anterior horn cell or peripheral nerve disorders (diabetic, arsenic, lead); myotonic dystrophy

1.3 Is your weakness
- persistent at all times?

Progressive muscular dystrophy; chronic polymyositis

- increasing as the day progresses?

Diurnal variation: in neuromuscular junction disorders

- variable from day to day?

Myasthenia gravis

- episodic? recurrent?

Myasthenia gravis; Eaton-Lambert syndrome; narcolepsy with cataplexy and sleep paralysis; transient ischemic attacks (may be accompanied by altered consciousness); intermittent electrolyte disturbances: hyper- or hypokalemia, hyper- or hypocalcemia, hyponatremia, hypophosphatemia, hypermagnesemia; familial periodic paralysis; multiple sclerosis

2 Character of the Weakness

2.1 Are you able to perform tasks of daily living? to drive a car? run to catch a bus? dress? shave? climb stairs? carry an object?

Fatigue: decreased energy, not true weakness. The patient with fatigue is able to perform a normal activity at least once but lacks the ability to perform a task repetitively. The patient with weakness experiences trouble on exercise or when he begins to move

3 Location and Type of the Weakness

3.1 Is the loss of strength
- generalized?

More likely systemic cause: endocrine, metabolic, infectious, drug-induced myopathy. Disorder of the motor system unlikely

- localized?

Myopathy of disuse; CNS involvement; neuropathy

3.2 Do you have a loss of strength in
- one extremity?

Monoplegia: paralysis of all muscles in one arm or leg

- the arm?

Cortical vascular lesion (thrombosis or embolus); cortical tumor or abscess; brachial plexus lesion

• the leg?	Crural monoplegia: any lesion of thoracic or lumbar cord: trauma, tumor, myelitis, multiple sclerosis
• the face, arm, leg, on one side of the body?	Hemiplegia, the most frequent distribution of paralysis: involvement of the descending motor tracts
• both legs?	Paraplegia: diseases of the spinal cord and the spinal roots or the peripheral nerves; spinal cord tumor; ruptured cervical disk; syringomyelia; multiple sclerosis; subacute combined degeneration; parasagittal tumors
3.3 Is the weakness • *symmetrical?*	Peripheral nerve lesion (alcoholic, vitamin B deficiency, nitrofurantoin, isoniazid therapy, lead, arsenic); Guillain-Barré syndrome; myopathy
• *asymmetrical?*	Lesion of the central nervous system; anterior horn cell lesion; multiple sclerosis; poliomyelitis; amyotrophic lateral sclerosis; polyneuropathies (diabetic, polyarteritis nodosa, sarcoidosis); entrapment neuropathy; may occur in myasthenia gravis
3.4 Which activities do you find difficult to perform?	Severity of weakness must be quantitated by evaluating alterations in functional abilities
3.5 Do you have difficulty in lifting objects? raising objects onto a shelf? shaving? washing, brushing your hair?	Proximal weakness of the upper extremities: myopathy; polymyositis; also in neuromuscular junction defect; inflammatory polyneuropathy; anterior horn cell disease
3.6 Do you have difficulty in turning doorknobs? picking up a pin? opening jars? fastening buttons?	Distal weakness of the upper extremities: peripheral nerve disease or anterior horn cell disorder; myotonic dystrophy
3.7 Do you have difficulty in walking? climbing and descending stairs? getting out of the bathtub? crossing your knees? rising from a chair?	Proximal weakness of the lower limbs: myopathy; muscular dystrophy; polymyositis; neuromuscular junction defect; inflammatory polyneuropathy
3.8 Have you noticed a tendency for your ankles to turn? a flopping of your feet? frequent tripping?	Distal weakness of the lower limbs: neuropathy; anterior horn cell disorder
3.9 Do you have difficulty in sitting up in bed?	Weakness of the trunk

4   Precipitating or Aggravating Factors

4.1   Does the weakness occur after
      • *a sustained effort?*   Myasthenia gravis
      • a large carbohydrate meal?   Hypokalemic periodic paralysis
      • fasting? rest following exercise?   Hyperkalemic periodic paralysis

5   Relieving Factors

5.1   *Does rest restore your muscular*   Myasthenia gravis
      strength?

6   Accompanying Symptoms

6.1   Do you have
      • *pain, tenderness, in your muscles?*   Peripheral neuropathy. Pain is not
                                                 prominent in myopathy; may occur in
                                                 inflammatory myopathies (polymyo-
                                                 sitis); polyarteritis nodosa

      • *numbness, tingling,* decreased or   Dysesthesia, hypalgesia, hypesthesia:
        painful sensations, in your   (with flaccid, areflexic paralysis): in-
        hands? feet?   volvement of mixed motor and sensory
                                                 nerves or affection of both anterior and
                                                 posterior roots. Distal ("stocking-and-
                                                 glove") sensory loss in peripheral nerve
                                                 diseases. Sensory changes exclude
                                                 myopathy as the cause of weakness

      • any impairment in the perception   If dissociated loss of pain and tempera-
        of pain? temperature? touch?   ture with preservation of touch: syrin-
                                                 gomyelia

      • twitchings in resting muscles?   Fasciculations: anterior horn cell lesion;
                                                 amyotrophic lateral sclerosis; benign
                                                 fasciculations

      • double vision?   Diplopia: myasthenia gravis (involve-
                                                 ment of ocular muscles)

      • difficulty swallowing? speaking?   Myasthenia gravis: weakness of lips,
        chewing?   tongue, palate, and pharynx
      • a defect in speech?   Aphasia: in hemiplegia: cortical or sub-
                                                 cortical lesion

6.2   In case of paraplegia: Do you have
      • bladder and bowel incontinence?   Bilateral lesions of the spinal cord with
                                                 bladder and bowel sphincter paralysis
                                                 (sphincters are spared in peripheral
                                                 nerve disease)

6.3   Do you have
      • a reduction in the size of some of   Muscular atrophy: lesion in the spinal
        your muscles?   cord, spinal roots, peripheral nerves, or
                                                 muscle; debilitating systemic disease;
                                                 disuse; senility

• no change in the size of your muscles?	Weakness without muscular atrophy: upper motor neuron lesion; lesion of the cerebral cortex; multiple sclerosis; spinal cord tumors early in their course; disorder of the neuromuscular junction (myasthenia gravis, drugs) or muscle (hypo- and hyperkalemia, hypercalcemia, hypothyroidism)
• an increase in the size of some of your muscles?	Congenital myotonia (without muscle weakness); pseudohypertrophy (calves) in Duchenne and Becker dystrophies
• pain in your joints?	Inflammatory myopathies; collagen-vascular disease; rheumatoid arthritis
• low back pain?	Intervertebral disk herniation with weakness in lower extremity
• a skin rash?	Systemic lupus erythematosus; dermatomyositis; scleroderma
• diarrhea? abdominal pain?	Polyneuropathy in: malabsorption, toxic exposure; polyarteritis nodosa
• fever? weight loss?	Underlying systemic condition

7   Iatrogenic Factors   See Etiology

8   Personal and Social Profile

8.1 What is your occupation?	Peripheral neuropathy due to lead, arsenic, n-hexane, methyl butyl ketone, acrylamide in: battery production, plumbing, smelting, painting, shoemaking, solvent use, insecticides
8.1a Have you been exposed to toxic products?	Polyneuropathy due to organophosphates (insecticides), dichlorophenoxyacetic acid (herbicides)
8.2 What is your alcohol consumption?	Alcohol, the most prevalent neurotoxin, is often not recognized as such by patients
8.3 Have you recently consumed home-canned vegetables? other tinned foods?	The possibility of botulism must be kept in mind; isolated cases of botulism can be missed
8.4 What is your sexual orientation?	Peripheral neuropathy in a homosexual man: herpes zoster, neuralgia from AIDS-related conditions, lumbosacral radiculitis of herpetic proctitis

9   Personal Antecedents Pertaining to the Weakness

9.1 Do you have any of the following conditions: diabetes? alcoholism? a thyroid disease? malignancy?

9.2   Have you recently had an infec-   Acute postinfectious polyneuropathy
tion? an operation? an immuniza-   (Guillain-Barré syndrome)
tion?

10   Family Medical History Pertaining to the Weakness

10.1   Are there other members of your   Muscular dystrophies: X-linked reces-
family who have weakness?   sive or autosomal dominant (myotonic
dystrophy); periodic paralysis: auto-
somal dominant; porphyria

PHYSICAL SIGNS PERTAINING TO WEAKNESS

Possible significance

Individual muscle testing — Objective evaluation of the pattern and degree of weakness

Spasticity; hyperactive tendon reflexes; extensor plantar reflex; no atrophy (or slight atrophy due to disuse); no fasciculations — Upper motor neuron paralysis: lesion of the corticospinal system

Atrophy; flaccidity; decreased or absent tendon reflexes; sensory loss and fasciculations may be present — Lower motor neuron paralysis; anterior horn cell lesion

Atrophy; flaccidity; decreased tendon reflexes; no sensory loss; no fasciculations — Some diseases of muscle: polymyositis; hyperthyroidism, muscular dystrophy

No atrophy; no alteration in tendon reflexes; no sensory loss — Diseases of the neuromuscular junction or muscle: myasthenia gravis, botulism; potassium or calcium disorders; thyroid myopathies; congenital myotonia

Distribution of Weakness

Weakness of individual muscles; marked atrophy — Lower motor neuron paralysis: lesion of one or more peripheral nerves, occasionally of spinal roots

Weakness affecting muscles in groups; no atrophy — Upper motor neuron lesion or supranuclear paralysis

Monoplegia without muscular atrophy — Upper motor neuron lesion; most likely in cerebral cortex; multiple sclerosis; early stage of spinal cord tumor

Monoplegia with atrophy	Lesion in the spinal cord, spinal roots, or peripheral nerves
• in the upper extremity	Brachial atrophic monoplegia in: syringomyelia, poliomyelitis, amyotrophic lateral sclerosis; brachial plexus lesion
• in the lower extremity	Lesion of the thoracic or lumbar cord or its roots and nerves
Hemiplegia	Almost always upper motor neuron lesion: involvement of the corticospinal pathways
Paraplegia	Lesion of the corticospinal tracts below the cervical cord; disease of the spinal cord and the spinal roots or of the peripheral nerves
Quadriplegia	Lesion in the cervical segment of the spinal cord
Weakness or sensory loss in a lower extremity; bilateral Babinski sign	Multiple sclerosis ("symptoms in one leg and signs in both")
Symmetrical distal weakness	Polyneuropathy
Symmetrical proximal weakness; normal or increased muscle bulk; preservation of reflexes	Myopathy
Increase in size and weakness of muscles	Pseudohypertrophy: Duchenne and Becker muscular dystrophy
Increased size and normal strength of muscles	Myotonia congenita
Ptosis; facial weakness; nasal or dysarthric speech; deep-tendon reflexes present; no sensory loss	Neuromuscular junction disorder: myasthenia gravis
Myotonia	Myotonic dystrophy
Skin rash; arthritis	Collagen-vascular disease with inflammatory myopathy: dermatomyositis, scleroderma, systemic lupus erythematosus
Dry, coarse, cool skin; delayed relaxation phase of the tendon reflexes	Hypothyroidism with myopathy
Cataract, baldness, gonadal atrophy	Myotonic dystrophy

†See the appendix on Laboratory Reference Values for the associated normal laboratory values.

LABORATORY TESTS PERTAINING TO WEAKNESS[†]

Test	Finding	Diagnostic Possibilities
Blood		
CK, AST, ALT, LDH, aldolase	Elevated	Active muscle destruction; myopathies
Potassium	Abnormal	Episodic kalemic paralyses; primary aldosteronism
Thyroid function tests	Abnormal	Thyroid myopathies

LABORATORY PROCEDURES PERTAINING TO WEAKNESS

Procedure	To Detect
Nerve conduction velocity studies	
Normal velocity	Spinal cord or muscle diseases (may be normal in alcoholic, diabetic, nutritional, uremic polyneuropathies)
Slow velocity	Segmental demyelination: peripheral neuropathies; inflammatory polyneuropathy (Guillain-Barré syndrome); entrapment neuropathies
Nerve biopsy*	To distinguish between segmental demyelinisation and axonal degeneration; to identify inflammatory neuropathies, amyloidosis, sarcoidosis
Muscle biopsy*	To distinguish between neurogenic and myopathic disorders; to identify muscular dystrophy, congenital myopathies, metabolic myopathies, polyarteritis nodosa
Electromyography*	To detect lesions affecting the anterior horn cell (fibrillations), peripheral nerves (denervation pattern), or muscle
Neostigmine or edrophonium test*	Increased muscle strength: myasthenia gravis
EEG, CT scan	Central nervous system lesion
Spine x-rays; computerized tomography	Involvement of spinal cord, nerve roots
Chest x-ray	Lung tumor, thymoma, with myasthenic state

*When indicated

SELECTED BIBLIOGRAPHY

Adams RD, Victor M: Motor paralysis; Diseases of the peripheral nerves; Principles of clinical myology: Diagnosis and classification of muscle diseases, in *Principles of Neurology*, 4th ed., pp. 37–53; 1028–1076; 1092–1103, New York: McGraw-Hill, 1989.

Eaton JM: Muscle disease—a primer. *Postgrad Med* 81(7):53–59, 1987.

Grob D: Acute neuromuscular disorders. *Med Clin North Am* 65:189–207, 1981.

Kagen LJ: Muscle weakness. Neuropathic or myopathic? *Hosp Pract* 20(9):82E–82U, 1985.

Osteoarticular System

40

Articular Pain

INTRODUCTION

Arthralgia   Joint pain in the absence of objective evidence of joint disease.
Arthritis   Joint pain with visible or palpable abnormality.

Joint pain is perceived as diffuse and poorly localized; when severe, it may be felt distally over most of the extremity; it may be referred to another anatomic location. Disorders of the joints are likely to be accompanied by pain on local movements, and the duration of the pain parallels that of the movement.

   Articular pain may be due to synovial tissue disease or to diseased cartilage and involvement of supporting structures. Inflammatory arthritides (rheumatoid arthritis, systemic lupus erythematosus) are characterized by accumulation of inflammatory cells in the synovial tissue and fluid. Acute inflammation in rheumatoid arthritis may result from immune complexes in synovial tissues and fluid, or cell-mediated damage. In the seronegative spondylarthritides such as ankylosing spondylitis and Reiter's syndrome, the enthesis (the transitional area of attachment of ligaments to bone) is the primary site of inflammation; the enthesopathies are commonly associated with the histocompatibility antigen HLA-B27. In infectious arthritis, the synovium is most commonly infected by the hematogenous spread of microorganisms from a primary site (skin, respiratory, or urinary tract), but occasionally no source can be found. Microorganisms may be introduced directly into the joint by a penetrating wound or intraarticular injection. Rheumatic fever occurs as a delayed sequel to pharyngeal infection with group A hemolytic streptococci. The acute inflammatory lesion in rheumatic fever is attributed to an immunologic mechanism. Microcrystalline synovitis (gout, pseudogout) is characterized by crystal formation within the synovial space, and an accompanying strong inflammatory reaction. Degenerative joint disease (osteoarthritis) is characterized by a chronic low-grade synovial inflammation and the presence in cartilage and supporting structures of alterations induced by continuous wear-and-tear processes; the proteoglycan content of osteoarthritic cartilage is diminished, although its rate of synthesis is increased.

ETIOLOGY

Monoarthritis

Acute

Crystal-induced: urate (gout); calcium pyrophosphate dihydrate (pseudogout); calcium hydroxyapatite
Trauma: tear of ligament or cartilage; meniscus injury; loose bodies

Chronic

Aseptic necrosis
Osteochondritis dissecans
Pigmented villonodular synovitis
Sarcoidosis
Foreign body
Neoplasms

Acute or Chronic

Infection: gonococcus, staphylococcus, streptococcus
Hemarthrosis
Mechanical internal derangement
Neurogenic arthropathy: diabetes, tabes
Onset of polyarthritis

Polyarthritis

Acute

Infection: bacterial (gonococcus, staphylococcus), viral (rubella, hepatitis); subacute bacterial endocarditis; Lyme arthritis
Rheumatic fever
Erythema nodosum
Serum sickness; drug reaction; Henoch-Schönlein purpura
Palindromic rheumatism
Sarcoidosis
Familial hypercholesterolemia

Chronic

Degenerative joint disease: osteoarthritis: primary, secondary
Inflammatory joint disease: rheumatoid arthritis (RA); ankylosing spondylitis; psoriatic arthropathy
Collagen-vascular diseases: systemic lupus erythematosus (SLE), polyarteritis nodosa, scleroderma, Sjögren's syndrome, mixed connective-tissue disease
Crystal-induced: gout, pseudogout

Acute or Chronic

Enteropathic arthropathy; Reiter's syndrome; Behçet's disease
Hypertrophic osteoarthropathy

Relapsing polychondritis
Whipple's disease; familial Mediterranean fever
Fibrositis; psychogenic rheumatism

Iatrogenic Causes of Articular Pain (Partial List)

Drug-Induced Gout

Diuretics: chlorothiazides, furosemide, ethacrynic acid; probenecid; sulfinpyrazone; allopurinol; antineoplastic drugs; cyclosporine; low doses of salicylate therapy

Drug-Induced Polyarteritis Nodosa

Sulfonamides, penicillin

Drug-Induced Serum-Sickness Type of Reaction

Penicillin, barbiturates, animal serums

Drug-Induced SLE and/or Positive Tests for Antinuclear Antibodies

Methyldopa; levodopa; phenytoin; penicillin; oral contraceptives; phenothiazines; hydralazine; procainamide; isoniazid; sulfonamides
Anticoagulant overdosage may produce acute hemarthrosis; too rapid withdrawal of corticosteroid therapy may induce arthralgia

HISTORY TAKING*

Possible meaning of a positive response

1   Location of the Pain

1.1 Where do you feel your pain? Point to the most painful spot with one finger	Helps determine whether the pain is primarily articular or periarticular (tendinitis, bursitis, fibrositis). Most arthritides are easily localized. Pain from tendinitis may be difficult to pinpoint
1.1a Does the pain radiate to other parts of your body?	Entrapment syndromes (carpal tunnel syndrome, herniated lumbar disk, cervical root compression)
1.2 How many joints are involved?	
• one?	Monoarticular process: infectious arthritis, crystal-induced monoarthritis, osteoarthritis, trauma; bursitis
• two to four joints?	Oligoarticular process: osteoarthritis, spondylarthropathies, enteropathic arthritis; periarthritis (tendinitis, bursitis, fibrositis) tends to involve only one, or a few, of the larger joints but spares the wrists, hands, and feet

*In this section, items in *italics* are characteristic clinical features.

• more than four joints?	Polyarticular process: RA; rheumatic fever; spondylarthropathies; viral arthritis; Reiter's syndrome; serum sickness

1.3   In which joint(s) do you have pain?

• large joints?	RA, spondylarthropathies
• hips and shoulders?	Peripheral joints most frequently affected in ankylosing spondylitis
• both shoulders and thighs?	Polymyalgia rheumatica
• sacroiliac joints? lumbar spine?	Ankylosing spondylitis; psoriatic arthropathy; Reiter's syndrome. Involvement of the axial skeleton is infrequent in rheumatoid arthritis (exception: the cervical spine)
• knees and hips?	Osteoarthritis: in weight-bearing joints; enteropathic arthritis
• wrists? elbows?	Inflammatory disease: RA; usually spared in osteoarthritis
• the small joints of hands or feet?	RA; may be involved in the polyarticular form of gout (with sparing of the great toe)
• *metacarpophalangeal?*	Rheumatoid arthritis (rarely affected in osteoarthritis)
• *proximal interphalangeal?*	Rheumatoid arthritis
• *distal interphalangeal?*	Osteoarthritis; psoriatic arthritis; commonly spared in RA
• a great toe?	Gout (the big toe is involved in 50 to 70 percent of initial attacks)
• the heels?	Reiter's syndrome; other spondylarthropathies (Achilles tendinitis)
• any of the above?	Acute rheumatic fever (knees, ankles: commonest); trauma

2   Mode of Onset and Chronology of the Pain

2.1 How long have you had joint pain?	Less than 6 weeks' duration: microcrystalline, infection, enteropathic arthritis, viral arthritis; acute rheumatic fever. More than 6 weeks: chronic process: RA, osteoarthritis. Several years' duration: rules out bacterial infections and malignant neoplasms

2.2   At what age did the joint condition appear?

• between 20 to 45?	RA; rheumatic fever is infrequent after age 20; SLE and Reiter's syndrome occur more frequently in the young
• *in a young man?*	Ankylosing spondylitis; gout; Reiter's syndrome
• after age 40?	Osteoarthritis (unusual before age 35)

	• in the elderly?	Osteoarthritis; polymyalgia rheumatica; gout; pseudogout; carcinomatous arthropathy; hypertrophic osteoarthropathy; neurogenic arthropathy; drug-induced gout or lupus
2.3	Was the onset of pain	
	• acute? (hours to days)	Infection; gout; pseudogout; rheumatic fever; onset of RA may be abrupt; any traumatic condition
	• gradual? (days to weeks to months)	RA; osteoarthritis; fibrositis
2.4	Is the joint condition	
	• intermittent? recurrent?	Gout; pseudogout; Reiter's syndrome; tendinitis, bursitis, fibrositis
	• constant? chronic? (more than 6 weeks)	Most significant rheumatic disorders; osteoarthritis; RA
2.5	Did the joint involvement	
	• appear and stay in one joint?	Gout; infection, gonococcal
	• appear simultaneously in several joints?	RA (especially in hands and feet); Reiter's syndrome
2.6	Does (did) the pain	
	• *"flit" from joint to joint? tend to leave one joint as a new one was affected?*	Migratory pattern: common in acute polyarthritis: acute rheumatic fever, gonococcal arthritis, drug sensitivity; erythema nodosum syndrome
	• *involve new joints, with persistence of the first affected?*	Additive pattern: RA, Reiter's syndrome

3   Character and Intensity of the Pain

3.1	Is your pain usually	
	• mild to moderate?	May be observed in rheumatoid arthritis
	• severe?	Traumatic conditions, gout, pseudogout, septic arthritis
3.1a	How many analgesic pills do you take?	
3.1b	Does the pain interfere with normal activities of daily living?	An indication of severity
3.1c	Does the pain ever disturb your sleep? awaken you?	Severe problem; bone and neurologic pain may also occur at night
3.2	What part of the 24-hour day is your pain worst?	
	• in the early morning hours?	RA; ankylosing spondylitis; tendinitis and bursitis
	• in the morning and evening?	Polymyalgia rheumatica
	• progressively worse as the day goes on?	Osteoarthritis (particularly in the weight-bearing joints)

3.3 Are your joints painful at rest?

RA; osteoarthritis (advanced stage); infectious arthritis; gout

4 Precipitating or Aggravating Factors

4.1 What makes your pain worse?
• movements?

Pain caused by any arthritis; osteoarthritis

• prolonged activity? excessive exercise? walking? stretching?

Osteoarthritis; tendinitis

• inactivity?

Fibrositis

4.2 Did the joint condition occur after
• *a trauma? a dietary or alcoholic excess?*

Acute attack of gout; trauma may also precipitate pseudogout

5 Relieving Factors

5.1 What makes your pain better?
• rest?

Osteoarthritis (pain at rest with severe disease); RA; most arthritides

• mild exercise?

RA; tendinitis; rest stiffness in osteoarthritis

• aspirin?

Most arthritides; RA; acute rheumatic fever

• colchicine?

Gout

5.1a Do salicylates fail to relieve your complaints?

Psychogenic rheumatism (in the absence of physical findings of arthritis)

6 Accompanying Symptoms

6.1 Are your joints swollen? tender? Are you unable to remove a ring? wear a watch?

Suggests significant swelling: may be due to synovial effusion or proliferation; periarticular involvement extending beyond the normal joint margins

6.1a Did the swelling appear
• simultaneously with the pain?

RA: swelling due to synovitis and accumulation of joint fluid; bursitis

• weeks to months after the pain?

Osteoarthritis: swelling due to proliferative changes in cartilage and bone

6.2 Do you have
• *a (generalized) stiffness, most severe in the morning?*

"Gelling" phenomenon: accentuation of the congestion and edema in synovium, joint capsule, and periarticular tissues resulting from inactivity; fibrositis syndrome

• wearing off within 15 minutes or less?

Osteoarthritis

• *lasting more than 30 minutes?* lasting up to 3 hours?

Characteristic of RA; ankylosing spondylitis; polymyalgia rheumatica (The duration of morning stiffness can be used as a fairly reliable index of rheumatoid activity)

6.3 Do you have limitation of motion? weakness? disability?

In most rheumatic disorders, particularly if the joints are inflamed: may be due to pain, muscle spasm, effusion, deformity, contracture; dermatomyositis; neurologic involvement in RA, vasculitis

6.3a Do you have difficulty
- holding a coffee cup? buttoning a shirt?
- putting on a coat? combing the hair?
- rising from a chair? putting on shoes and stockings?

Disability involving the hands: RA; tendinitis; peripheral neuropathy
Proximal weakness may be found in any disorder affecting the shoulders or hips; polymyalgia rheumatica; polymyositis; nerve root impingement

6.4 Do you have
- fever?

Acute rheumatic fever; infection: gonococcal, septic arthritis; gout; SLE (fever is absent in osteoarthritis and infrequent in chronic polyarthritis)

- with chills?
- weight loss? fatigue? pain in your muscles?

Bacteremia with acute polyarthritis
Underlying systemic disorder: collagen-vascular disease; subacute bacterial endocarditis; neoplasm. Weight loss may be profound in RA (systemic signs are absent in osteoarthritis)

- skin lesions?

Psoriatic arthritis; SLE; scleroderma; Reiter's syndrome; Lyme arthritis; rheumatic fever; erythema nodosum; gonorrheal arthritis; juvenile RA

- chronic diarrhea? gastrointestinal complaints?

Arthritis associated with: scleroderma; inflammatory bowel disease; Whipple's disease; salmonella; vasculitis; gastrointestinal shunts

- difficulty swallowing?
- shortness of breath? cough? expectorations?

Dermatomyositis; scleroderma
Pulmonary lesions associated with RA, SLE, polymyositis, dermatomyositis, sarcoidosis, Churg-Strauss disease, Caplan's syndrome, necrotizing vasculitis, lung carcinoma

- hemoptysis?

Bronchogenic carcinoma with hypertrophic osteoarthropathy

- chest pain?

SLE (pleurisy and pericarditis); rheumatic fever; RA; ankylosing spondylitis; scleroderma; polymyositis

- back pain?

Ankylosing spondylitis; spondylitis is common in psoriatic arthritis, Reiter's syndrome, colonic arthritis

- an eye condition? burning, redness, discharge?

Episcleritis associated with RA; conjunctivitis in Reiter's syndrome; keratitis sicca in Sjögren's syndrome; anterior uveitis in ankylosing spondylitis, sarcoidosis

• pain in your fingers when exposed to cold?	Raynaud's phenomenon: SLE, scleroderma, Sjögren's syndrome; may occur in RA
• pain on urination? a urethral discharge?	Gonococcal arthritis; Reiter's syndrome

7   Iatrogenic Factors   See Etiology

8   Personal and Social Profile

8.1	Sex and race of the patient?	Gout and the spondylarthropathies are more common in men; rheumatoid arthritis and fibrositis are more common in women. Polymyalgia rheumatica is more frequent in whites; sarcoidosis is more frequent in blacks
8.2	What are your living conditions at home?	May reveal physical inconveniences present in the home
8.3	Have you recently had any sexual contact(s)?	3 to 17 days prior to the arthritis: gonococcal arthritis (disseminated gonorrhea is the most frequent etiology of joint infection in young, sexually active patients; may cause polyarthritis prior to localization to a monoarticular form); Reiter's syndrome
8.3a	What is your sexual orientation?	Joint pains in a homosexual man: tenosynovitis of disseminated gonococcal infection; arthritis of hepatitis B
8.4	Have you ever worked in a coal mine?	Coal workers with RA have an increased incidence of an interstitial lung disease ("rheumatoid pneumoconiosis" or "Caplan's syndrome")

9   Personal Antecedents Pertaining to the Articular Pain

9.1	Have you ever had x-rays, a biopsy, of your joints? When? With what results?	
9.2	Prior to the onset of joint pain, did you have	
	• a sore throat?	A group A hemolytic streptococcal infection is usually noted about 2 weeks prior to acute rheumatic fever
	• any injection of serum?	Serum sickness; hepatitis B with arthritis
	• a rubella infection?	Polyarthralgia or polyarthritis synchronous with rubella
	• an operation? a trauma?	Gout; pseudogout
	• a trauma to the involved area?	Posttraumatic arthritis

• an emotional stress? a physical stress?	Gout, fibrositis, psychogenic rheumatism; enteropathic arthropathies
9.3 Have you ever had	
• similar attacks in the past?	Gout; pseudogout; Reiter's syndrome (RA is less episodic)
• an episode of renal colic?	Gouty renal disease
9.4 Do you have a blood abnormality?	Acute polyarthralgia or polyarthritis occurs in sickle cell anemia; hemoglobinopathies may be associated with septic arthritis, avascular necrosis of bone

10   Family Medical History Pertaining to the Articular Pain

10.1 Is there a family history of	
• joint pain?	Gout, RA, ankylosing spondylitis, osteoarthritis of the distal interphalangeal joints (Heberden's nodes) have a familial aggregation
• psoriasis?	30 percent of patients with psoriatic arthritis give a family history of psoriasis

PHYSICAL SIGNS PERTAINING TO ARTICULAR PAIN

	Possible significance
Joint swelling with	
• fluctuation or bulging	Effusion within the joint space
• a boggy, nonfluctuant feeling	Soft-tissue swelling; synovial thickening: RA, gout
• a hard, irregular enlargement	Hypertrophy of cartilage or bone; osteophytes in osteoarthritis
Periarticular swelling	Disorder of periarticular structures: bursitis, tendinitis, cellulitis
• with sharply defined borders	Over bony prominences: bursal effusion
Direct pressure over the joint elicits	
• pain	Arthritis; inflammatory joint disease
• no pain	Involvement of periarticular tissues: bursitis, tendinitis
Contractures	An indication of antecedent synovial inflammation
Swollen joint, with overlying skin	
• red and warm	Acute rheumatic fever; RA; other inflammatory joint diseases; gout; pyogenic infection (local heat is absent in chronic inflammation)
• not discolored	Osteoarthritis
Symmetric involvement	Frequent in rheumatoid arthritis; polymyalgia rheumatica; viral arthritis; SLE; crystal-induced arthritis

Asymmetric involvement	Osteoarthritis; crystal-induced arthritis; spondylarthropathies; Lyme arthritis; psoriatic arthritis; Reiter's syndrome; enteropathic arthropathies
Crepitation on motion	Irregularity in the articulating surfaces: granulation tissue in RA; osteophytes and disorganized cartilage in osteoarthritis; may also arise from the soft tissues
Joint deformity	Indicates a long-standing pathologic process. May result from ligament destruction, soft tissue contracture, bony enlargement, ankylosis, erosive disease, or subluxation: RA; chronic gout; hemophilic arthritis; occasionally: osteoarthritis
• ulnar deviation of the fingers at the metacarpophalangeal joints	Frequently observed deformity in RA
Limitation of motion	May be caused by pain, muscle spasm or guarding, effusion distending the capsule, deformity, or contracture; disorder of tendon, muscle, or nerve
Specific tender sites or trigger points; tender subcutaneous nodules	Fibrositis
Atrophy and weakness of muscles	
• adjacent to the affected joints	Primary joint disease (atrophy of skeletal muscles in RA often parallels the severity of the joint disease)
• generalized	Primary muscle disorder; polymyositis
Subcutaneous swellings	
• over pressure points, over the extensor surface of the elbows	Rheumatoid nodules: in 20 to 30 percent of patients with RA
• in margin of ear, periarticular areas	Tophi of gout: in 13 to 25 percent of gouty patients
• nodules at the	
• dorsal margins of the distal interphalangeal joints	Heberden's nodes in osteoarthritis
• proximal interphalangeal joints	Bouchard's nodes in osteoarthritis
Fever	Acute rheumatic fever; collagen-vascular disease; juvenile RA (Still's disease); gout; infectious arthritis
Skin	
• psoriatic lesions; nail lesions	Psoriatic arthropathy
• butterfly rash of the face	Systemic lupus erythematosus
• villaceous (heliotrope) rash on the eyelids, cheeks, forehead	Dermatomyositis
• petechiae	Henoch-Schönlein purpura; SLE; subacute bacterial endocarditis

- various cutaneous manifestations | Rheumatic fever; Reiter's syndrome; gonococcal arthritis; polyarteritis nodosa; allergic angiitis; derma-tomyositis; SLE; scleroderma; rheuma-toid arthritis; rubella arthritis; hepatitis-associated arthritis; Lyme disease
- mucocutaneous lesions (glans penis, mouth, palms and soles) | Reiter's syndrome
- painful red tender nodules on the legs | Erythema nodosum
- ulcerations of oral mucosae and/or genitalia | Behçet's syndrome; Stevens-Johnson syndrome

Splenomegaly	In 5 to 10 percent of patients with RA; Felty's syndrome (with neutropenia)
Lymphadenopathy; splenomegaly	Felty's syndrome; juvenile RA; SLE
Wheezes; pleural effusion	Pulmonary lesions associated with RA, SLE, sarcoidosis, Churg-Strauss disease
Neurologic abnormalities; loss of pro-prioception	Neurogenic arthropathy: diabetes melli-tus, tabes dorsalis

LABORATORY TESTS PERTAINING TO ARTICULAR PAIN[†]

Test	Finding	Diagnostic Possibilities
Blood		
RBCs	Normocytic hypochromic an-emia	Rheumatoid arthritis (RA)
	Hemolytic an-emia	SLE; other collagen-vascular dis-eases
	Normal hemato-crit, hemoglobin	Osteoarthritis
WBCs	Leukocytosis	Infectious arthritis; microcrystalline arthropathy; juvenile RA; RA (occasionally)
	Leukopenia	SLE; Felty's syndrome
ESR	Normal	Osteoarthritis; fibrositis
	Elevated	Not specific: inflammatory muscu-loskeletal disorders; RA; polymyal-gia rheumatica

[†]See the appendix on Laboratory Reference Values for the associated normal laboratory values.

Test	Finding	Diagnostic Possibilities
Uric acid	Increased	Gout; hematologic disorders; diuretics; etc.
Rheumatoid factor (antibodies to IgG)	Positive(1 : 320)	Not specific: RA (75 percent); SLE (20 to 30 percent); infectious diseases; etc.
	Negative	Osteoarthritis; crystal-induced arthropathy; ankylosing spondylitis; Reiter's syndrome; psoriatic arthritis; colonic arthritis
Antinuclear antibodies*	Positive	SLE; RA (10 to 20 percent)
HLA-B27 antigen*	Present	Ankylosing spondylitis; Reiter's syndrome; psoriatic arthritis; colonic arthritis
Antistreptolysin O*	Abnormal	Acute rheumatic fever
Serum complement*	Normal	RA
	Decreased	SLE; RA (with extraarticular disease)

Synovial Fluid Analysis

Indicated in acute monoarthritis or when a septic or crystal-induced arthropathy is suspected

WBC/mm^3 (Normal <200)	<3000 (mononuclear cell predominance)	Noninflammatory synovial fluid: osteoarthritis, SLE, trauma
	3000 to 50,000 (polymorphonuclear leukocyte predominance)	RA, gout, other inflammatory arthritides
	>50,000 (polymorphonuclear leukocyte predominance)	Septic arthritis
	Hemorrhagic	Traumatic arthritis; hemophilia
Protein, g/100 mL (Normal 1 to 4)	1 to 4.5	Osteoarthritis
	3 to 6	Inflammatory effusion: RA, septic, etc.

*Should only be carried out when there is clinical evidence to suggest a specific diagnosis

Test	Finding	Diagnostic Possibilities
Gram's stain; culture	Positive	Septic arthritis
Glucose (Normal blood glucose level)	Normal	Noninflammatory: osteoarthritis, trauma
	Reduced	Inflammatory effusion; septic arthritis
Crystals	Present	Gout (monosodium urate); pseudogout (calcium pyrophosphate dihydrate)

LABORATORY PROCEDURES PERTAINING TO ARTICULAR PAIN

Procedure	To Detect
Joint x-rays	Juxtaarticular erosions, periarticular osteoporosis: RA
	Marginal sclerosis, bony spurs and bridges: osteoarthritis
	Punched-out defects in bone adjacent to joints: chronic gout
	Calcification of fibrocartilage and articular hyaline cartilage: pseudogout
	Periostitis: hypertrophic osteoarthropathy; Reiter's syndrome
Synovial biopsy*	Tuberculosis; sarcoidosis; hemochromatosis; amyloidosis; pigmented villonodular synovitis; synovial tumor; etc.

*When indicated

SELECTED BIBLIOGRAPHY

Berg E: The acutely swollen joint. *Postgrad Med* 75(1):62–75, 1984.
Bluestone R: The patient who hurts all over. *Postgrad Med* 72(6):71–79, 1982.
Polley HF, Hunder GG: *Rheumatologic interviewing and physical examination of the joints,* 2nd ed. Philadelphia: Saunders, 1978.
Snyderman R (ed): Advances in rheumatology. *Med Clin North Am* 70(2):215–496, 1986.
White RH: The patient with aches and pains. *Postgrad Med* 81(5):216–226, 1987.

INTRODUCTION

Local Pain Caused by any pathologic process which impinges upon or irritates sensory nerve endings in mesodermal tissues: periosteum, capsule of apophyseal joints, fascia, muscles, annulus fibrosus, and ligaments. It usually results from low back strain or muscle spasm. The pain thresholds of these structures are variable: the periosteum is most sensitive, followed by ligaments and fibrous joint capsules, tendons, fascia, and muscles in that order; bone for the most part is insensitive. Pain arising from secondary (protective) muscular spasm may be associated with many disorders of the spine and is usually related to local pain.

Referred Somatic Pain May be projected from the spine into areas related to the lumbar and upper sacral dermatomes (thighs, legs, calves). Decreased sensory and motor function in the lower extremities is never found in association with referred somatic pain.

Referred Pain from Visceral Disease Pain arising in pelvic and abdominal viscera may be referred to the spine. The pain of pelvic diseases is referred to the sacral region; lower abdominal diseases are referred to the lumbar region (centering around L2 to L4), and upper abdominal diseases to the lower thoracic spine (T8 to L1 to L2).

Radicular Pain Sharp pain radiating from a central position near the spine to some part of the lower extremity and caused by distortion, stretching, compression or irritation of a spinal root. A space-occupying lesion in the spinal cord or in the intervertebral foramen may be responsible.

Protrusion of lumbar intervertebral disks is the major cause of severe and chronic or recurrent low back pain; facet joint irritation can also produce a pain pattern simulating that of a ruptured disk.

ETIOLOGY

Mechanical
    Low back strain* or derangement, acute or chronic; poor muscle tone; chronic postural strain; scoliosis
    Trauma: compression fracture: vertebral body or transverse process; previous surgery
    Congenital anomalies: spondylolysis, spondylolisthesis; lumbosacral anomaly, spina bifida
    Protrusion of lumbar intervertebral disks;* spondylotic spurs (unilateral spondylosis); unilateral facet syndrome; lumbar adhesive arachnoiditis
    Osteoarthritis;* spinal stenosis
Infections: acute pyogenic; tuberculosis; epidural and subdural abscess

*Common cause

Systemic inflammatory diseases: ankylosing spondylitis; Reiter's syndrome; psoriatic arthritis; enteropathic arthritis
Metabolic disorders: osteoporosis; osteomalacia; Paget's disease
Neoplastic: primary or metastatic; multiple myeloma; lymphoma
Referred pain: retroperitoneal structures; pelvic organs; diseases of the colon; tumor
Nonorganic:* fibrositis; compensation hysteria; malingering; anxiety; depression

Iatrogenic Causes of Low Back Pain

Anticoagulants: may cause sudden lumbar pain due to retroperitoneal bleeding
Chronic corticosteroid therapy: osteoporosis with vertebral collapse

HISTORY TAKING*

Possible meaning of a positive response

1   Location and Radiation of the Pain

1.1   Where do you have pain?

Local pain is always felt in or near the affected part of the spine

1.1a   Please indicate the site of the pain.

It may be difficult for the patient to localize the pain accurately with words; he or she may be more specific by pointing to the site of the pain

1.2   Do you have pain
• in the midline (over the lower lumbar area)?
• in one (or both) sacroiliac joint(s)?

Local back pain: may have its origin in any of the underlying structures
Sacroiliac strain; ankylosing spondylitis (in young males)

1.3   Does the pain radiate
• from the abdomen through to the back?
• *from a central position near the spine to some part of the lower extremity?*

Referred pain from visceral disease

Radicular pain ("sciatica"): disk disease; primary degenerative joint disease of the spine; spondylolisthesis; ankylosing spondylitis

1.3a   How far distally does the pain extend?

The extent of radiation in many instances may be used as a rough index of the severity of the lesion

---

*In this section, items in *italics* are characteristic clinical features, and items in **boldface** are potentially life-threatening or urgent conditions.
**Useful screening question for ankylosing spondylitis

1.3b Does the pain radiate into

* *the posterior part of the thigh, the calf, to the heel, sole of the foot, and 4th and 5th toes?*

"Sciatica": L5 to S1 disk and lesion of the first sacral root. In most patients with sciatica, only one leg is involved, and in subsequent attacks, the sciatica is confined to the same leg

* *the hip, groin, posterolateral thigh, lateral calf, dorsum of the foot, first or second and third toes?*

Sciatica: L4 to L5 disk; lesion of the 5th lumbar root

* the anterior part of the thigh and knee?

L3 to L4 disk and lesion of the 4th lumbar root (rare)

2 Mode of Onset and Chronology of the Pain

2.1 When did the pain appear?
* first episode before age 40?** Ankylosing spondylitis
* in middle and later life? (age over 45) Osteoarthritis; underlying systemic disorder; osteoporosis

2.2 How long have you had pain in your back?
* acute and self-limited episode? Low back derangement or strain
* longer lasting, chronic pain? Disk disease
  * at least 3 months?** (In a man under age 40): ankylosing spondylitis

2.3 Was the onset of the pain
* sudden? rapid? Mechanical or infectious origin of the pain; injury to soft tissue in the lower part of the back; vertebral body collapse in severe osteoporosis

* gradual? insidious?** Ankylosing spondylitis; systemic disorder; pain from disk disease may develop insidiously

2.4 Do you have recurring episodes of back pain? Protrusion of intervertebral lumbar disk; recurrent acute strains (any cause of chronic or recurring low back pain can produce an acute attack)

* with insidious onset of each episode of backache?
* each episode lasting months? } Spondylarthropathy

2.5 Has the pain
* remained the same? Stabilized process
* worsened? Evolutive process. Insidiously progressive back pain in an older patient: tumor, infection

3 Character and Intensity of the Pain

3.1   Is the pain
      • mild? moderate to severe? se-   An individually variable factor which
        vere, unbearable?   should be interpreted with caution. The
                                                possibility of exaggeration or prolonga-
                                                tion of pain for purposes of compensa-
                                                tion or other personal reasons should be
                                                kept in mind

3.2   Does the pain
      • make you unable to work? to en-   ⎫
        gage in social activities?   ⎬   Useful indexes to the degree of severity
      • confine you to bed? interfere   ⎭   of pain
        with sleep?

3.3   Is the back pain
      • dull, aching in character? slow in   Local pain produced by stimuli within
        onset, long in duration? diffuse?   deep skeletal structures (ligaments, fas-
                                                cia, muscles, periosteum)

3.4   Is the back pain
      • steady? constant in duration?   Local pain (may be intermittent):
                                                strain; lumbar disk (early stage); osteo-
                                                porosis
      • aching? deep? diffuse? steady?   Referred pain from the spine or from
                                                visceral disease
      • unremittent, severe, and pro-   Neoplasm (vertebral tumor); pyogenic
        gressive?   or tuberculous infection of the spine
      • intermittent, recurrent?   Ruptured disk causing instability of the
                                                spine; ankylosing spondylitis; fibrositis
      • throbbing?   Pain caused by neoplasms

3.5   If a distal radiation is present, is the
      radiated pain

      • *sharp*, lancinating, intense?   ⎫   Radicular type of pain: distortion,
      • well localized? rapid in onset?   ⎬   stretching, irritation, or compression of
                                            ⎭   a spinal nerve root
      • dull, aching, steady? deep? poor-   Referred pain from spinal structures
        ly localized?
      • mild?   Spinal cord lesion (associated with
                                                neurologic abnormalities)

4   Precipitating or Aggravating Factors

4.1   Did the pain accompany or follow
      • a trauma, an injury to the back?   The most frequent cause of low back
                                                pain; herniated lumbar disk; low back
                                                strain; a vertebral fracture must be ex-
                                                cluded; in the elderly patient: osteopor-
                                                osis, with collapse or wedging of a ver-
                                                tebra

- a strenuous use of the back? lifting a heavy object?
- unaccustomed heavy work?
- a bending forward motion? your getting up from bed?

Injury to soft tissue in the lower back: lumbosacral or sacroiliac strain; disk disease, facet joint irritation

4.1a In case of a trauma prior to the onset of pain, when did it occur?

Persistence of acute symptoms beyond 72 h is highly indicative of some serious underlying process other than mechanical derangement and requires hospitalization

4.2 Did the pain appear spontaneously?

In many cases of ruptured intervertebral disk, no trauma is recalled

4.3 Is the pain caused or exacerbated by
- moving the trunk? active use of the back?

Local pain; acute strain; lumbar disk disease (sudden displacement of nuclear material); osteoarthritis; infection of the vertebral column

- walking?

Intermittent spinal claudication from spinal stenosis (with paresthesias and weakness in the legs)

- prolonged weight bearing?

Structural abnormalities; spondylolisthesis

- *coughing? sneezing? straining at stool?*

Nerve root compression; radicular pain; lumbar disk lesion; local pain may also be aggravated

- bending with the knees extended? lifting a heavy object from the floor with the trunk bent?

Lumbar disk disease; local pain: traumatic strain

- maintaining a particular posture over a period of time?

Postural back pain with inadequate musculature

- sitting?

Disk herniation

- emotional tension?

Fibrositis

- rest? inactivity?

Spondylarthropathy: ankylosing spondylitis; fibrositis

4.4 Is the pain unaffected by movement of the spine?

Referred pain from visceral disease

4.5 Does the pain occur or worsen
- *in the early morning upon arising?*
- at night?

Ankylosing spondylitis

Destructive lesion: neoplastic; infectious (septic arthritis; osteomyelitis); Paget's disease; osteomalacia; spinal cord tumor; ankylosing spondylitis

4.6 For the female patient with pain in the sacral region: Does the pain appear

- before and/or during the menstruation?
- when you have been standing for several hours?

Endometriosis involving the uterosacral ligaments

Malposition of the uterus; fibroma of the uterus (the pelvis is seldom the site of a disease which causes obscure low back pain)

5 Relieving Factors

5.1 Is the pain relieved or improved by
- bed rest?

Local mechanical back disorder: herniated disk; traumatic, strain; osteoarthritis; radicular pain

- lying on a firm bed? on the floor?

Lumbar disk disease: decrease of the vertebral loading of the spine

- lying supine with the knees flexed? or on one side?

Decreasing the tension and pressure of the nerve root: disk disease

- *sitting?*

Spinal claudication (spinal stenosis)

- mild activity? "loosening up" in the morning?

May be observed in osteoarthritis; fibrositis

- by trying to curl up?

Underlying systemic disorder: visceral disease: pancreatic neoplasm, posterior penetrating ulcer

- movement? exercise?**

Ankylosing spondylitis

5.2 Is the pain unrelieved by recumbency? rest?

Visceral pain; destructive, neoplastic or infectious disease of the spine; ankylosing spondylitis

6 Accompanying Symptoms

6.1 If the pain has appeared immediately after a trauma to the back
- can you move your legs?

A **vertebral fracture** must be excluded

6.1a Do you have any muscle weakness? loss of sensation in the limbs? urinary incontinence? inability to void?

Vertebral fracture: **spinal cord lesion**

6.2 If the pain was precipitated by a minor trauma, did you
- feel a "sudden snap" in the lower part of the back?
- experience the sensation of something "tearing", "giving way" in the back?

In lumbar disk lesion: sudden rupture of the defective annulus due to sudden rise in the tension in the nucleus and backward displacement of nuclear material

6.3 In case of chronic and/or recurring low back pain, do you have

• *numbness, tingling of either or both lower extremities?*
• any weakness, wasting of a muscle in a lower extremity?

May accompany radicular pain arising from compression and irritation of nerve roots; disk disease; osteoarthritis; congenital smallness of the lumbar canal with multiple spondylitic caudal radiculopathy; a space-occupying lesion in the spinal cord or in the intervertebral foramen may be responsible

6.4 Do you have
• fever? a general malaise? fatigue?

Ankylosing spondylitis. Acute pain in the back may occur in any febrile disorder; infectious lesion of the spine; underlying systemic disorder. (Absent in osteoarthritis)

• any stiffness of your back and limitation of motion?
  • increased by exercise?

Local pain; strain; lumbar disk disease (In referred pain from visceral disease, there is no stiffness and motion is of full range)

  • especially marked in the morning?** (produced by inactivity? relieved by activity?)

Ankylosing spondylitis

• difficulty, burning on urination? frequency of urination?

Reiter's syndrome with spondylarthropathy; carcinoma of prostate with metastases to the lower part of the spine

• (female patient) a vaginal discharge?

Gynecologic disease causing low back pain

• pain in other joints?

Occurs in 25 percent of patients with ankylosing spondylitis; osteoarthritis

• a skin condition?

Psoriasis with spondylarthropathy

• an eye condition?

Conjunctivitis: Reiter's syndrome with spondylitis. Anterior uveitis: ankylosing spondylitis

• chronic diarrhea?

Spondylitis may be associated with ulcerative colitis, Crohn's disease, Whipple's disease (rarely)

• bowel and bladder dysfunction? incontinence?

Acute cauda equina compression: may be due to a centrally herniating disk

• an increase of weight?

Aggravating factor in traumatic and degenerative disorders of the spine

• a loss of weight?

Neoplasm; tuberculosis of the spine

7   Iatrogenic Factors   See Etiology

8   Personal and Social Profile

8.1 Age and sex of the patient?

Low back pain in:
a young patient: muscle or ligament strain, injury; spondylarthropathy; herniated disk

an elderly patient: osteoarthritis, osteoporosis, malignant lesion

a postmenopausal woman: compression vertebral fracture from osteoporosis.

Reiter's disease, ankylosing spondylitis,
and back injuries: more common in
males

8.2   What is your occupation?   Increased incidence of disk disease in
                                              occupations where heavy lifting is re-
                                              quired: truck drivers, material handlers,
                                              nurses

8.2a Are you suing for compensation for   The pain may be exaggerated or pro-
      your back pain?   longed because of psychologic factors,
                                              especially when there is the possibility
                                              of personal gain (compensation)

9   Personal Antecedents Pertaining to the Low Back Pain

9.1   Have you ever had
      • an x-ray of your spine? a my-
        elography?   spinal   surgery?
        When? With what results?
      • multiple lumbar operations and   Lumbar adhesive arachnoiditis
        myelograms?

9.2   Have you had diarrhea before your   Enterobacterial infection; inflammatory
      backache?   bowel disease preceding spondylarth-
                                             ropathy

10   Family Medical History Pertaining to the Low Back Pain

10.1 Are there any members of your   Family occurrence of ankylosing spon-
      family who have arthritic diseases?   dylitis, of psoriasis
      a skin disease?

PHYSICAL SIGNS PERTAINING TO LOW BACK PAIN*

	Possible significance
Inability to move the legs	Fractured spine
Fever; flaccid paraplegia; localized pain with percussion and palpation of the spine	Epidural abscess with compression of the spinal cord
Muscle spasm and tenderness in involved area	Herniated disk; osteoarthritis; ankylosing spondylitis; lumbosacral strain
Localized tenderness on percussion or pressure over the involved area	Tumor; infection; osteoporosis with vertebral compression

*In this section, items in **boldface** are potentially life-threatening or urgent conditions.

Tenderness on palpation of the sacroiliac joints; paravertebral muscle spasm and tenderness; loss of lumbar lordotic curve	Sacroiliitis: in the early stages of ankylosing spondylitis
Painful lateral compression of the pelvis	Sacroiliac disease: associated with osteoarthritis, ankylosing spondylitis
Painful and limited straight-leg-raising maneuver	Positive Lasègue's sign: disease of lumbosacral joints; herniated lumbar intervertebral disk; lumbosacral roots involvement
Difference in midline measurements from sacrum to T12, in flexion and extension, less than 7 cm	Diminished lumbar flexion; chronic phase of ankylosing spondylitis
Motor, sensory, and reflex changes in the lower extremities	Nerve root involvement: ruptured lumbar intervertebral disk; osteophytic spur; spinal lesion
Diminished chest expansion (<5 cm)	Costovertebral joint involvement in ankylosing spondylitis
Aortic regurgitation murmur	Ankylosing spondylitis: in 3 percent of patients
Tenderness over the costovertebral angle	Renal disease; adrenal disease; injury to the transverse processes of the first or second lumbar vertebra
Full range motion of the spine; no local signs; no stiffness of the back	Referred pain from visceral disease (colon, diverticulitis, tumor of the colon, gynecologic disorder)
Abdominal, rectal, and pelvic examination	May reveal gastrointestinal, urologic, and gynecologic diseases extending to the spine or causing referred pain

LABORATORY TESTS PERTAINING TO LOW BACK PAIN[†]

Test	Finding	Diagnostic Possibilities
Blood		
ESR	Elevated	Infection of the vertebral column; multiple myeloma; ankylosing spondylitis
	Normal	Osteoarthritis
Protein electrophoresis; immunoglobulin electrophoresis	Abnormal	Multiple myeloma; collagen-vascular diseases

[†]See the appendix on Laboratory Reference Values for the associated normal laboratory values.

Test	Finding	Diagnostic Possibilities
Alkaline phosphatase	Normal	Osteoporosis; multiple myeloma
	Elevated	Metastatic carcinoma; Paget's disease
Acid phosphatase	Elevated	Metastatic carcinoma of prostate
HLA-B27 antigen*	Positive	Ankylosing spondylitis; Reiter's syndrome; enteropathic arthropathy; psoriatic arthritis

*When indicated

LABORATORY PROCEDURES PERTAINING TO LOW BACK PAIN

Procedure	To Detect
Lumbar spine x-rays	Osteophytic overgrowth, spur formation, bridging of vertebrae: osteoarthritis
	Disk narrowing: disk herniation (x-ray may be normal)
	Sacroiliac arthritis, syndesmophytes, "bamboo spine": ankylosing spondylitis
	Bone destruction: neoplasm, tuberculosis, neuropathic disorders
	Collapse; wedging of a vertebra: osteoporosis (nonspecific abnormality)
	Vertebral fracture; spondylolisthesis; spondylolysis; Paget's disease
X-ray of other bones and joints	Malignancy, osteoporosis, etc.
Myelography*	Disk herniation; spinal cord tumor
Bone scan	Hot spots: fractures; neoplastic and inflammatory lesions
Computerized tomography (CT);* magnetic resonance imaging (MRI)*	Destructive lesions of the vertebral bodies and posterior elements; presence of a paravertebral soft tissue mass; disk herniation; narrow canal
Psychiatric evaluation*	Depression; malingering; compensation hysteria

*When indicated

SELECTED BIBLIOGRAPHY

Boachie-Adjei O: Evaluation of the patient with low back pain. *Postgrad Med* 84(3):110–119, 1988.
Curd JG, Thorne RP: Diagnosis and management of lumbar disk disease. *Hosp Pract* 24(9):135–148, 1989.
Frymoyer JW: Back pain and sciatica. *N Engl J Med* 318:291–300, 1988.
Hadler NM: The patient with low back pain. *Hosp Pract* 22(10A):17–22, 1987.

42
Pain in the Lower Extremities

INTRODUCTION

Pain in the lower extremities may result from diseases of the skin and of the musculo-skeletal, vascular, and nervous systems. Superficial pain (skin and adjacent structures) is well localized and is associated with tenderness and hyperalgesia. The pain from trauma is due to mechanical stimulation of nerve endings. In bacterial infections, rapidly forming edema increases local tissue pressure and causes pain in skin already made hyperalgesic by chemical factors associated with injury. Deep pain originates in fascia, vessels, periosteum, joints, and supporting structures; it is often poorly localized and dull, and may be associated with muscle rigidity and deep tenderness. The pain from ischemia in skeletal muscles (arteriosclerosis) may be produced by the action on sensory nerve endings of metabolites accumulating in the muscles or by changes in the nerves from ischemia. The pain of joint involvement is related to inflammation of the synovial membranes. Pain due to diseases of the peripheral nerves may be associated with areflexia and distal or other sensory impairment. Irritation and compression of nerve roots by a herniated nucleosus pulposus or osteoarthritis can cause pain in the lower extremities. Pain from the deep muscles of the back or from the vertebrae may be the source of pain referred to the extremity. Referred pain is usually well localized.

ETIOLOGY

Skin and Soft Tissues

Acute trauma to the skin
Cellulitis: bacterial and fungal infections; lymphangitis
Erythema nodosum

Articular and Periarticular Structures

Arthritis: acute pyogenic arthritis; gout; rheumatoid arthritis; rheumatic fever; osteoarthritis; posttraumatic condition; hypertrophic osteoarthropathy
Bursitis; tendinitis; ruptured popliteal (Baker's) cyst

Bone and Periosteum

Fracture; osteomyelitis; tumors

Muscles

Acute suppurative myositis; polymyositis, dermatomyositis; polymyalgia rheumatica
Muscle strain, trauma, or tear
Nocturnal muscle cramps

Vascular

Arterial disorders: arterial occlusion: acute (thrombosis, embolism, cholesterol emboli, injury); chronic (arteriosclerosis obliterans, thromboangiitis obliterans)

Venous disorders: varicose veins; venous thrombosis: superficial, deep; chronic
    venous insufficiency; postphlebitic syndrome
Lymphedema
Erythromelalgia

Neurologic

Polyneuropathy; mononeuropathy multiplex (polyarteritis nodosa, diabetes)
Nerve root compression: ruptured lumbar intervertebral disk; osteoarthritis; spinal
    cord neoplasm
Entrapment neuropathy: meralgia paresthetica
Reflex sympathetic dystrophies; causalgia
Interdigital neuroma; glomus tumor

Iatrogenic Causes of Pain in the Lower Extremities

Oral contraceptives with or without venous thrombosis
Corticosteroids: avascular necrosis of head of femur; increased liability to septic
    arthritis
Penicillin, sulfonamides, iodides, bromides, oral contraceptives: erythema nodosum
Clofibrate: calf cramps
Faulty intramuscular injection: sciatic neuritis
Anticoagulants: muscle hematoma

HISTORY TAKING*

Possible meaning of a positive response

1   Location and Radiation of the Pain

1.1   Where do you have pain?
    • in a joint?
        • hip?

Osteoarthritis; rheumatoid arthritis; ankylosing spondylitis; acute trauma; septic arthritis [infectious arthritis affects
large joints (hips, knees) more fre-
quently]; polymyalgia rheumatica;
neoplasm; avascular necrosis of the
femoral head; referred pain: pelvic inflammatory disease

        • knee?

Osteoarthritis (the commonest source of
major disability in osteoarthritis); meniscus tear; knee sprain; rheumatoid
arthritis; septic arthritis; gout, pseudogout; neuropathic; ruptured Baker's
cyst. Occasionally, pain from the hip
may be felt only in the knee

*In this section, items in *italics* are characteristic clinical features, and items in **boldface** are
potentially life-threatening or urgent conditions.

• ankle? foot?	Traumatic injury, sprain (may affect any joint); neuropathic, diabetes (pain, when present, is mild)
• *great toe?*	Gout
• small joints of foot? (metatarsophalangeal, toes)	Rheumatoid arthritis [pseudogout does not affect the small joints of (hands and) feet]
• in an area adjacent to a joint?	Periarticular structure: bursitis, tendinitis
• in the thigh?	Arthritis of hip; avascular necrosis of hip; arthritis of knee; meralgia paresthetica; herniated lumbar disk; trauma; fracture; fibrositis; myositis; polymyalgia rheumatica; intermittent claudication; psoas abscess; primary or metastatic tumors; Paget's disease
• in the calf?	Trauma; fractured bone; bone disease: osteomyelitis, tumor, Paget's disease; vascular occlusion, chronic or acute; intermittent claudication; thrombophlebitis; ruptured popliteal cyst; spontaneous rupture of plantaris tendon (sudden onset of severe pain during exertion); Achilles tendinitis; peripheral neuropathy, multiple sclerosis; night cramps; restless legs syndrome; erythema nodosum; arthritis of knee, ankle. Calf cramps in: dehydration, hyponatremia, hypothyroidism, thyrotoxic myopathy; uremia; hypomagnesemia; amyotrophic lateral sclerosis
• in both feet?	If acute pain: cholesterol emboli arising from ulcerating plaques in the aorta
• in the foot? toes?	Ischemic rest pain due to chronic arterial occlusion
• in the soles?	Plantar neuralgia; Morton's neuroma; tarsal tunnel syndrome; plantar fasciitis in Reiter's syndrome
• in the forefoot?	Rheumatoid arthritis; psoriasis; hallux valgus deformity
• in the heel?	Achilles tendinitis in Reiter's syndrome; ankylosing spondylitis; enteropathic arthropathy; idiopathic heel spurs; Achilles bursitis; fascial strain
• along the limb in a linear fashion? crossing over joint and muscle areas?	Lesion of nerve or blood vessel; herniated intervertebral disk; neuropathy; deep-vein thrombosis; arterial occlusion
1.2 *Do you have back pain radiating to your limb?*	Radicular pain

- *in the lateral region of the thigh, calf? to the dorsum of the foot?*

  Lesion of the fifth lumbar root: herniation of disk between the fourth and fifth lumbar vertebrae

- *in the posterior part of the thigh? calf? to the heel and plantar surface of the foot?*

  Lesion of the first sacral root: herniation of disk between the fifth lumbar and the first sacral vertebrae

- in the anterior part of the thigh and knee?

  Lesions of the fourth and third lumbar roots (rarer)

2 Mode of Onset and Duration of the Pain

2.1 How long have you had pain in your leg?

2.2 Was the onset of pain
- sudden?

  Acute arterial occlusion (large to medium-sized vessels); acute infectious process, articular or nonarticular; in calf: spontaneous rupture (during exercise) of plantaris tendon; in both feet: cholesterol emboli arising from ulcerating plaques in the aorta; gout; trauma; nocturnal muscle cramps

- gradual? (several hours)

  (Onset may be sudden): venous thrombosis; cellulitis; lymphangitis; arthritis; disk disease; osteomyelitis

- gradual? (days to months)

  Chronic arterial occlusion; bursitis, tendinitis, fibrositis; rheumatoid arthritis; osteoarthritis; erythema nodosum; neuropathy; erythromelalgia; causalgia; interdigital neuroma

- months to years?

  Primary varicose veins; postphlebitic syndrome

2.3 Is the pain in your leg chronic? recurrent?

  Varicose veins; venous thrombosis (if there is a continuing risk factor: carcinoma, immobilization, antithrombin III or protein C deficiency); chronic venous insufficiency

3 Character and Intensity of the Pain

3.1 Is your pain
- *sharp? shooting?* burning?

  Nerve lesions: posterior nerve roots, peripheral neuropathy

- dull? diffuse?

  Venous or lymphatic disorders (the pain of venous thrombosis is not characteristic: it may be either an ache or a cramp, sharp or dull, and severe or mild)

- aching?

  Muscle or joint problems

- throbbing?

  Pain arising in the bones

3.2   Is the pain

• severe?	Arterial occlusion; osteomyelitis; ruptured synovial cyst; nocturnal muscle cramps; gout; venous thrombosis; arthritis; muscle tear. In the hip: acute trauma; septic arthritis
• mild to moderate?	Deep-vein thrombosis; muscle or joint pain (osteoarthritis, rheumatoid arthritis); bursitis; tendinitis; cellulitis; lymphangitis

4   Precipitating or Aggravating Factors

4.1   In case of articular pain: Do you have pain in your joint

• only with movement? walking? climbing stairs?	Hip and knee: osteoarthritis (early stage) Knee: posttraumatic internal joint derangement
• on prolonged standing?	Hip and knee: osteoarthritis
• at rest?	Rheumatoid arthritis; osteoarthritis (advanced stage)

4.1a Is the pain induced or made worse with weight bearing?	Hip and knee: osteoarthritis
4.1b In case of pain in the knee: Is the pain worse after sitting, kneeling? climbing stairs?	Chondromalacia patellae

4.2   In case of nonarticular pain: Is the pain induced or made worse

• *by sneezing? coughing? straining at stool?* bending? lifting?	Disorders of the vertebral column or of the posterior nerve roots (ruptured lumbar intervertebral disk)
• by elevation of your leg? exposure to cold?	Pain of ulceration; ischemic rest pain; chronic arterial occlusion
• by dependency?	Venous obstruction
• by exercise? movement?	Chronic arterial occlusion; postphlebitic syndrome; venous thrombosis; osteomyelitis; muscle strain
• at night?	Nocturnal muscle cramps (not symptoms of arterial disease of any kind; more frequent in pregnant women, the middle aged, and the elderly); chronic arterial occlusion; involvement of bone; neoplasm of the hip, tuberculosis; varicose veins
• by weight bearing?	Venous thrombosis
• by rest?	Ischemic pain (felt in the toes and metatarsal joints): in severe chronic arterial insufficiency, multiple levels of occlusion

• by prolonged standing?	Chronic venous insufficiency; varicose veins; lymphedema; origin of pain in the lumbar spine or feet; postphlebitic syndrome
• by movements of the back?	Disorder of the spine or hip

4.3   *Is your pain induced by walking?*   Intermittent claudication: chronic arterial occlusion (the pain of intermittent claudication is unilateral at first and may become bilateral at any time); also in musculoskeletal disorders; pseudoclaudication from cauda equina compression in spinal stenosis

4.3a   Where do you have pain on walking?

• in the calf?	Occlusion of popliteal artery or higher
• *at the instep? the arch of the foot?*	Thromboangiitis obliterans: involvement of vessels of the leg with sparing of the femoral and iliac arteries
• in the thigh, buttock, and calf?	Occlusion of common femoral artery or iliac arteries
• with low back pain? numbness or weakness in the legs?	Pseudoclaudication syndrome: spinal stenosis due to spondylosis or congenital narrowing

4.3b   How long are you able to walk, at an average pace on level ground, before the pain appears?   The walking distance required to produce pain is usually constant at any stage of the chronic arterial occlusion. Symptoms of cauda equina pseudoclaudication are less stereotypic

• half an hour?	Early stage of chronic arterial occlusion
• between one-half and two blocks?	Most frequently in chronic arterial occlusion
• 50 to 100 steps?	Advanced stage of the disease

5   Relieving Factors

5.1   Is the (nonarticular) pain relieved by

• elevation of your leg?	Venous thrombosis; chronic venous insufficiency, postphlebitic syndrome
• dependency? • (at night) by dangling your leg over the side of the bed?	(Rest) pain due to chronic arterial occlusion

5.2   In case of pain induced by walking: Is your pain relieved by

• *sitting?*	Pseudoclaudication
• rest?	
• *promptly?* (1 to 2 min)	Chronic arterial occlusion with intermittent claudication

• gradually? Does the pain persist for longer than 10 min after you have stopped walking?

Pseudoclaudication syndrome; degenerative hip and/or knee joint disease; probably not chronic arterial occlusion

5.3   In case of pain in the foot: Does the pain improve with weight bearing? as the day progresses?

Rheumatoid arthritis

6   Accompanying Symptoms

6.1   In case of hip pain: Do you have:
• inability to walk? limping?

Osteoarthritis, necrosis of hip; hips may be affected in ankylosing spondylitis (painless limp in neuropathic arthropathy)

• difficulty in arising from a chair? from a kneeling position? putting on shoes and stockings?

In almost all moderate to severe disease of the hip

6.2   In case of knee pain: Do you have
• a feeling of locking, snapping at times?
• pain on squatting? on running up and down stairs?

Posttraumatic internal joint derangement: involvement of medial meniscus; ligament tear; loose body

6.2a   Is your painful knee swollen? red? hot?

Infection: septic, gonococcal arthritis; crystal-induced arthritis. May accompany a ruptured popliteal cyst

6.2b   Is your swollen knee relatively painless?

Intermittent hydrarthrosis: recurrent joint effusion, usually in young women at menstruation

6.3   In case of hip or knee pain: Do you have stiffness after prolonged immobility?

Intra- or extraarticular disorder; rheumatoid arthritis; tendinitis, bursitis

6.4   In case of acute nonarticular pain: Has the pain been followed by coldness? numbness? tingling? muscle weakness?

Acute arterial occlusion (thrombosis or embolism)

6.5   In case of acute nonarticular pain: Is the leg pain accompanied by
• local swelling?

Cellulitis; lymphangitis; superficial thrombophlebitis; acute venous thrombosis; rupture of plantaris tendon; ruptured popliteal cyst (pseudothrombophlebitis); severe muscle strain; muscle tear; muscle hematoma; bone lesions, fracture; exacerbation of postphlebitic syndrome

• no swelling?
• tender red nodules on the legs?

Arterial insufficiency; neurogenic pain
Erythema nodosum

6.6 Do you have
     • fever? chills?   Acute sepsis; septic arthritis; acute
                                          osteomyelitis; erythema nodosum;
                                          acute suppurative myositis

     • *numbness, tingling in the limb?* Nerve root compression: herniated
                                          lumbar intervertebral disk

     • skin ulcerations?   Chronic arterial occlusion; multiple
                                          sites of vascular occlusion; thromboan-
                                          giitis obliterans

     • swollen leg(s)?   Venous thrombosis; chronic venous in-
                                          sufficiency; postphlebitic syndrome

     • (male patient) pain on urination? ⎫
     • (female patient) a vaginal dis-   ⎬ Gonococcal arthritis or tendinitis
       charge?   ⎭

     • sexual impotence?   With hip, thigh, and buttock claudica-
                                          tion: Leriche syndrome: distal aortoiliac
                                          occlusion

7   Iatrogenic Factors   See Etiology

8   Personal and Social Profile

8.1 Do you smoke?   Adverse effect on occlusive arterial dis-
                                          ease

8.2 What is your sexual orientation?   In a homosexual man: joint pains:
                                          tenosynovitis of disseminated gonococ-
                                          cal infection, arthritis of hepatitis B;
                                          localized nerve pain: herpes zoster,
                                          neuralgia of AIDS-related conditions

9   Personal Antecedents Pertaining to the Pain

9.1 Have you ever had an x-ray of your
     joints? bones? When? With what
     results?

9.2 Have you recently had
     • a trauma to your limb?   Deep-vein thrombosis; cellulitis; post-
                                         traumatic arthritis; acute attack of gout;
                                         infection introduced into the body by
                                         the trauma
                                         Hip: fracture; posttraumatic avascular
                                         necrosis of head of femur
                                         Knee: torn ligament or meniscus; loose
                                         bodies; a knee trauma or arthritis may
                                         precede a ruptured popliteal cyst

     • unusual exercise or activity?   Muscle strain or trauma (pain usually in
       (jogging, hiking, tennis, squash?) both legs)
     • an operation? a prolonged im-   Risk factors for deep-vein thrombosis
       mobilization? carcinoma? preg-
       nancy?

9.3 Do you have
  • a heart disease? atrial fibrilla-   **Acute embolic arterial occlusion**
    tion?
  • diabetes?   Neurogenic limb pain; chronic arterial
                                              occlusion

PHYSICAL SIGNS PERTAINING TO PAIN IN THE LOWER EXTREMITIES

Possible significance

Local swelling, warmth, erythema, fever; open wound	Infectious process: cellulitis, with or without lymphangitis
Swollen, red, warm, tender joint(s)	Acute pyogenic arthritis; posttraumatic; rheumatoid arthritis; gout; crystal-induced arthritis; rheumatic fever
Cold, pale limb; motor weakness; loss of sensation; absent pulses; no swelling • with irregular heart rhythm	Acute arterial occlusion: embolism, thrombosis, injury Atrial fibrillation with arterial embolism
Palpable pulse disappearing with exercise; absent pulse(s); cool limb, extremity becoming pale on elevation; trophic changes in skin and nails; ulceration	Chronic arterial occlusion: atherosclerosis of large and medium-sized arteries
After a period of elevation of the leg: • flushing time >20 s • venous filling time >30 s	} Severe arterial obstruction; inadequate collateral circulation
Absent pulses with warm, normally colored extremity	Chronic arterial occlusion with adequate collateral blood flow
Cyanotic mottling of the skin of the feet	Livedo reticularis (with symmetric rest pain in the feet: cholesterol emboli from the aorta)
Tender cords in the path of veins; erythema of the overlying skin; no prominent leg swelling	Superficial-vein thrombosis
Leg edema; tenderness in the calf muscles; calf cyanosis, calf pain with dorsiflexion of the foot (Homan's sign)	Deep-vein thrombosis; ruptured popliteal cyst (clinical diagnosis of deep-vein thrombosis is uncorrect in up to 50 percent of cases)
Localized tenderness in the calf	Torn calf muscle
Bone tenderness • with fever, chills, local swelling	Fracture; malignancy Osteomyelitis
Warm, tender, red nodules over the tibial areas	Erythema nodosum: associated with infection (streptococcal, tuberculous, fungal), sarcoidosis, inflammatory bowel disease, oral contraceptives

Palpable, tender temporal artery	Polymyalgia rheumatica (with pain in the limbs)
Absent ankle and knee jerks; sensory impairment; tenderness of deep tissues	Polyneuropathy
Low back and leg pain	Ruptured lumbar intervertebral disk; osteoarthritis, with nerve root compression
• with weakness of the extensors of the great toe and of the foot; difficulty in walking on the heels; no reflex change; sensory deficit in the lateral leg and mediodorsal aspect of the foot; limitation of straight-leg raising	Lesion of the fifth lumbar root
• with diminished to absent ankle reflex, weakness of plantar flexors, difficulty in walking on the toes, sensory deficit in the lateral border and sole of the foot and toes; limitation of straight-leg raising	Lesion of the first sacral root

LABORATORY PROCEDURES PERTAINING TO PAIN IN THE LOWER EXTREMITIES

Procedure	To Detect
Lumbosacral spine x-rays	Intervertebral disk herniation; primary or metastatic neoplasm
Joint and bone x-rays	Fracture; rheumatoid arthritis; osteoarthritis; gout; pseudogout; osteomyelitis; primary or metastatic tumor
Doppler ultrasound and plethysmography	Proximal vein thrombosis
Contrast venography	The "gold standard" for diagnosis of deep venous thrombosis
Arthrogram*	Pseudothrombophlebitis (ruptured popliteal cyst)
Doppler ultrasound;* arteriography*	Peripheral arterial disease; location and extent of the occlusive involvement in chronic or acute arterial occlusion
CT scan*; myelography*	Intervertebral disk herniation; spinal cord tumor
Nerve conduction studies;* electromyography;* muscle biopsy*	Lesions of the anterior horn cells, muscle, peripheral nerves
Joint fluid analysis*	See Chapter 40 "Articular Pain"

*When indicated

SELECTED BIBLIOGRAPHY

Katerndahl DA: Calf pain mimicking thrombophlebitis. *Postgrad Med* 68(6):107–115, 1980.

Mann RA: Pain in the foot. *Postgrad Med* 82(1):154–162, 167–174, 1987.

Strandness DE Jr: Vascular diseases of the extremities, in Wilson J, Braunwald E, Isselbacher KJ et al (eds). *Harrison's Principles of Internal Medicine,* 12th ed., chap. 198, New York: McGraw-Hill, 1991.

43

Pain in the Neck and Shoulder

INTRODUCTION

Local Pain   Caused by any pathologic process which impinges upon, or irritates, sensory nerve endings in periosteum, synovial membranes, muscles, annulus fibrosus, and ligaments.

Referred Pain   Produced by stimulation of sensory nerve endings in the structural soft tissues which support the cervical spine and which are part of the cervical disk complex.

Radicular (root) Pain   Caused by distortion or compression of a spinal root.

Pain arising from the cervical spine is experienced in the neck and back of the head, but may be projected to the shoulder and arm. The pain of herniated nucleosus pulposus is deep and poorly localized to the level of the spine where the disk rupture has occurred. It is usually associated with evidence of neurologic involvement. Nerve roots may also be involved in osteoarthritis of the cervical spine.

Pain of brachial plexus origin (abnormalities of the thoracic outlet) is felt in and around the shoulder, in the supraclavicular region, or between the shoulders; it is associated with neurologic and circulatory abnormalities in the arm.

Shoulder pain resulting from a tear in the rotator cuff or from a calcific tendinitis may radiate into the arm or hand, but is not associated with peripheral sensory, motor, and reflex changes. Apart from acute traumatic lesions, 85 to 90 percent of painful disability of the shoulder is due to nonarticular disorders of tendons, bursas, tendon sheaths, and the musculotendinous cuff.

ETIOLOGY

Neck Pain

Fibrositis; chronic cervical muscle spasm
Osteoarthritis: cervical spondylosis
Acute cervical strain; torticollis (stiff neck); sternocleidomastoid tendinitis
Herniated cervical disk
Rheumatoid arthritis; ankylosing spondylitis
Tumors: local; metastatic
Whiplash injury
Polymyalgia rheumatica
Osteomyelitis

Pain in the Shoulder

Local: rotator cuff tear; calcific tendinitis; adhesive capsulitis
Subacromial or subdeltoid bursitis
Vertebral column: fractures; arthritis; protruded disk
Osteoarthritis

Neurovascular
  Compression (thoracic outlet) syndromes: cervical rib syndrome, scalenus anticus
    syndrome, costoclavicular syndrome, hyperabduction syndrome
  Shoulder-hand syndrome: idiopathic; secondary: trauma, stroke
Peripheral nerves: trauma; tumors; neuropathy
Spinal cord: syringomyelia; herpes zoster; tumors
Carpal tunnel syndrome; synovitis of elbow with nerve entrapment
Referred viscerogenic pain in the shoulder
  Thorax: cardiac, pericardial, aorta, diaphragm lesions
  Abdomen: biliary tract disease, diaphragm

HISTORY TAKING*

Possible meaning of a positive response

1   Location and Radiation of the Pain

1.1 Where do you have pain?	The patient usually can indicate the site of origin
• anterior neck pain?	Thyroid; intrathoracic disease with referred pain to the neck; ischemic heart disease
• in the neck and back of head?	Pain arising fron the cervical spine; cervical osteoarthritis
• in the neck, shoulder, arm?	Tear of the rotator cuff; tendinitis; abnormalities of the thoracic outlet (pain of brachial plexus origin). Pain in the deltoid area usually reflects disease of the neck and shoulder; it is rarely viscerogenic
• in and around the shoulder?	
• with pain in the supraclavicular region? between the shoulders?	Pain resulting from abnormalities of the thoracic outlet
1.2 Does the pain radiate	
• from the neck to the shoulder(s)? the arm(s)?	Cervical nerve root involvement: herniated cervical disk; osteoarthritis
• from the neck to the suboccipital or postauricular region? the mid- or upper portions of the neck laterally?	Almost certainly excludes lower cervical nerve root compression
• from the shoulder to the arm? the hand?	Thoracic outlet syndrome; may occur in calcific tendinitis
• from the trapezius ridge, the top of the shoulder to the anterior upper part of the arm? radial forearm? thumb?	Ruptured cervical disk (disk lesion between the fifth and sixth cervical vertebrae, sixth cervical root)

*In this section, items in *italics* are characteristic clinical features.

- from the wrist to the forearm and shoulder?

Carpal tunnel syndrome: the pain may be referred to the forearm and the shoulder and neck regions

2 Mode of Onset and Duration

2.1 How long have you had pain?
   - hours to days?

Neck: acute cervical strain; whiplash injury
Shoulder: acute process: calcific tendinitis, subacromial bursitis

   - weeks to months?

Neck: subacute or chronic process: herniated cervical disk; osteoarthritis; fibrositis
Shoulder: chronic process: adhesive capsulitis, shoulder-hand syndrome

2.2 Was the onset of pain

   - abrupt? sudden?

Neck: herniated cervical disk. Shoulder: calcific tendinitis (onset may be subacute)

   - gradual ? insidious?

Neck: cervical osteoarthritis; polymyalgia rheumatica
Shoulder: adhesive capsulitis

3 Character and Intensity of the Pain

3.1 Is the pain
   - dull? aching? constant?

Neck: pain caused by muscle or joint disorder; chronic cervical muscle spasm
Shoulder: adhesive capsulitis; also in chronic form of calcific tendinitis; skeletal pain

   - severe? interfering with sleep?

Shoulder: calcific tendinitis: night pain may be prominent

3.2 In case of pain in the neck projected to the arm: *Is the radiated pain sharp? shooting?*

Pain associated with cervical nerve root lesion; radicular pain of cervical disk disease; coincidental involvement of nerve roots in osteoarthritis

4 Precipitating or Aggravating Factors

4.1 Is your neck pain induced or enhanced by
   - the performance of certain tasks? certain positions?

Pain arising from the cervical spine; abnormalities of the thoracic outlet

   - hyperextension of the neck?

Cervical nerve root compression; ruptured cervical disk; osteoarthritis

   - coughing? sneezing?

Ruptured cervical disk

   - activity? motion?

Neck: mechanical pain: disk lesion, osteoarthritis

• inactivity?	Fibrositis; chronic cervical muscle spasm
• worse in the morning?	Arthritis; polymyalgia rheumatica

4.2 Is the pain in the shoulder increased by

• motion of the shoulder? internal rotation? abduction? extension?	Lesion of the tendinous structures about the shoulder; tear of the tendon cuff; calcific tendinitis; adhesive capsulitis
• inserting your arm into a coat sleeve?	
• certain positions of the arm? elevation of the arm above the chest level? the performance of certain tasks with arm?	Thoracic outlet syndrome
• activity? exertion?	Tendinitis; coronary insufficiency (especially if the upper extremities are not being used)
• coughing? sneezing?	Ruptured cervical disk

4.2a Is the pain in the shoulder worse at night? — Lesion of the tendinous structures about the shoulder: calcific tendinitis; bursitis; rupture of the rotator cuff

5 Relieving Factors

5.1 Is your neck pain relieved by

• rest? the recumbent position? flexion of the neck?	Cervical nerve root compression
• movement? activity?	Fibrositis

6 Accompanying Symptoms

6.1 Do you have

• stiffness, limitation of mobility of the neck?	Pain arising from the cervical spine; osteoarthritis, ruptured cervical disk, fibrositis
• stiffness, limitation of mobility, wasting of the muscles, of the shoulder?	Intrinsic disease of the shoulder: bursitis, tendinitis, adhesive capsulitis ("frozen shoulder"); rheumatoid arthritis (stiffness is absent in referred pain to the shoulder)

6.1a Is the stiffness worse in the morning? — Almost any disorder of the cervical spine

6.2 Do you have difficulty

• looking behind? turning the head while driving a car?	Cervical spine involvement with impaired range of motion
• hair combing? putting on a coat? taking dishes from the cupboard? reaching into a hip pocket for a wallet?	Abnormality within the shoulder joint, its capsule, or overlying tendons

6.3   *Do you have numbness, tingling, weakness, in your arm? hand?*

With neck pain: cervical nerve root compression

With shoulder pain: thoracic outlet syndrome. Sensory or other neurologic changes in the arm indicating disease of the nerve roots, plexus, or peripheral nerves are absent when shoulder pain is due to calcific tendinitis

6.4   Do you have
 • pain and/or swelling in other joints?

With neck pain: rheumatoid arthritis (may produce compression of the spinal cord: rare); spinal rheumatoid arthritis is rarely confined to the spine

 • a swollen hand? painful on motion?

Shoulder-hand syndrome (reflex dystrophy); occasionally thoracic outlet syndrome

6.5   Do you have
 • headaches?

Patients with long-standing chronic nuchal muscle spasm or rheumatoid arthritis of the spine often develop occipital headaches; temporal arteritis may cause pain in the occipital and upper cervical regions

 • fever?

Infection of cervical vertebra

 • episodes of vertigo? visual impairment?

With neck pain: compression of the vertebral arteries by degenerative spurs in the spinal canal may compromise the blood supply to the brain

 • a weakness in your legs? disturbance of your gait? (ataxia)

Compression of the spinal cord by cervical disk or by bony ridges formed in the spinal canal; primary neurologic disease: syringomyelia; amyotrophic lateral sclerosis; tumor

 • *pain in your fingers when they are immersed in cold water?*

With shoulder pain: unilateral Raynaud's phenomenon may occur in thoracic outlet syndrome

7   Personal and Social Profile

7.1   What is your profession?

Persons in certain occupations (draftsmen, typists, clerks) are liable to chronic spasm of the posterior cervical muscles (fibrositis). Continuous use of the arm above the head (dress saleswomen, painters, librarians) predisposes to bursitis or tendinitis of the shoulder. Thoracic outlet syndrome may result from repetitive shoulder movements, such as those used to play violin, work on an assembly line, operate a video display terminal

8   Personal Antecedents Pertaining to the Pain in the Neck and/or Shoulder

8.1   Have you ever had an x-ray of your neck? your shoulder? When? With what results?

8.2   Have you recently sustained
  • a trauma to the neck? a car accident?

Acute cervical strain; whiplash injury: injury to the ligaments and muscles (the pain may appear 48 to 72 hours after the accident)

  • sudden hyperextension of the neck? diving? forceful manipulations?

Ruptured cervical disk

8.3   Have you recently had
  • a trauma to your shoulder? heavy work? unusual or vigorous exercise? sport activities?

Rotator cuff tear

  • prolonged immobilization of the joint?

Adhesive capsulitis

8.4   Do you have a neurologic disease? rheumatoid arthritis? osteoarthritis?

PHYSICAL SIGNS PERTAINING TO PAIN IN THE NECK AND SHOULDER

Possible significance

Tenderness and limitation of motion of the neck

Disease of the ligaments, muscles, or apophyseal joints in the cervical spine; osteoarthritis

Swollen, red, warm, tender joint

Acute pyogenic arthritis, posttraumatic, crystal-induced arthritis

Shoulder pain with
  • loss of radial pulse in bracing and pulling down on shoulders, abducting arm over head, or during Adson's test*
  • pallor on elevating the arm

Thoracic outlet syndrome

  • supraclavicular palpable abnormality

Aneurysm of the subclavian artery, cervical rib, tumor causing the thoracic outlet syndrome

Neck and shoulder pain radiating into the arm, with weakness, deep-tendon reflex, and sensory changes in the arm

Involvement of nerve roots: osteoarthritis of the cervical spine; ruptured cervical disk

*Adson's test: the patient holds a full breath with the head tilted back or turned toward the affected side

Shoulder pain with tenderness and limitation of extension, abduction, rotation; no sensory, motor, and reflex changes

Tear of the rotator cuff; calcific tendinitis; adhesive capsulitis

Shoulder pain with trophic and vasomotor changes of the hand

Thoracic outlet syndrome

LABORATORY PROCEDURES PERTAINING TO PAIN IN THE NECK AND SHOULDER

Procedure	To Detect
Cervical spine x-rays	Osteoarthritis; rheumatoid arthritis; ruptured cervical disk; cervical rib with thoracic outlet syndrome
Shoulder x-rays	Linear calcific deposits: calcific tendinitis
Chest x-rays	Thoracic outlet anomalies; superior sulcus (Pancoast's) tumor of the lung
Myelogram,* CT scan*	Encroachment on the spinal cord; spondylosis (bony ridges in the spinal canal)
Contrast arthrography*	Rotator cuff tear
Joint fluid analysis*	See Chapter 40 "Articular Pain"

*When indicated

SELECTED BIBLIOGRAPHY

Bonafede RP, Bennett RM: Shoulder pain. *Postgrad Med* 82(1):185–193, 1987.
Nakano KK: Neck pain, in Kelley WN, Harris ED Jr, Ruddy S et al (eds). *Textbook of Rheumatology*, 2nd ed., pp. 416–435, Philadelphia: Saunders, 1985.
Thornhill TS: The painful shoulder, in Kelley WN, Harris ED Jr, Ruddy S et al (eds). *Textbook of Rheumatology*, 2nd ed., pp. 435–448, Philadelphia: Saunders, 1985.

44

Pain in the Upper Extremities

INTRODUCTION

Pain in the upper extremities may result from diseases of the skin and of the musculo-skeletal, vascular, and nervous systems. Any agent (mechanical, chemical, thermal) causing inflammation, swelling, ischemia, or destruction of pain-sensitive tissues may be painful. Superficial pain (caused by bacterial infection, trauma, burns) is well localized and is associated with tenderness and hyperalgesia. Deep pain arising from vessels, fascia, joints, periosteum, and supporting structures is often poorly localized and dull, and may be accompanied by muscular rigidity and deep tenderness. The pain due to disorders of the joints (acute or chronic process) is usually related to inflammation of the synovial membrane. Pain from ischemic skeletal muscles is due to the action on sensory nerve endings of metabolites accumulating in the muscles or changes in the nerves themselves. Painful intermittent vasospasm in the hands, initiated by exposure to cold (Raynaud's phenomenon), is attributed to digital artery closure secondary to either a vasoconstrictive mechanism (in young female patients) or obstruction by atherosclerosis. Pain caused by diseases of the peripheral nerves or by entrapment neuropathy (carpal tunnel syndrome) is usually accompanied by motor, reflex, and other sensory changes. Irritation of the cervical nerve roots (herniated nucleosus pulposus, osteoarthritis) can cause pain in the upper extremities. Pain in the upper limb caused by compression of the neurovascular bundle as it leaves the thorax (thoracic outlet syndrome) is frequently associated with evidence of vascular compression. Pain originating from intrathoracic structures (ischemic heart disease) may radiate to the inner surfaces of the arm.

ETIOLOGY

Skin and Soft Tissues

Cellulitis: bacterial and fungous infection; lymphangitis
Acute trauma to the skin

Articular and Periarticular Structures

Arthritis: acute pyogenic arthritis; rheumatoid arthritis; rheumatic fever; osteoarthritis; gout; posttraumatic; hypertrophic osteoarthropathy
Bursitis; tendinitis

Bones and Periosteum

Osteomyelitis; fractures; tumors

Muscles

Acute suppurative myositis; polymyositis, dermatomyositis; polymyalgia rheumatica; fibrositis

Neurologic

Polyneuropathy, mononeuropathy; carpal tunnel syndrome
Cervical nerve root compression: protruded cervical disk; osteoarthritis; spinal cord disorder
Brachial plexus disorders: thoracic outlet syndromes; superior sulcus tumor of the lung

Vascular/Hematologic

Raynaud's phenomenon; phlebitis; thromboangiitis obliterans; erythromelalgia

Iatrogenic Causes of Raynaud's Phenomenon

Beta-blocking drugs; ergotamine preparations; methysergide; cytotoxic drugs; oral contraceptives

HISTORY TAKING*

Possible meaning of a positive response

1   Location of the Pain?

1.1 Where do you have pain?	
• in a joint?	Pain resulting from an articular disorder is perceived as coming directly from the joint, not from the bones between the joints
• elbows? wrists?	Rheumatoid arthritis (frequently symmetric); septic arthritis; pseudogout; gout; trauma
• *metacarpophalangeal joints?*	Rheumatoid arthritis; occasionally in gout
• *proximal interphalangeal joints?*	Rheumatoid arthritis (nontender Bouchard's nodes in osteoarthritis)
• *distal interphalangeal joints?*	Osteoarthritis (Heberden's nodes; often painless); psoriatic arthritis
• *carpometacarpal joint of thumb?*	Osteoarthritis
• in an area adjacent to a joint?	Periarticular structures; tendinitis, bursitis, bone
• at an elbow?	Epicondylitis (tennis elbow): due to repetitive wrist extension or pronation-supination
• at a wrist?	Tenosynovitis; tuberculous synovitis

*In this section, items in *italics* are characteristic clinical features, and items in **boldface** are potentially life-threatening or urgent conditions.

- in the arm? forearm? (nonarticular)

Origin of pain in: skin, muscle, bone, vessels, nerves: nerve entrapment (carpal tunnel syndrome); thoracic outlet syndrome; herniated cervical disk; peripheral neuropathy. Pain due to lesions of muscle is usually felt over the muscle belly, not at the areas of insertion near the joints or tendons

- in the hand?

Arthritis; tendinitis; trauma, entrapment neuropathy at neck, elbow, wrist (carpal tunnel syndrome); peripheral neuropathy; thoracic outlet syndrome; vascular occlusion; Raynaud's phenomenon; erythromelalgia (rare); lymphangitis

- *in the first three fingers?*

Carpal tunnel syndrome: compression of the median nerve at the wrist

- at the ulnar aspect of the hand?

Lesion of the ulnar nerve (commonly at the elbow) or of the brachial plexus

- *in the fingers? at the finger tips?* (on exposure to cold)

Raynaud's phenomenon or disease

- along the limb in a linear fashion? crossing over joint and muscle areas?

Lesion of nerve or blood vessels: nerve root compression; thoracic outlet syndrome; peripheral nerve lesion; referred pain, ischemic heart disease

- *the tip of the shoulder, the anterior upper part of the arm, the radial forearm, the thumb?*

Fifth to sixth cervical disk disease: involvement of the sixth cervical root

- *the shoulder blade, pectoral region, posterolateral upper arm, dorsal forearm and elbow, index and middle finger?*

Sixth to seventh cervical disk disease: involvement of the seventh cervical root

- the posteromedial part of the arm and forearm?

Involvement of the eighth cervical root

2   Mode of Onset of the Pain

2.1   How long have you had pain in your arm? limb?

2.2   Was the onset of pain
- sudden? (minutes to hours)

Acute infectious process; trauma; gout; acute arterial occlusion

- gradual? (hours to days)

Lymphangitis; arthritis; tendinitis; bursitis; fibrositis; rheumatoid arthritis

3   Character of the Pain

3.1   Is the pain
- moderate?

Rheumatoid arthritis; osteoarthritis; tennis elbow; fibrositis

• aching?	Muscle or joint problem
• shooting? sharp?	Nerve lesion; cervical root pain (herniated protruded cervical disk; cervical spondylosis; cervical intraspinal lesion)
• burning?	Carpal tunnel syndrome; erythromelalgia (rare)
• severe?	Arthritis (at rest); osteomyelitis (with motion); gout; infection; trauma
• throbbing?	Pain arising from bone

4 Precipitating or Aggravating Factors

4.1 In case of articular pain: Is the pain
- present only with movements? — Osteoarthritis (early stage)
- present at rest? — Rheumatoid arthritis; osteoarthritis (later stage)
- increased by motion? activity? — Any disorder of the joints; tennis elbow; fibrositis

4.2 In case of nonarticular pain: Is the pain in your arm induced or made worse
- *by sneezing? coughing?* hyperextension of the neck? shaving under the chin? — Cervical nerve root pain: herniated protruded cervical disk; cervical spondylosis
- upon rotating the head? on laterally flexing the neck? — Cervical spine lesion
- on general exertion? — Referred pain: **ischemic heart disease** (inner arm)
- when elevating the arm above the head? bracing the shoulders? — Thoracic outlet syndrome

4.3 If the pain is localized to the first three fingers: Does the pain occur
- when grasping an object for a prolonged time?
- at night?

Carpal tunnel syndrome (more frequent in women): frequently bilateral

4.4 In case of pain in the fingers: Is the pain induced by
- *exposure to cold?* — Raynaud's phenomenon (70 to 90 percent of patients are women)

5 Relieving Factors

5.1 In case of nonarticular pain: Is the pain relieved by
- flexion of the neck? — Cervical nerve root compression
- *nitroglycerin? rest?* — **Ischemic heart disease** with referred pain

5.2 In case of pain in the fingers: Is the pain relieved
     • by heat?   Raynaud's phenomenon
     • by shaking the hand?   Carpal tunnel syndrome

6   **Accompanying Symptoms**

6.1 In case of articular pain: Is the joint swollen?   Infectious arthritis (in large joints); crystal-induced arthritis (gout, pseudo-gout); rheumatoid arthritis

6.1a Are you unable to remove a ring? wear a watch? slip the hand into an old glove?   Clues to diffuse swelling of the hand: rheumatoid arthritis; scleroderma; polymyositis; Raynaud's disease; neurovascular compression syndrome; superior vena cava syndrome; lymphatic obstruction

6.1b Are you unable to drive a car? to dress? eat?   Related to pain rather than restricted motion at the elbow (the shoulder is able to compensate for most limitation of motion at the elbow)

6.1c Are you unable to lift with the hands? shave? sew? open jars?   Disability related to affections of the hand

6.1d Is the disability
     • greatest in the morning?   Rheumatoid arthritis
     • worse with prolonged use of the joint?   Osteoarthritis

6.2 In case of nonarticular pain: Is the involved area swollen? red?   Cellulitis, with or without lymphangitis

6.3 Is the arm swollen? discolored?   Occasionally in the thoracic outlet syndrome, with venous occlusion; phlebitis; lymphangitis; cellulitis

6.4 Do you have
     • fever? chills?   Septic arthritis; acute osteomyelitis; cellulitis; acute suppurative myositis
     • *numbness, tingling,* burning in the arm?   Nerve root compression syndrome; thoracic outlet syndrome; peripheral neuropathy
     • chest pain on exertion?   **Ischemic heart disease** with referred pain in the arm
     • bloody expectorations? cough?   Lung tumor with hypertrophic osteoarthropathy; superior sulcus (Pancoast's) tumor involving the brachial plexus

7   **Iatrogenic Factors   See Etiology**

8   Personal and Social Profile

8.1   What is your occupation?

Thoracic outlet syndrome from repetitive shoulder movements: work on an assembly line; keyboard operation
Carpal tunnel syndrome due to repetitive wrist motion: sewing, operating computers
Raynaud's syndrome can occur in chain saw or pneumatic drill operators; vinyl chloride exposure

8.2   What is your sexual orientation?

Localized nerve pain in a homosexual man: herpes zoster, neuralgia of AIDS-related conditions

9   Personal Antecedents Pertaining to the Pain

9.1   Have you recently had
   • a trauma, an injury to the affected area?

Posttraumatic arthritis or muscular pain; portal of entry for infecting agent: cellulitis, acute suppurative myositis, septic arthritis

   • intravenous cannulations?

Thrombophlebitis

   • a trauma to the neck? a "whiplash" injury?

May cause radicular symptoms

   • injections into the shoulder muscles? an infectious disease?

May precede acute brachial plexus neuropathy

   • unusual or vigorous exercise?

Rotator cuff tear with pain radiating into the arm

PHYSICAL SIGNS PERTAINING TO PAIN IN THE UPPER EXTREMITIES

	Possible significance
Local swelling, warmth, erythema; fever	Infectious process; cellulitis with or without lymphangitis
Tender, swollen, red, warm joint(s)	Acute pyogenic arthritis; posttraumatic; crystal-induced arthritis; rheumatoid arthritis; rheumatic fever
Weakness and sensory loss in the first middle three fingers; tenderness on pressure over the carpal ligament; atrophy of the thenar eminence; positive Tinel's sign (tingling sensation in the fingers on tapping the median nerve at the wrist)	Carpal tunnel syndrome: most commonly in middle-aged women; may be caused by tenosynovitis at the wrist or result from trauma, amyloidosis, hypothyroidism
Bone tenderness	Fracture; malignancy
• with fever, chills, local swelling	Osteomyelitis

Color changes in the fingers brought about by putting the patient's hands into ice water for a few minutes	Raynaud's phenomenon; may occur in: collagen-vascular disease, rheumatoid arthritis; arteriosclerosis; thromboangiitis obliterans; cryoglobulinemia; occupational trauma; thoracic outlet syndrome; drugs
Clubbing	Hypertrophic osteoarthropathy: lung carcinoma
Palpable tender temporal artery	Associated polymyalgia rheumatica (with pain in the limbs)
Pain in the arm and the neck	Osteoarthritis of the cervical spine; ruptured cervical disk, with involvement of cervical nerve root
• with sensory impairment in the tip of the shoulder, anterior upper part of the arm, radial forearm, thumb; weakness in flexion of the forearm; absent biceps and supinator reflexes; retained triceps reflex	Protruded disk between the fifth and sixth cervical vertebrae: involvement of the sixth cervical root
• with sensory impairment in the second and third fingers; weakness in extension of the forearm and in the hand grip; absent triceps reflex; retained biceps and supinator reflexes	Protruded disk between the sixth and seventh vertebrae: involvement of the seventh cervical root

LABORATORY PROCEDURES PERTAINING TO PAIN IN THE UPPER EXTREMITIES

Procedure	To Detect
Cervical spine x-rays	Osteoarthritis; intervertebral disk herniation; cervical rib with thoracic outlet syndrome
Chest x-ray	Superior sulcus tumor of the lung (Pancoast's syndrome)
Joint and bone x-rays	Rheumatoid arthritis; osteoarthritis; fracture; osteomyelitis; tumor, primary or metastatic; hypertrophic osteoarthropathy
Joint fluid analysis*	See Chapter 40 "Articular Pain"

*When indicated

Procedure	To Detect
Nerve conduction studies*	Neuropathies; thoracic outlet syndromes; carpal tunnel syndrome (delayed conduction at the wrist)
Electromyography*	Lesions of anterior horn cells, muscle, peripheral nerves
Muscle biopsy*	Myopathies vs. neuropathies
Angiography;* venography;* ultrasonography*	Location and extent of occlusive vascular involvement
CT scan*; myelography*	Intervertebral disk herniation; spinal cord tumor

*When indicated

SELECTED BIBLIOGRAPHY

Adams RD, Victor M: Pain in the back, neck, and extremities, in *Principles of Neurology*, 4th ed., pp. 155–180, New York: McGraw-Hill, 1989.
Stabile MJ, Warfield CA: Differential diagnosis of arm pain. *Hosp Pract* 25(1):55–64, 1990.
Stabile MJ, Warfield CA: The pain of peripheral vascular disease. *Hosp Pract* 23(3):99–107, 1988.

Hematologic-Metabolic Disorders

45
Anemia

INTRODUCTION

Anemia   Reduction in red blood cell (RBC) mass; hemoglobin concentration below 14 g/dL in males, below 12 g/dL in women.

Physiologically, anemia may be defined as a reduction in oxygen-carrying capacity of the blood as reflected by its hemoglobin concentration. Anemia may develop as the result of inadequate production of RBCs. This may be due to a decrease in the number of functioning erythroid stem cells (aplastic anemia, marrow fibrosis). Impaired production of RBCs may also result from abnormal maturation of erythroid cells. A defect in hemoglobin synthesis may be due to iron deficiency, a defect in the synthesis of heme (sideroblastic anemia), or globin (thalassemia). Maturation disorders due to deficiency of vitamin B_{12} or folic acid result in megaloblastic anemias and reflect impaired DNA synthesis involving all replicating tissues.

Anemia may result from excessive destruction of RBCs. A shortening of erythrocyte survival occurs in hemolytic anemias, which may be inherited or acquired. Inherited hemolytic disorders usually result from intrinsic (or intracorpuscular) defects and include hemoglobinopathies (sickle cell anemia), enzymopathies, and membrane defects (hereditary spherocytosis with undue rigidity of the red cells). Acquired hemolytic anemias usually reflect extrinsic (extracorpuscular) defects. In antibody-mediated, idiopathic or secondary, hemolysis (positive Coombs' antiglobulin test), presence of either IgG or complement renders the red cell vulnerable to phagocytosis. Coombs-negative hemolytic anemias may result from mechanical damage to red cells (microangiopathic hemolytic anemia, "heart valve hemolysis").

Anemia may also appear as the result of acute blood loss. Iron deficiency due to chronic blood loss (from pelvic organs in women and from the gastrointestinal tract in men) is probably the most common form of anemia.

On the basis of the three erythrocyte indexes [mean corpuscular volume (MCV), mean corpuscular hemoglobin concentration (MCHC), mean corpuscular hemoglobin (MCH)], anemias may be classified into normocytic, microcytic, and macrocytic anemias.

ETIOLOGY

Normocytic (MCV: 80–100 fl)

Acute blood loss
Chronic systemic diseases: infections; rheumatoid arthritis; collagen-vascular dis-
   orders; chronic renal disease; malignancy; leukemias; lymphomas; myxedema
Bone marrow metastases
Bone marrow aplasia
Hemolytic anemias
   Extrinsic abnormalities
      Immune-mediated: collagen-vascular diseases; drugs; infections; lymphocytic
         malignancies
      Mechanical damage: prosthetic heart valves; microangiopathic hemolytic ane-
         mia; disseminated intravascular coagulation (DIC)
      Direct toxic effect: drugs, poisons; malaria; septicemia
   Intrinsic abnormalities
      Hereditary spherocytosis; glucose-6-phosphate dehydrogenase (G-6-PD) de-
         ficiency; sickle-cell anemia; hemoglobin variants; paroxysmal nocturnal
         hemoglobinuria

Microcytic (MCV <80 fl)

Iron deficiency; chronic blood loss
Thalassemias
Sideroblastic anemias
Occasionally microcytic: anemia of chronic disease; hemoglobinopathies

Macrocytic (MCV >100 fl)

Megaloblastic anemia
   Vitamin B_{12} deficiency: pernicious anemia; malabsorption; dietary deficiency
      (rare); transcobalamin II deficiency
   Folic acid deficiency: inadequate intake; malabsorption; increased requirements
      (pregnancy, malignancy)
   Antimetabolites; orotic aciduria; some refractory anemias
Nonmegaloblastic macrocytic anemias
   Liver disease; acute blood loss (reticulocytosis); hemolytic anemias; aplastic an-
      emias; alcoholism

Iatrogenic Causes of Anemia (Partial List)

Megaloblastic Anemia

Folate antagonists; cotrimoxazole; methotrexate; phenytoin; barbiturates; oral contraceptives; primidone; trimethoprim; triamterene

Immune Hemolytic Anemia

Methyldopa; cephalosporins; levodopa; penicillins; quinidine; sulfonamides; mefenamic acid; melphalan; isoniazid; rifampin; insulin; chlorpromazine; phenacetine; dapsone; procainamide

Hemolytic Anemia (In Glucose-6-Phosphate Dehydrogenase Deficiency)

Nitrofurantoin; aspirin; phenacetin; quinidine; vitamin C; cotrimoxazole; probenecid; procainamide; sulfonamides; sulfones; antimalarials; chloramphenicol; nalidixic acid

Aplastic Anemia

Analgesics; antimetabolites: alkylating agents; phenytoin; mephenytoin; trimethadione; carbamazepine; chloramphenicol; gold salts; phenylbutazone; quinacrine; penicillamine; sulfonamides; (ionizing radiation)

Peptic Ulceration and/or Gastrointestinal Blood Loss

Aspirin; nonsteroidal anti-inflammatory agents; anticoagulants; corticosteroids

HISTORY TAKING*

Possible meaning of a positive response

1   Mode of Onset and Duration

1.1 How long have you been aware that you have anemia?

Since birth: thalassemia, other hemoglobinopathies (patients may be unaware of mild to moderate lifelong anemias until they have a routine blood test or develop symptoms during pregnancy or after a severe febrile infection). At late middle-age or elderly: pernicious anemia. Any age: iron deficiency; folate deficiency

1.2 Do you know the most recent date at which a blood examination indicated that you had no anemia?

Implies the absence of congenital anemia. Anemia of recent onset: acquired disease

1.2a Have you ever been rejected/accepted as a volunteer blood donor?

Helps to date the onset of anemia

*In this section, items in *italics* are characteristic clinical features, and items in **boldface** are potentially life-threatening or urgent conditions.

1.3 How was your anemia detected?
   • at a routine checkup examina-   Anemia may be initially asymptomatic
     tion?   if insidious in onset. Individuals with
                                       mild anemia are often asymptomatic
   • because you were sick?   The degree to which symptoms occur
                                       depends on the rapidity of the onset of
                                       anemia, its severity, the patient's age
                                       and cardiovascular status. In otherwise
                                       healthy   individuals   symptoms   are
                                       usually present when hemoglobin falls
                                       below 7 or 8 g/100 mL

1.4 Has the anemia developed
   • rapidly?   Bleeding or hemolysis
   • gradually?   Marrow failure; vitamin B_{12} deficiency

1.5 Is the anemia chronic or recurrent?   Hereditary disease; chronic or episodic
                                           bleeding

2 Accompanying Symptoms

2.1 Do you have
   • fatigue? shortness of breath, pal-   May occur in mild or chronic anemia.
     pitations following exercise?   Decrease in hemoglobin prevents max-
                                          imum O_2 flow to tissues, with decreased
                                          exercise tolerance
   • shortness of breath, palpitations   Severe anemia; tachycardia: cardiac
     at rest? a pounding pulse?   adjustment to anemia; when hemoglo-
                                          bin is less than 7.5 g/100 mL, resting
                                          cardiac output usually increases with
                                          increased heart rate and stroke volume
                                          Rapidly developing anemia
   • dizziness or faintness upon aris-
     ing from a sitting or recumbent
     position? extreme fatigue?
   • chest pain on exertion? pain in   Angina pectoris, intermittent claudica-
     the calves when walking?   tion may become manifest in anemic
                                         patients with underlying organ disease
   • headaches? dizziness? vertigo?   Cerebral hypoxia due to marked ane-
     roaring in the ears? restlessness? mia
     irritability? difficulty sleeping or
     concentrating?
   • a humming sound in your head?   Rapid blood flow through cranial arter-
                                         ies indicating significant anemia
   • loss of appetite? abdominal dis-   Gastrointestinal symptoms of severe
     comfort? indigestion? nausea?   anemia attributable to shunting of
     bowel irregularities?   blood away from the splanchnic bed
   • black, tarry stools? blood on your **Gastrointestinal bleeding:** the most
     stools?   common cause of chronic iron de-
                                         ficiency in men

• diarrhea?	Neoplasm of the colon and rectum underlying the anemia; intestinal malabsorption: folate or vitamin B_{12} deficiency (folate deficiency is the more common, because folate stores are adequate for only 6 months, whereas vitamin B_{12} stores are sufficient for 3 to 6 years after deprivation)
• a change in your stool habits?	Neoplasm of colon and rectum
• *epigastric pain? relieved by food? antacids?*	Peptic ulcer with chronic blood loss
• episodic abdominal pain?	Acute hemolysis; painful vasoocclusive episodes in sickle cell anemia; gallstones (develop frequently in patients with chronic hemolytic disorders)
• burning sensations of the tongue?	Pernicious anemia; iron-deficiency anemia; folate deficiency
• sores around the angles of the mouth?	Angular cheilosis: iron-deficiency anemia
• painful ulcers in your mouth? a sore throat?	Aplastic anemia with neutropenia and infection of oral mucosa
• difficulty swallowing?	Dysphagia in Plummer-Vinson syndrome: chronic iron-deficiency anemia, postcricoid esophageal webs; mucosal ulcerations in aplastic anemia
• *a craving for ice? starch? clay?*	Pica: compulsive ingestion of unusual non-nutritive substances: may be a manifestation of iron-deficiency anemia or may impair iron absorption and lead to iron deficiency
• difficulty walking? unsteadiness of gait? numbness, tingling ("pins-and-needles") in the hands, toes?	Ataxia, loss of position sense, paresthesias: in vitamin B_{12} deficiency with subacute combined degeneration
• a weight loss?	Carcinoma; leukemia; lymphoma
• fever?	Systemic inflammation; infection; leukemia; lymphoma or other neoplasm; collagen-vascular disease; infection complicating anemia
• chills?	Accompany severe hemolytic process
• a bleeding tendency?	The disorder producing the anemia is not confined to the RBCs (aplastic anemia with pancytopenia); presence of additional disturbance of the other marrow elements or of the liver; the anemia itself may be due to the blood loss resulting from a disorder of hemostasis

- cough? hemoptysis?

    Infection or neoplasm of the lung may be causes of the anemia; pulmonary bleeding in idiopathic pulmonary hemosiderosis

- back pain? bone pains?

    Congenital hemolytic anemias (sickle cell anemia): infarction of bone and bone marrow; malignancies; multiple myeloma; patients with sickle cell anemia have a predisposition to *Salmonella* osteomyelitis

- bone tenderness?

    Myeloid metaplasia; leukemia; multiple myeloma

- a darkening of your urine resembling tea or cola?

    Blood or hemoglobin: may signify urinary tract disease or hematologic problem. Hematuria: in sickle cell trait; hemoglobinuria: intravascular hemolysis. Bilirubin does not occur in the urine in uncomplicated hemolytic anemia; dipyrroles (products of bilirubin degradation) may appear in the urine and darken its color during periods of increased hemolysis

- *darkly discolored urine in the morning, clearing during day?*

    Paroxysmal nocturnal hemoglobinuria (gross hemoglobinuria may be present only intermittently)

2.2   For the female patient: What is the frequency, the duration of your periods?

    Estimated iron losses of menstruation: 20 to 30 mg per month

2.2a How many pads or tampons per day, per period, do you use? more than 4 pads per day or 12 per period?

2.2b Have you noticed the appearance of clots in the blood lost during menstruation?

    Increased menstrual blood loss: the single most common cause of iron deficiency in temperate countries

2.2c Do you have vaginal bleeding between your periods? abnormal menstruations?

    Menstrual disorders, both amenorrhea and increased bleeding, are common in, and may aggravate, iron-deficiency anemia

3   Iatrogenic Factors   See Etiology

4   Personal and Social Profile

4.1   Ethnic background of the patient?

    Sickle cell trait: in about 8 percent of American blacks. G-6-PD deficiency; in about 10 percent of American blacks. Thalassemia: in patients of Mediterranean or Far Eastern extraction

4.2	What is your daily diet? (described meal by meal)	Inadequate diet may produce nutritional folate deficiency. The patient may deliberately deceive the physician because of embarrassment over eating habits or financial restrictions
4.2a	Do you follow any particular diet?	Identifies individuals who follow "fad" diets, any type of unusual diet, who exclude important foods from their diet
4.3	What is your alcohol intake?	Alcohol is probably the most common toxin associated with anemia. Alcoholism associated with folate deficiency, sideroblastic anemia
4.4	What is (was) your present (past) occupation?	Aplastic anemia due to benzene, ionizing radiation in: chemists, furniture refinishing, cleaning, degreasing, radiation workers
4.5	Do you have any hobbies? sport activities?	(Drugs and) chemicals may produce hemolytic or aplastic anemia. Iron deficiency from chronic GI blood loss has been documented in long-distance runners
4.6	Do you often use cleaning fluids? insecticides? any paints? hair dyes? deodorants? depilatories?	May produce blood dyscrasias (may be overlooked by the patient)
4.7	Have you ever lived in, or traveled to, tropical countries? Vietnam?	Endemic areas of malaria

5 Personal Antecedents Pertaining to the Anemia

5.1	Have you ever had past examinations of your blood? stools? bone marrow? x-rays of your stomach? bowel? When? With what results?	
5.2	Do you have any of the following conditions:	
	• a peptic ulcer?	Iron-deficiency anemia due to chronic blood loss
	• past surgery on the stomach? the intestine?	Iron-deficiency anemia following subtotal gastrectomy: iron malabsorption, persistent bleeding. Megaloblastic anemia after partial or total gastrectomy, anastomoses, ileal resection
	• a recent trauma? operation?	Causes of blood loss due to soft tissue bleeding (e.g., fractured hip in the elderly)

• chronic leg ulcers?	Sickle cell anemia; rarely in hereditary spherocytosis and other long-standing hemolytic anemias
• constant or episodic jaundice? yellowing of the skin or eyeballs?	Inherited hemolytic anemia
• gallstones?	Bilirubin stones in congenital hemolytic anemias: increased excretion of bile pigment through the hepatobiliary system
• a chronic GI disease?	Folate malabsorption in nontropical sprue
• a chronic liver condition?	Anemia in alcoholic cirrhosis may result from acute and chronic GI blood loss, coexistent folic acid deficiency, hypersplenism, and a direct suppressive effect of alcohol on the bone marrow
• a thyroid condition?	Anemia of hypothyroidism: usually normocytic; macrocytosis can usually be attributed to folic acid or B_{12} deficiency
• a chronic infection?	The anemia of chronic inflammation is due to impaired iron metabolism, decreased erythrocyte lifespan, and inadequate marrow response to the mild hemolysis
• a chronic condition of the joints?	Autoimmune hemolytic anemia is associated with SLE or with B cell neoplasms (chronic lymphocytic leukemia); rheumatoid arthritis with impaired iron metabolism; sickle cell disorders
• a chronic renal disease?	Normochromic, normocytic anemia in chronic renal failure: depressed erythropoiesis due to diminished biosynthesis of erythropoietin by the diseased kidney and to the effects of retained toxins on bone marrow
5.3 For the female patient: How many pregnancies (abortions) have you had? When?	Iron losses of pregnancy are estimated at 500 mg
5.4 Have you recently been hospitalized?	Extensive diagnostic phlebotomy may result in iron-deficiency anemia, particularly in patients with low iron stores (menstruating women)

6   Family Medical History Pertaining to the Anemia

6.1 Are there any members of your family who have
 • anemia? jaundice? gallstones? a splenectomy?

A positive family history suggests an inherited red cell disorder; pernicious anemia; sickle cell trait; G-6-PD deficiency; thalassemia; hereditary spherocytosis

PHYSICAL SIGNS PERTAINING TO ANEMIA*

Possible significance

Pallor of the palms, nail beds, oral mucous membranes, palpebral conjunctivas

The most evident sign of anemia; skin color is affected by the thickness of the epidermis, pigmentation, blood flow, fluid content of the subcutaneous tissues

Pallor of the palmar creases

Hemoglobin below 7 g/100 mL

Jaundice

Hemolytic anemia; liver disease

Petechiae

Acute leukemia; aplastic anemia; autoimmune hemolysis with idiopathic thrombocytopenic purpura

Pallor; cold, clammy skin; **clinical shock**
 • systolic blood pressure <100 mmHg
 • pulse rate of 100 or more beats per minute

Acute hemorrhage; blood loss of 2000 mL
Blood loss of 1000 mL or more
Blood volume probably less than 80 percent of normal

Tachycardia; systolic ejection murmur (most marked at the pulmonic area)

Increased cardiac output (hemoglobin less than 7.5 g/100 mL); traumatic hemolysis

Heart murmur; fever; splenomegaly

Subacute bacterial endocarditis with anemia of chronic desease

Sternal tenderness

Leukemia; multiple myeloma

Fever

Infection; malignancy; lymphoma; collagen-vascular disease

Lymphadenopathy

Lymphoma; leukemia; infection; metastatic carcinoma

Splenomegaly

Infectious disease; hemolytic anemia; collagen-vascular disease; neoplastic disorder

*In this section, items in *italics* are characteristic clinical features, and items in **boldface** are potentially life-threatening or urgent conditions.

Maxillary prominence ("chipmunk" facies); frontal bossing	Severe congenital hemolytic anemias with expansion of red marrow within the maxillary bones
Nail changes: brittleness, longitudinal ridging, flattening	Chronic iron-deficiency anemia; spooning (koilonychia) is rare
Smooth tongue	Glossitis: vitamin B_{12}, folate, or iron deficiency
Chronic leg ulcers	Sickle cell anemia; rarely in other hemolytic anemias
In the lower legs: weakness, incoordination, loss of position sense, abnormal tendon reflexes; unsteady gait	Degeneration of the dorsal and lateral columns of the spinal cord in vitamin B_{12} deficiency
Rectal and pelvic examination	May reveal: hemorrhoids, tumor or infection causing anemia

LABORATORY TESTS PERTAINING TO ANEMIA[†]

Evaluation of any patient with anemia requires a careful interpretation of a peripheral blood film and of the three erythrocyte indexes: mean red cell volume (MCV), mean corpuscular hemoglobin concentration (MCHC), mean corpuscular hemoglobin (MCH)

Test	Finding	Diagnostic Possibilities
Blood		
Blood smear	Poikilocytosis	Disordered erythropoiesis: iron-deficiency anemia; thalassemia
	Spherocytes	Hereditary spherocytosis; acquired immunohemolytic anemia
	"Teardrop" RBCs	Myelophthisic anemias; myelofibrosis
	Target cells	Sickle cell disease; hemoglobin C, D, E, etc.; thalassemia; liver disease; postsplenectomy state
	Schistocytes, helmet cells	Microangiopathic or traumatic type of hemolytic anemia; malignant hypertension; uremia
	Sickle cells	Sickle cell syndromes
	Rouleaux	Dysproteinemia; multiple myeloma

[†]See the appendix on Laboratory Reference Values for the associated normal laboratory values.

Test	Finding	Diagnostic Possibilities
Reticulocyte count	Normal or decreased	Bone marrow failure; iron deficiency; vitamin B_{12} deficiency; folic acid deficiency; uremia; chronic inflammation
	Increased	Hemolysis; response to acute blood loss; recovery from impaired erythropoiesis; myelophthisic anemia
Iron	Decreased ⎫	
Iron-binding capacity (IBC)	Increased ⎬	Iron-deficiency anemia
	Iron and IBC decreased	Infections; malignancy; uremia; chronic illnesses
	Iron increased, IBC decreased	Thalassemia; hemolysis
Haptoglobin	Decreased	Hemolysis
Sickle cell preparation	Positive	To detect sickle cell anemia
Hemoglobin electrophoresis	Abnormal	To detect hemoglobinopathies (C, D, etc.)
Coombs' test	Positive	Immunohemolytic anemia
Erythrocyte enzyme assays	Abnormal	Red cell enzymes deficiencies
Unconjugated bilirubin	Increased	Hemolysis; internal bleeding
Lactate dehydrogenase	Increased	Hemolysis
Ferritin	Decreased	Iron-deficiency anemia
	Increased	Anemia of chronic disease; liver disease
WBCs and/or platelets	Decreased	Anemia is part of a more general hematologic problem, e.g., aplastic anemia, leukemia

Test	Finding	Diagnostic Possibilities
WBCs	Hypersegmented neutrophils	Vitamin B_{12} deficiency; folic acid deficiency
	Leukopenia	Vitamin B_{12} and folic acid deficiency; aplastic anemia
	Immature	Leukemia

Stool

Occult blood	Positive	Chronic blood loss
Bone marrow examination*		May reveal: aleukemic leukemia; multiple myeloma; lymphoma; maturation defect: megaloblastic anemia; bone marrow failure; metastatic lesions
Bone marrow biopsy		To detect tumor cells; granulomas; fibrosis

*Indicated in any unexplained anemia

SELECTED BIBLIOGRAPHY

Beutler E: The common anemias. *JAMA* 259:2433–2437, 1988.

Christensen DJ: Diagnosis of anemia. *Postgrad Med* 73(1):293–300, 1983.

Williams WJ: Approach to the patient, in Williams WJ, Beutler E, Erslev AJ et al (eds). *Hematology,* 4th ed., pp. 3–8, New York: McGraw-Hill, 1990.

Wintrobe MM: The approach to the patient with anemia, in Wintrobe MM, Lee GR, Boggs DR et al (eds). *Clinical Hematology,* 8th ed., pp. 529–558, Philadelphia: Lea & Febiger, 1981.

46

Bleeding Tendency

INTRODUCTION

Hemostasis   The process which spontaneously arrests the flow of blood from vessels carrying blood under pressure.

Primary Hemostasis   The rapid formation of platelet plugs at sites of injury.

Secondary Hemostasis   The formation of fibrin resulting from reactions of the plasma coagulation system.

The hemostatic mechanism involves the blood vessels, the platelets, and the plasma coagulation factors. The initial event of primary hemostasis is adhesion of platelets to areas of the vessel wall in which the subendothelium has been exposed by endothelial cell disruption or injury. After adhesion, platelets become activated and, under the influence of mediators like adenosine diphosphate and thromboxane A_2, recruit additional circulating platelets to bind to the adherent platelet monolayer and form a platelet aggregate. There are two activation pathways of the coagulation system: the intrinsic or contact pathway, which involves factors XII, XI, and VIII, and the extrinsic or tissue factor-mediated pathway, which involves tissue factor and factor VII. Both pathways result in the activation of factor X. Activated factor X converts prothrombin to thrombin in a reaction that is accelerated by activated factor V. Thrombin then converts fibrinogen to fibrin. The interaction of activated factors VIII, IX, and X; the interaction of the tissue factor–factor VII complex with factor X; and the conversion of prothrombin to thrombin require phospholipid and calcium. The coagulation mechanism is regulated by antithrombin and the protein C-protein S system.

A bleeding tendency may be caused by vascular abnormalities, platelet disorders, and plasma coagulation factor abnormalities (coagulopathies). Vascular defects are common, but they seldom lead to serious bleeding. Platelet defects may be qualitative (inherited or acquired) or quantitative. Thrombocytopenia is the most common serious bleeding disorder involving platelets. In idiopathic thrombocytopenic purpura, a platelet-bound IgG antibody is generally involved in the mechanism of platelet destruction. Coagulopathies may be primary (congenital) or secondary to some underlying disease. The congenital disorders are often familial and almost always involve a single coagulation factor. The defect may be due to a total lack of the molecule (e.g., afibrinogenemia) or, more often, to a defective function of the molecule (e.g., hemophilia). Secondary or acquired coagulopathies are far more common than the inherited disorders. They usually involve multiple coagulation factors. Liver diseases and vitamin K deficiency are major causes of lack of production or defective synthesis of coagulation factors. Disseminated intravascular coagulation, another common problem, results from pathologic activation of the hemostatic mechanism within the circulation because of introduction of foreign material into the bloodstream.

Precise diagnosis of a bleeding tendency requires specialized laboratory evaluation.

ETIOLOGY

Vascular Purpura

Vasculitis: Henoch-Schonlein purpura; drugs; infections: meningococcal, rickettsial
Congenital: hereditary hemorrhagic telangiectasia; Ehlers-Danlos syndrome
Miscellaneous: senile purpura; infections; scurvy; Cushing's syndrome; multiple myeloma; macroglobulinemia; cryoglobulinemia; amyloidosis

Thrombocytopenia

Decreased production
   Marrow aplasia; marrow fibrosis; marrow infiltration with malignant cells; cytotoxic drugs, chemicals, radiation
Increased destruction
   Immunologic (autoantibodies to platelet antigens): idiopathic thrombocytopenic purpura, viral agents, bacterial sepsis, systemic lupus erythematosus (SLE); drugs
   Nonimmunologic: disseminated intravascular coagulation; microangiopathic hemolytic anemia; thrombotic thrombocytopenic purpura (TTP); vasculitis, hemolytic uremic syndrome; acute infections, sepsis; prosthetic heart valves
Sequestration: splenomegaly
Intravascular dilution: massive transfusion; loss by hemorrhage

Qualitative Platelet Defects

Platelet adhesion defects (von Willebrand's disease); platelet aggregation defects (Glanzmann's thrombasthenia); platelet release defects (drugs, uremia)

Coagulation Defects

Congenital
   Hemophilia: A (factor VIII deficiency); B (factor IX deficiency)
   Deficiency of each of the following factors: I (fibrinogen), II (prothrombin), V, VII, X, XII (Hageman: asymptomatic), XIII
Acquired
   Vitamin K deficiency: obstructive jaundice, hepatocellular disease, intestinal malabsorption, drugs, nutritional
   Disseminated intravascular coagulation: shock, infections, burns, amniotic fluid embolism, retained dead fetus, neoplasms
   Multiple myeloma; macroglobulinemia
   Fibrinolytic states: administration of streptokinase, urokinase; liver disease; surgery for prostatic cancer
   Circulating anticoagulants

Iatrogenic Causes of Bleeding Tendencies (Partial List)

Vascular Abnormalities

Atropine; corticosteroids; iodides; penicillin; phenacetin; quinine; sulfonamides

Thrombocytopenia

Suppression of platelet production: cotrimoxazole; myelosuppressive drugs; thiazides; estrogens

Immunologic platelet destruction: digitoxin; nonsteroidal anti-inflammatory agents; heparin; phenytoin; gold salts; methyldopa; quinidine; quinine; rifampin; sedatives; stibophen; sulfonamides

Platelet Dysfunction

Aspirin; clofibrate; dextran; penicillins; dipyridamole; indomethacin; phenylbutazone; dextran; sulfinpyrazone

Impaired Coagulation

Heparin; oral anticoagulants

HISTORY TAKING*

Possible meaning of a positive response

1 Mode of Onset and Duration

1.1 When did the bleeding symptoms appear?
- at birth?

Large cephalohematomas: more common in acquired bleeding disorders: hemorrhagic disease of the newborn; may occur in hemophilia

- from the umbilical stump? following circumcision?

Hemorrhagic disease of the newborn; hypofibrinogenemia; factor XIII deficiency. Uncommon in the other hereditary coagulation disorders

- *until you began to walk?* in childhood?

Congenital defect of a single factor: hereditary bleeding disorders, hemophilia; hemarthroses in hemophilia do not develop until 3 to 4 years of age; idiopathic thrombocytopenic purpura (ITP)

- in adolescence? during military service?

Hereditary bleeding disorder, if mild, may manifest itself in adolescence

- during adulthood?

Recent onset indicates an acquired bleeding disorder, usually defects of multiple factors; most disorders of vessels and platelets; hereditary hemorrhagic telangiectasia: usually symptomatic in early adulthood or middle age

*In this section, items in *italics* are characteristic clinical features, and items in **boldface** are potentially life-threatening or urgent conditions.

1.2   In case of bleeding of recent onset, did it appear
    • abruptly?

Acute disseminated intravascular coagulation (DIC); acute ITP; allergic purpura; intoxication; rickettsial and meningococcal infections (purpura); thrombotic thrombocytopenic purpura (TTP); drug reactions; Henoch-Schönlein purpura

    • chronically?

Chronic ITP; senile purpura; chronic DIC; circulating anticoagulants

2   Location of Bleeding

Can suggest a platelet or plasma coagulation defect

2.1   Do you bleed or bruise easily in several sites?

Suggests a general bleeding tendency

2.2   Where is the bleeding localized?
    • *in superficial sites? skin, mucous membranes* (GI, GU tracts)?

Primary hemostatic defect: disorders of platelets or blood vessels often cause mucosal or superficial bleeding

    • *in deep subcutaneous tissues, muscles, joints, body cavities?*

Plasma coagulation defect. Subcutaneous and deep hematomas and hemarthroses are characteristic of hereditary coagulation disorders, most commonly hemophilia A or hemophilia B

2.3   Do you bleed from the gums? the nose? Is there blood in your urine? Have you ever vomited blood? passed black, tarry stools?

Spontaneous bleeding from bodily orifices may complicate any significant hemorrhagic diathesis. Some patients with primary hemostatic defects, especially von Willebrand's disease, may have recurrent GI hemorrhage. However an underlying local lesion may be responsible

2.3a Do your gums bleed easily when you brush your teeth?

Localized gum disorder or severe platelet deficiency; scurvy

2.4   Do you bruise or bleed easily into the muscles?

von Willebrand's disease; DIC

3   Severity of Bleeding

The amount of blood lost usually is exaggerated by the patient

3.1   Do you have
    • single, localized bleeding spots on the skin?

Vascular malformation: hereditary hemorrhagic telangiectasia; areas of vasculitis: Henoch-Schönlein purpura

- multiple, small generalized bleeding spots?
- larger areas of discoloration?

Petechiae: any of the platelet or vascular disorders

Ecchymoses: coagulation defect (also in vascular or platelet disorder); DIC. Bruises greater than 3 cm in diameter, especially if spontaneous, suggest a bleeding diathesis

3.2 For the female patient: What is the duration of your periods?

3.2a Do you have vaginal bleeding between your periods? clots in your menstrual blood?

Menorrhagia (prolonged and increased menstrual flow) and menometrorrhagia (prolonged menstrual flow with irregular intermenstrual bleeding): usually due to gynecologic disorders; however may be the sole complaint in women with mild thrombocytopenia, von Willebrand's disease, or autosomally inherited coagulation disorders

4   Precipitating or Aggravating Factors

4.1 Does your bleeding appear
- *spontaneously?* without perceptible trauma?

Petechiae and/or ecchymoses due to platelet or vascular disorder usually appear spontaneously; may occur in hereditary coagulation disorder, when trauma is so slight as to go unnoticed by the patient; hemarthroses (in hereditary coagulation disorder) often develop without significant trauma

- *following a trauma?*

Bleeding in coagulation disorders (also in purpuric syndromes)

4.2 Does the bleeding after trauma or surgery come on
- *immediately?*

Purpuric (vascular or platelet) syndrome

- *hours or days after injury?*

Plasma coagulation disorder with temporary hemostatic efficacy of normal platelet plug formation

4.2a Is the bleeding after a trauma or surgery
- *shortlived?*
- *persistent?*

Purpuric syndrome
Plasma coagulation disorder

4.3 Do you bleed from superficial minor cuts? scratches? razor nicks?

If persistent, profuse bleeding: disorder of platelet or vessel (inadequacy of primary hemostasis); seldom in patient with coagulation disorder

4.4 Do you bruise or bleed under the   Significant: suggests a hemostatic dis-
     skin (hematoma) at the sites of in-   order
     jections? immunizations?

5 Relieving Factors

5.1 In case of external bleeding: Is the
     bleeding
     • *readily, promptly controlled by local*   Purpuric syndrome: vascular or platelet
       measures?   defect
     • *unaffected by local therapy?*   Coagulation disorder

6 Accompanying Symptoms

6.1 Do you have
     • fever? malaise?   Underlying disorder; leukemia with
                                                 thrombocytopenia; TTP; infectious dis-
                                                 ease; septicemia with purpura

     • pain, swelling in your joints?   Hemarthroses in hemophilia; SLE with
                                                 thrombocytopenia
     • pain in the joints and the abdo-   Allergic (Henoch-Schönlein) purpura
       men?
     • pain in the bones?   Multiple myeloma (with or without
                                                 amyloidosis) with vascular purpura,
                                                 platelet dysfunction, or coagulation fac-
                                                 tor abnormality
     • chronic diarrhea?   Malabsorption with vitamin K de-
                                                 ficiency
     • black, tarry stools? bloody urine?   Bleeding from the GI or GU tract in a
                                                 patient with a hemorrhagic diathesis
                                                 should be ascribed to an organic lesion
                                                 until proved otherwise

6.2 *Is the healing of wounds slow? pro-*   Factor XIII deficiency; hereditary afibri-
     tracted? with abnormal scar forma-   nogenemia; dysfibrinogenemias
     tion?

7 Iatrogenic Factors   See Etiology

                                                 The importance of exhaustive interro-
                                                 gation regarding drug use cannot be
                                                 overemphasized

7.1 Do you take
     • aspirin? other nonsteroidal anti-   Inhibit platelet cyclooxygenase and
       inflammatory drugs?   suppress normal platelet aggregation;
                                                 may provoke bleeding in a patient with
                                                 a preexisting hemostatic defect
     • anticoagulants with any other   Some drugs may potentiate the anti-
       drugs?   coagulant effects of coumarins

8 Personal and Social Profile

8.1 What is your profession?	Interrogation regarding chemical exposure must be exhaustive. The development of thrombocytopenia in an adult should arouse suspicion of a possible toxic action of chemical(s) on bone marrow
8.1a Do you have any hobbies?	
8.1b Do you think that you are exposed to any chemical agents?	
8.2 What is your sexual preference?	Bruises in a homosexual man or a drug addict: AIDS-related condition: idiopathic thrombocytopenic purpura; Kaposi's sarcoma (may mimic purpura or may be purpuric before becoming nodular)
8.2a Do you use drugs?	

9 Personal Antecedents Pertaining to the Bleeding Tendency

9.1 Have you ever bled following a trauma? an accident? tooth extraction? minor surgery (tonsillectomy, circumcision)? childbirth?	Underlying hemostatic disorder
9.1a *Was the bleeding disproportionate to the injury?*	Characteristic of a hemostatic defect
9.1b Did the bleeding persist for days or weeks?	If bleeding after a dental procedure persists for 3 days or more: hemorrhagic diathesis
9.1c Did you need blood transfusions? How many?	A rough guide to the severity of the postsurgical or posttraumatic bleeding
9.2 *Have you ever had a major trauma, surgery, and/or multiple tooth extractions without abnormal bleeding?*	Evidence against a hereditary hemorrhagic disorder; present bleeding is acquired
9.3 In case of prior pregnancy: Was there any severe bleeding during delivery?	von Willebrand's disease; thrombocytopenia; DIC; hereditary deficiency of factor II, V, VII, or X (autosomal recessive; rare)
9.4 Do you have	
• a liver disease?	Decreased synthesis of factors II, V, VII, IX, X, XI, fibrinogen; chronic DIC and fibrinolysis may occur in chronic liver disease
• a renal disease?	Platelet dysfunction in uremia, induced by (a) dialyzable substance(s)

• hemophilia? treated with blood product transfusions?

AIDS-related immunothrombocytopenic purpura

9.5   Have you ever had
      • acute episodes of abdominal pain?

In hemophilia: **retroperitoneal hemorrhage;** bleeding into the psoas sheath may mimic appendicitis; **hemorrhage into the bowel** may be confused with intestinal obstruction; Henoch-Schönlein purpura

• recurrent GI bleeding?

Common in hereditary hemorrhagic telangiectasia; Henoch-Schönlein purpura

• an intracranial hemorrhage?
  • spontaneously?

The most serious complication of ITP (in 1 percent or less of the patients), usually subarachnoid

  • following a minor trauma?

May occur in coagulation disorders: subdural, epidural, or intracerebral

9.6   In the female patient: Are you pregnant?

Both ITP and TTP occur with higher frequency in pregnancy; complications of pregnancy may cause DIC

10   Family Medical History Pertaining to the Bleeding Tendency

10.1 *Are there any members of your family who have bleeding tendencies?*

Hereditary coagulation disorder (85 percent are due to factor VIII deficiency). Since bleeding can be mild, lack of a family history of bleeding does not exclude an inherited hemostatic disorder. Approximately 30 percent of patients with hemophilia give a negative family history. The family history is usually negative in the autosomal recessive traits

• one of your parents?

Hereditary hemorrhagic telangiectasia; von Willebrand's disease: autosomal dominant. Excludes hemophilia A or B in the patient

• maternal uncles? male siblings?

Hemophilia A and B : X-chromosome-linked recessive inheritance

10.2 Are (were) your parents related?

An autosomal recessive disease may emerge when both asymptomatic parents are heterozygotes: most likely to occur with consanguinity

PHYSICAL SIGNS PERTAINING TO THE BLEEDING TENDENCY*

	Possible significance
Cutaneous bleeding not blanching on pressure	Purpura: collections of blood in the skin
Dilated capillaries blanching on pressure	Hereditary hemorrhagic telangiectasia, where the blood is within the capillary dilatation; telangiectasia may cause bleeding without any hemostatic defect
Pinpoint lesions, around the feet, ankles, legs, not blanching on pressure	Petechiae: leakage of red cells through capillaries in dependent regions; severe thrombocytopenia; vascular defect
Palpable, tender, pruritic purpura	Acute vasculitis
Larger subcutaneous collections of blood, bruises	Ecchymoses: leakage of blood from small arterioles and veinules; vascular or platelet disorder (may be seen in the coagulation disorders: usually large and solitary)
Local deeper and palpable extravascular masses	Hematomas: subcutaneous extravasation of blood: coagulation disorder
Purpura and periarticular swelling	Henoch-Schönlein purpura
Purpura and splenomegaly	Thrombocytopenia due to hypersplenism: liver disease with portal hypertension; congestive splenomegaly (very rare in ITP)
Purpura with anemia; lymphadenopathy; fever	Acquired bleeding disorder; leukemia
Purpura with neurologic abnormalities, fever	Thrombotic thrombocytopenic purpura
Hemorrhage into synovial joints; joint deformities; ankyloses	Repeated hemarthroses: virtually diagnostic of a severe hereditary coagulation disorder (factor VIII and IX deficiency); rare in other plasma coagulation defects or in purpuric syndromes

*In this section, items in *italics* are characteristic clinical features.

Jaundice	Liver disease with impaired hepatic synthesis of coagulation proteins; biliary tract obstruction with impaired absorption of vitamin K and deficiency of factors II, VII, IX, X
Purpura, ecchymoses; bleeding from venipuncture wounds, from skin suture sites; multiple bleeding sites	Disseminated intravascular coagulation (DIC)
Abnormal scar formation	Hereditary afibrinogenemia; dysfibrinogenemia; factor XIII deficiency
Funduscopic examination: small retinal hemorrhages	Common in thrombocytopenic and other purpuric disorders; rare in hereditary coagulation disorders

LABORATORY TESTS PERTAINING TO THE BLEEDING TENDENCY[†]

Test	Finding	Diagnostic Possibilities
Bleeding time		A sensitive measure of platelet function
	Prolonged	Vascular defect; thrombocytopenia (platelet count less than 100,000/mm^3); qualitative platelet defect; von Willebrand's disease
	>15–20 min	Greatly increased risk of bleeding
Platelet count		Correlates well with the propensity to bleed
	Normal	Qualitative platelet abnormality; thrombasthenia; platelet release defects; von Willebrand's disease; coagulopathies
	50,000–100,000/mm^3	Bleeding occurs only with severe trauma or other stress
	<50,000/mm^3	Easy bruising; skin purpura with minor trauma; bleeding after mucous membrane surgery
	<20,000/mm^3	Spontaneous bleeding; intracranial or other spontaneous internal bleeding

[†]See the appendix on Laboratory Reference Values for the associated normal laboratory values.

Test	Finding	Diagnostic Possibilities
Prothrombin time	Normal	Deficiency of factors VIII, IX, XI, XII, or XIII; thrombocytopenia; von Willebrand's disease
	Prolonged	Abnormality of tissue factor-dependent pathway and common pathway coagulation systems: deficiency of factors VII, II, V, or X; vitamin K deficiency; DIC; hypofibrinogenemia; dysfibrinogenemia; heparin or coumarin effect; liver failure
Partial thromboplastin time	Normal	Deficiency of factors VII or XIII; thrombocytopenia
	Prolonged	Abnormality of intrinsic and common pathway coagulation systems: deficiency of factors XII, high-molecular-weight kininogen, prekallikrein, XI, IX, VIII, II, V, or X; DIC; von Willebrand's disease; vitamin K deficiency; heparin or coumarin effect; liver failure; hypofibrinogenemia; dysfibrinogenemia
Thrombin time	Normal	Deficiency of factors XII, XI, VIII, IX, VII, II, V, or X
	Prolonged	DIC; dysfibrinogenemia; liver failure; presence of heparin; hypofibrinogenemia
Fibrinogen	Decreased	DIC; liver failure; hypofibrinogenemia
Fibrin degradation products assay	Abnormal	DIC; fibrinogenolysis; liver disease; dysfibrinogenemia
Clot lysis rate	Rapid	Alpha$_2$ plasmin inhibitor

SELECTED BIBLIOGRAPHY

Williams WJ: Classification and clinical manifestations of disorders of hemostasis, in Williams WJ, Beutler E, Erslev AJ et al (eds). *Hematology,* 4th ed., pp. 1338–1342, New York: McGraw-Hill, 1990.

Wintrobe MM: The diagnostic approach to the bleeding disorders, in Wintrobe MM, Lee GR, Boggs DR et al (eds). *Clinical Hematology,* 8th ed., pp. 1045–1071, Philadelphia: Lea & Febiger, 1981.

47
Enlarged Thyroid Gland

INTRODUCTION

Goiter Generalized enlargement of the thyroid, whether diffuse, irregular, or nodular.

Generalized enlargements of the thyroid (with the right lobe tending to enlarge more than the left) are associated with normal, increased, or decreased hormone secretion, depending upon the underlying disturbance. Simple (nontoxic) goiter is defined as any enlargement of the thyroid gland that does not result from an inflammatory or neoplastic disease and that is not initially associated with thyrotoxicosis or myxedema. It may be due to impaired thyroid hormone synthesis, such as iodine deficiency, ingestion of a goitrogen, or an abnormality in a hormone biosynthetic pathway. In most cases its cause cannot be determined. Decreased hormone synthesis appears to increase the responsiveness of the gland to thyrotropin (TSH) that remains within the normal range. The resulting increased functioning thyroid mass and cellular activity overcome mild impairment of hormone synthesis; the patient is clinically euthyroid, though goitrous. Although the gland may first enlarge diffusely, it typically evolves into a multinodular goiter as areas of the thyroid undergo degenerative changes.

Impairment in the ability to synthesize adequate quantities of thyroid hormone leads to hypersecretion of TSH and hence goiter. If this compensatory response is inadequate, goitrous hypothyroidism results with reduced secretion of both thyroxine (T4) and triiodothyronine (T3). The commonest cause of goiter with hypothyroidism is chronic thyroiditis (Hashimoto's disease), in which autoimmune factors play a prominent role. Hypothyroidism secondary to decreased secretion of thyrotropin, due to either pituitary or hypothalamic disease, is associated with a small thyroid gland.

Thyrotoxicosis is the clinical state resulting from the excess production of T3, T4, or both. The most common cause is a diffuse toxic goiter (Graves' disease). The hyperproduction of T4 and T3 is thought to result from thyroid stimulation by circulating IgG auto-antibodies that bind to the thyrotropin receptor of the thyroid gland. Another common form of hyperthyroidism is toxic multinodular goiter, in which localized areas of the gland become autonomous and function excessively. Thyroiditis may also result in thyrotoxicosis with enlargement of the thyroid gland.

Focal enlargement of the thyroid may be due to a cyst, a benign adenoma, or carcinoma.

ETIOLOGY

Goiter Associated with Euthyroidism

Simple nontoxic goiter* (endemic, sporadic)
   Iodine deficiency; goitrogens; defective thyroid hormone synthesis
Thyroiditis: acute, subacute (euthyroid phase)
Thyroid neoplasms: benign; malignant

*Common cause

Goiter Associated with Hyperthyroidism

Diffuse toxic goiter* (Graves' disease)
Toxic multinodular goiter*
Toxic adenoma
Iodine-induced hyperthyroidism
Ingestion of excessive amounts of thyroid hormone
Subacute thyroiditis: granulomatous (de Quervain); lymphocytic (silent)
TSH-secreting pituitary tumor

Goiter Associated with Hypothyroidism

Chronic (Hashimoto's) thyroiditis*
Heritable biosynthetic defects
Iodine deficiency; naturally occurring goitrogens
Drug-induced
Iodine excess in patients with underlying thyroid disease
Subacute throiditis (chypothyroid phase)

Iatrogenic Causes of Goiter With or Without Thyroid Dysfunction

Amiodarone; antipyrine; aniline derivatives; cobalt; isoniazid; iodides; lithium; para-aminosalicylic acid; phenylbutazone; propylthiouracil, methimazole; sulfonamides; iodinated contrast agents

HISTORY TAKING*

Possible meaning of a positive response

1   Mode of Onset and Evolution

1.1   How long have you known that you have a swelling in your neck?

May be difficult to determine exactly when onset is insidious. The patient with multinodular goiter is often asymptomatic and the goiter is discovered on a routine physical examination

1.1a   How long have you had complaints?

Multinodular goiters are present for 5 to 10 years before toxicity becomes evident. The symptoms of diffuse toxic goiter usually begin gradually. Early symptoms of hypothyroidism are nonspecific and of insidious onset

1.2   Was the onset of the swelling
• acute? (hours to days)

Hemorrhage into a thyroid nodule, cyst, or tumor; pyogenic thyroiditis

*In this section, items in *italics* are characteristic clinical features.

• subacute? (days to weeks)	Subacute thyroiditis; thyroid carcinoma
• gradual, insidious? (months to years)	Nontoxic goiter; hypothyroidism; Graves' disease; thyroid adenomas

1.3 If the swelling has been present for years: Has its volume

• remained unchanged?	Nontoxic goiter
• recently increased?	
• gradually and without tenderness?	Thyroid carcinoma; a continuing enlargement of one of the nodules in multinodular goiter raises the suspicion of malignancy
• rapidly, with local pain?	Hemorrhage into a nodule; de Quervain's thyroiditis; rapid growth of a thyroid nodule increases the probability of malignancy

2 Precipitating or Aggravating Factors

2.1 Have you recently had an emotional stress?	It has been suggested that psychological trauma may trigger the onset of overt hyperthyroidism (controversial)
2.2 What is your consumption of iodide?	In a patient with multinodular goiter, ingestion of excess iodide may result in thyrotoxicosis (jodbasedow phenomenon)
2.3 Prior to the appearance of the swelling, did you have fever? malaise? a sore throat?	Subacute thyroiditis frequently occurs 2 to 3 weeks after viral upper respiratory infection (influenza virus, coxsackievirus, adenovirus)

3 Accompanying Symptoms

3.1 *Do you have sensitivity to cold?* decreased sweating? Do you sleep with more blankets on the bed? Do you have a preference for warm weather?	Cold intolerance in hypothyroidism
3.2 *Do you find hot weather intolerable?* Do you prefer a cooler environment?	
3.2a Do you sleep with fewer blankets? kick off the covers while asleep?	Heat intolerance in Graves' disease
3.2b Do you have excessive sweating?	Hyperdynamic circulatory state in hyperthyroidism
3.3 Do you feel nervous? irritable? fidgety?	Nervousness is the most common symptom of Graves' disease; irritability and emotional lability may lead to deteriorating domestic or occupational relationships

3.4 Do you have palpitations? continuous? episodic?

Sinus tachycardia; chronic or paroxysmal atrial fibrillation (paroxysmal supraventricular tachycardia and flutter
are rare in hyperthyroidism); cardiovascular symptoms of hyperthyroidism
predominate in older subjects

3.5 Do you have easy tearing? especially on exposure to wind or
cold? a gritty foreign body sensation in the eyes? a blurred vision?

Common complaints in Graves' in-
filtrative ophthalmopathy

3.5a Have friends observed that your
eyes were prominent?

Proptosis of Graves' disease

3.6 Do you have
  • an increased appetite?
  • a decreased appetite?
  • a gain in weight? with anorexia?

  • a loss of weight? despite increased appetite?
  • frequent bowel movements?

Hyperthyroidism
Hypothyroidism; thyroid carcinoma
Hypothyroidism; gross obesity is never
a feature of hypothyroidism per se
Hyperthyroidism

Increased gastrointestinal motility in
hyperthyroidism; increased frequency
of defecation and softening of the stools
are often present in Graves' disease
(frank diarrhea is uncommon); medullary carcinoma of thyroid

  • constipation?

Decreased peristaltic activity in hypothyroidism

  • muscle aching? cramps? stiffness?

Hypothyroid myopathy; cramps usually
occur in patients in whom the hypothyroidism is of rapid onset or in patients
with a rapid change from a hyperthy-
roid to a hypothyroid state (after surgery for Graves' disease, a second
radioactive iodine treatment for hyperthyroidism, vigorous antithyroid drug
therapy)

  • paresthesias in the hands?

Carpal tunnel syndrome in hypothyroidism

  • weakness? difficulty in climbing
stairs? rising from a chair?
  • a wasting of some of your muscles?

(Proximal) myopathy in Graves' disease: affects men with thyrotoxicosis
more commonly than women

  • fatigue?
  • hair loss?

Hypo- as well as hyperthyroidism
Hyperthyroidism; also in hypothyroidism

  • swollen legs?

Congestive heart failure or pretibial
myxedema of Graves' disease over the
dorsum of the legs or feet

- diminished menstrual flow?

Oligomenorrhea is common in hyperthyroidism; may progress to amenorrhea

- excessive and irregular menstruation?

Frequent in younger women with hypothyroidism: failure of ovulation; decreased secretion of progesterone, endometrial proliferation with menorrhagia

- a deeper voice? coarsening or huskiness of the voice?

Hypothyroidism: accumulation of mucopolysaccharides in the vocal cords or oropharynx

- hoarseness?

Compression of the recurrent laryngeal nerve: suggests thyroid carcinoma (extension beyond the capsule of the gland); also in subacute thyroiditis; rare in simple goiter

- any difficulty in
  - breathing?

Compression and displacement of the trachea by the enlarged thyroid in multinodular goiter. Dyspnea on effort is common in hyperthyroidism: reduced vital capacity resulting from weakness of the respiratory muscles

  - swallowing?

Dysphagia due to compression and displacement of the esophagus by a massively enlarged thyroid; also in carcinoma; chronic thyroiditis; subacute thyroiditis

  - hearing?

Hypothyroidism; defect of thyroid hormone synthesis with congenital deafness

- excessive sleepiness?

Hypothyroidism

- depression?

Rather than appearing agitated, the elderly patient with hyperthyroidism may be depressed

- decreased memory? decreased ability to calculate?

May be observed in the elderly with hypothyroidism. Rarely psychiatric symptoms may dominate the clinical picture in hypothyroidism ("myxedema madness")

3.7 In case of sudden or gradual and painful swelling in the thyroid gland: *Does the pain radiate to the lower jaw? ear? occiput? with chills? malaise?*

Subacute granulomatous (de Quervain's) thyroiditis; thyroid cancer

3.8 Have you noticed a swelling at another site in your neck?

Local metastasis of a thyroid carcinoma

4 **Iatrogenic Factors   See Etiology**

5   Personal and Social Profile

5.1   What is your occupation?

Ingestion of excess thyroid hormone ("factitious thyrotoxicosis") should be considered in medical or paramedical personnel with symptoms of hyperthyroidism and a nonpalpable thyroid gland

6   Personal Antecedents Pertaining to the Enlarged Thyroid Gland

6.1   Have you ever had previous thyroid tests? radioactive uptake? scan? When? With what results?

6.2   Did you have x-ray therapy to the head or neck in childhood?

May be followed later in life by thyroid disease, including carcinoma

6.3   Do you have any of the following conditions:
  • a thyroid condition? thyroid surgery? a cardiac disease? an eye disease?

7   Family Medical History Pertaining to the Enlarged Thyroid Gland

7.1   Does someone in your family have a thyroid condition? a goiter?

Familial predisposition to Graves' disease, Hashimoto's thyroiditis, myxedema, congenital defects of thyroid hormone synthesis, medullary carcinoma of the thyroid

PHYSICAL SIGNS PERTAINING TO THE ENLARGED THYROID GLAND*

Possible significance

Enlarged thyroid; systolic thyroid bruit; fine tremor; warm moist thin skin; tachycardia; wide pulse pressure; stare; lid lag; lid retraction
  • separation of the fingernail from the nailbed

Hyperthyroidism; one third of elderly patients with Graves' disease will not have a detectable goiter

Onycholysis (Plummer's nail): common in hyperthyroidism

Proptosis; chemosis; ophthalmoplegia

Ophthalmopathy of Graves' disease

Raised thickened area on legs or feet

Pretibial myxedema in Graves' disease

Thyroid palpable (or absent); somnolent patient; dry, sparse hair; dry, thickened, cool skin; periorbital puffiness; macroglossia; enlarged heart; bradycardia; prolonged tendon reflex relaxation time

Hypothyroidism

*In this section, items in **boldface** are potentially life-threatening or urgent conditions.

Solitary thyroid nodule	Toxic or nontoxic adenoma; malignancy
Enlarged, firm, irregular thyroid	Multinodular goiter, toxic or nontoxic; Hashimoto's thyroiditis; cancer in a multinodular goiter
Jugular venous distention; suffusion of the face when the patient's arms are raised above the head	Pemberton's sign: large retrosternal goiter
Hard, fixed gland, or nodules	Malignancy
Fever; enlarged, tender thyroid	Acute or subacute thyroiditis
Mass in the thyroid; marfanoid habitus; mucosal neuromas	Medullary carcinoma of the thyroid and pheochromocytoma: multiple endocrine neoplasia, type III
Proximal muscular weakness and atrophy	Chronic thyrotoxic myopathy; may occur in overt or masked hyperthyroidism
Stridor; dyspnea	Tracheal obstruction: massively enlarged thyroid; simple (nontoxic) goiter; retrosternal goiter; carcinoma

LABORATORY TESTS PERTAINING TO THE ENLARGED THYROID GLAND[†]

Test	Finding	Diagnostic Possibilities
Blood		
T4 concentration	Elevated	Hyperthyroidism; increased thyroxine-binding globulin (TBG)
	Decreased	Hypothyroidism; decreased TBG
T3 concentration	Elevated	Hyperthyroidism; T3-toxicosis
	Decreased	Hypothyroidism
Resin T3 uptake; free T4; free T4 index	Elevated	Hyperthyroidism
	Decreased	Hypothyroidism
Sensitive TSH assay	Elevated	Hypothyroidism, thyroprivic and goitrous varieties
	Decreased	Pituitary or hypothalamic hypothyroidism; thyrotoxicosis

[†]See the appendix on Laboratory Reference Values for the associated normal laboratory values.

Test	Finding	Diagnostic Possibilities
Thyrotropin-releasing hormone (TRH) stimulation test	Subnormal or no response	Pituitary hypothyroidism; thyrotoxicosis
	Supranormal response	Primary (thyroidal) hypothyroidism
Antimicrosomal antibodies; anti-thyroglobulin antibodies	High titers	Hashimoto's disease; Graves' disease

LABORATORY PROCEDURES PERTAINING TO THE ENLARGED THYROID GLAND

Procedure	To Detect
Thyroid scan	Areas of increased or decreased function within the thyroid; retrosternal goiter; ectopic thyroid tissue; functioning metastases of thyroid carcinoma
Thyroid echography	Thyroid cysts vs. solid nodules
X-rays of chest, trachea	Deviation or compression of trachea; retrosternal goiter
Needle biopsy or aspiration	Evaluation of thyroid nodules

SELECTED BIBLIOGRAPHY

Hamburger JI: The various presentations of thyroiditis. *Ann Intern Med* 104:219–224, 1986.

Ingbar SH: Diseases of the thyroid, in Wilson J, Braunwald E, Isselbacher KJ et al (eds). *Harrison's Principles of Internal Medicine,* 12th ed., chap. 316, New York: McGraw-Hill, 1991.

Kaplan MM, Larsen PR (eds): Thyroid disease. *Med Clin North Am* 69(5):847–1120, 1985.

Larsen PR: The thyroid, in Wyngaarden JB, Smith LH Jr (eds). *Cecil Textbook of Medicine,* 18th ed., pp. 1315–1340, Philadelphia: Saunders, 1988.

48
Fever of Unknown Origin

INTRODUCTION

Fever of Unknown Origin (FUO)   An illness of 3 weeks' duration, with temperature exceeding 101°F (38.3°C) on several occasions, and no established diagnosis after 1 week of intensive study.

Temperature may range in healthy adults from 97.8 to 99.2°F (36.5 to 37.4°C). There is a normal diurnal variation in body temperature, the lowest oral reading being in the early morning, and the highest [99°F (37.2°C) or more] between 6 P.M. and 10 P.M. The febrile patterns of most diseases tend to follow this normal diurnal temperature variation. An oral temperature above 99°F (37.2°C) in a subject at bedrest should be regarded as indicating a disease.

Fever may be produced by many stimuli: bacteria and their endotoxins, viruses, yeasts, spirochetes, immune reactions, hormones, and drugs. These exogenous pyrogens stimulate certain cells, principally neutrophils and mononuclear macrophages, to synthesize and release an endogenous pyrogen (EP), identical to interleukin-1 (IL-1). EP/IL-1 initiates many of the reactions termed collectively the "acute phase response" and acts on the thermoregulatory centers in the anterior hypothalamus to produce fever.

The majority of obscure fevers ultimately prove to be atypical manifestations of commoner diseases rather than of unusual illnesses.

ETIOLOGY

Infections (30–40 Percent)

Granulomatous infections: disseminated tuberculosis, atypical mycobacterial infections; deep-seated fungus infections
Bacterial endocarditis
Intraabdominal abscess: subphrenic, pancreatic, splenic, pelvic; appendicitis; diverticulitis
Hepatobiliary infection: cholecystitis; cholangitis; liver abscess
Urinary tract infection; intrarenal abscess; perinephric abscess; chronic pyelonephritis; prostatic abscess
Sinusitis; osteomyelitis
Bacteremia: gonococcemia; meningococcemia; brucellosis
Viral, rickettsial, and chlamydial infections: infectious mononucleosis; cytomegalovirus; human immunodeficiency virus (HIV) infection; hepatitis; group B coxsackie virus; psittacosis
Parasitic diseases: amebiasis; malaria; toxoplasmosis
Spirochetal infections: leptospirosis; relapsing fever

Neoplasms (20–30 Percent)

Carcinoma: kidney, lung, pancreas, liver, large bowel; atrial myxoma; unknown primary; metastatic; lymphoma

419

Collagen-Vascular Diseases (10–15 Percent)

Giant cell arteritis (polymyalgia rheumatica); systemic lupus erythematosus (SLE); Still's disease; hypersensitivity vasculitis; polyarteritis nodosa; Wegener's granulomatosis; rheumatic fever

Miscellaneous (10–20 Percent)

Sarcoidosis; granulomatous hepatitis; inflammatory bowel disease; familial Mediterranean fever; pulmonary emboli; subacute thyroiditis; retroperitoneal hematoma; hemolytic states; drug fever; habitual hyperthermia; factitious fever

Undiagnosed (5–10 Percent)

Iatrogenic Causes of Fever (Partial List)

Antibiotics: penicillins, novobiocin, amphotericin B, cephalosporins; asparaginase; p-aminosalicylic acid; hydralazine; antihistamines; iodides; procainamide; arsenicals; isoniazid; rifampin; bleomycin; laxatives (phenolphthalein); quinidine; barbiturates; sulfonamides; phenytoin; methyldopa; thiouracils; captopril; cimetidine
Intravenous or intraarterial catheter infections; infected arteriovenous fistulas

HISTORY TAKING

Possible meaning of a positive response

1   Mode of Onset and Duration

1.1   How long have you had fever?

As the duration of fever increases, infection becomes less likely

• for more than 6 months?

Granulomatous hepatitis; Still's disease of adults; habitual hyperthermia (in young women); factitious fever

1.2   Was the onset of fever
• abrupt?

Malaria; many pyogenic or viral infections

• gradual?

Subacute and chronic infections: typhoid fever, brucellosis, tuberculosis

2   Pattern of Fever

Specific fever patterns have little significance in the diagnosis of FUO

2.1   At what site do you measure your temperature?
• oral?

Normal average temperature: 98.6°F (37.0°C)

• axillary?

Normal average temperature: 97.6°F (36.5°C)

• rectal?

Normal average temperature: 99.6°F (37.5°C)

2.2 What are the averages, the maximum readings?
- low-grade fever?

Disseminated fungal infection. In a patient past middle age, even low-grade fever should be regarded as indicating an organic disease

- high fever?

Urinary tract infection caused by gram-negative bacilli, meningococcemia; tuberculosis; malaria; drug fever

- extremely high fever? greater than 106°F (41.1°C)?

Consider factitious fever (in adults)

2.3 At what time of the day do you have fever? the highest temperature?

In most patients with fever higher levels of temperature usually occur in the evening

- morning temperature higher than evening temperature?

Miliary tuberculosis

2.4 Is your temperature always above 100°F (37.7°C)?
- with little or no variations throughout the day?

Sustained fever: psittacosis, typhoid fever, typhus; endocarditis; drug fever

- with an elevation of 1°F or more that abates each day, but never returns to normal?

Remittent fever: accentuation of the normal diurnal temperature pattern; bacterial endocarditis; brucellosis; malignancy (this type of fever is seen in most cases and is not characteristic)

2.5 Does your temperature fall to normal each day?

Intermittent fever: bacterial endocarditis; falciform malaria; tuberculosis

2.6 Do you have wide swings in temperature (remittent or intermittent)?

Hectic fever (usually with chills and sweats): occult pyogenic abscess; malaria; lymphoma; collagen-vascular disease; pyelonephritis; ascending cholangitis

2.7 Do you have febrile periods of several days, with one or more days of normal temperature between episodes?

Relapsing, or recurrent, fever: non-falciparum malaria; visceral leishmaniasis; relapsing fever *(Borrelia recurrentis)*; brucellosis; rat-bite fever *(Spirillum minus)*; Haverhill fever *(Streptobacillus moniliformis)*; chronic meningococcemia; filariasis; cholangitis; subacute bacterial endocarditis; Hodgkin's disease ("Pel-Ebstein fever"); drug reaction; inflammatory bowel disease; familial Mediterranean fever

3   Precipitating or Aggravating Factors

3.1 Prior to the onset of the fever, did you have a boil? a tooth extracted? any genitourinary procedure?

Bacteremia; subacute bacterial endocarditis

4   Accompanying Symptoms

4.1   Do you tolerate your fever well?

In disseminated tuberculosis, the fever is usually intermittent and well tolerated by the patient, who may be unaware of its presence despite peaks to 103 to 105°F (39.4 to 40.5°C)

4.2   Do you have
   • repeated shaking chills? (with teeth chattering, bed shaking)?

Pyogenic infection with bacteremia; bacterial endocarditis (especially staphylococcal); pylephlebitis; pelvic thrombophlebitis; intermittent biliary duct obstruction; malaria; pyelonephritis; rat-bite fever; brucellosis; drug reaction; neoplasms; lymphoma; collagen-vascular disorders; intermittent administration of antipyretics; acute hemolytic crises

   • excessive sweats?

A common response to infection, marking the falling, or defervescent, phase of fever

   • during the night?

Miliary tuberculosis; Hodgkin's disease; in a homosexual man: AIDS-related condition, lymphoma

   • a loss of weight?

Fever accelerates many metabolic processes and is accompanied by interleukin-1-mediated muscle wasting and weight loss: neoplasm; tuberculosis. If weight unchanged despite fever of long duration: factitious fever, habitual hyperthermia (usually in young, psychoneurotic women)

   • trouble breathing? cough? dyspnea? vague chest discomfort?

Miliary tuberculosis; multiple pulmonary emboli (pulmonary sarcoidosis is usually a nonfebrile disease). In an AIDS-patient: *Pneumocystis carinii* pneumonia, cytomegalovirus, *Mycobacterium avium-intracellulare*

   • headaches?

Giant cell arteritis; typhoid fever; brucellosis; sinusitis

   • fever blisters?

Herpes labialis: reactivation of latent herpes simplex virus infection by elevation in temperature. In: pneumococcal infections, streptococcosis, malaria, meningococcemia, rickettsioses

   • pain in your joints?

Collagen-vascular disease; rheumatic fever; polymyalgia rheumatica; sarcoidosis; drug fever; bronchogenic tumor; familial Mediterranean fever; Lyme disease; atrial myxoma

• pain in the muscles?	Polyarteritis nodosa; polymyalgia rheumatica; trichinosis; brucellosis
• pain in the chest?	Multiple pulmonary emboli; familial Mediterranean fever
• pain in the abdomen?	Cholangitis with intermittent biliary fever; biliary obstruction due to stone; perinephric abscess; hypernephroma; Crohn's disease; gynecologic infection; dissecting aortic aneurysm; familial Mediterranean fever
• pain in the back?	Vertebral osteomyelitis; perinephric abscess
• bone pain?	Osteomyelitis; (non-Hodgkin) lymphoma
• a sore throat?	Infectious mononucleosis; retropharyngeal abscess; streptococcal tonsillitis followed by rheumatic fever
• discomfort in the jaw muscles with chewing? a blurred vision?	Polymyalgia rheumatica
• frequent or painful urination?	Urinary tract infection
• (in a male patient): dysuria? rectal pain?	Prostatic abscess
• altered bowel habits? diarrhea?	Crohn's disease; ulcerative colitis; typhoid fever; schistosomiasis; amebiasis
• a skin rash?	Gonococcal infection; sarcoidosis; polyarteritis nodosa; lymphoma; rheumatic fever; Rocky Mountain spotted fever
• swollen glands?	Lymphoma; leukemia; drug fever: sarcoidosis; malignant histiocytosis; Still's disease
• a sequence of various illnesses? influenza, stroke, urinary tract infection, arthritis?	Subacute bacterial endocarditis; atrial myxoma

5 Iatrogenic Factors   See Etiology

	Drug fever is an important cause of cryptic fever. A drug well tolerated for many years may abruptly induce a reaction, including fever
5.1 Do you take corticosteroids? other immunosuppressive agents?	Patients especially vulnerable to infection
5.2 Did you recently receive any antibiotics	
• before the onset of your fever?	Drug fever
• after the onset of your fever?	May modify the clinical picture; may mask subacute bacterial endocarditis. Allergy to one of the antibiotics may become superimposed on the fever of an underlying infection

6   Personal and Social Profile

6.1   Have you recently been exposed to a person with tuberculosis? to an Asian immigrant?

Mycobacterial infections are more common among blacks, Native Americans, southeast Asians, and individuals from outside the U.S.

6.2   Have you recently traveled to tropical or developing countries?

Amebic liver abscess; typhoid fever. Malaria: Asia, Africa, some areas of South and Central America. Schistosomiasis: Caribbean islands, Africa, Far East

6.2a   Have you been in Vietnam?

Malaria in a Vietnam war veteran

6.3   Where do you live?

Southwest United States: coccidioidomycosis. Southwest US, Pacific Northwest, Texas: tick-borne relapsing fever. Mississippi River Valley: histoplasmosis

6.4   What is your profession?

In farmers, veterinarians, slaughterhouse workers: brucellosis. In workers in the plastic industry: polymer-fume fever. Exposure to beryllium can lead to a febrile illness. (Female) health care workers: factitious fever

6.5   Do you have any contact with domestic or wild animals? birds?

Brucellosis; birds, pigeons: psittacosis

6.5a   Have you had
   • a rat bite within the last 10 weeks?

Rat bite fever

   • a tick bite within the last 2 weeks?

Rocky Mountain spotted fever

6.6   Did you ever ingest
   • unpasteurized milk? cheese?
   • poorly cooked pork?

Brucellosis
Trichinosis

6.7   Do you use narcotics?

In intravenous drug users: bacterial endocarditis, frequently on the tricuspid valve; human immunodeficiency virus (HIV) infection; AIDS-related condition

6.8   What is your sexual orientation?

Fever in a homosexual man: HIV infection: AIDS-related condition; syphilis, opportunistic infection, cytomegalovirus with or without *Pneumocystis*; lymphoma. In AIDS-patients, *Mycobacterium avium-intracellulare* infection is a common preterminal event

7 Personal Antecedents Pertaining to the FUO

7.1 Have you ever had a tuberculin skin test? tuberculosis?

7.2 Do you have any of the following conditions: hematologic or other malignancy? diabetes mellitus? AIDS? (acquired immunodeficiency syndrome); neutropenia? sickle cell anemia?

Patient may become infected with unusual opportunistic pathogens or may fail to respond normally to common infectious agents

• a valvular heart disease?

Subacute bacterial endocarditis (uncommon in patients with pure mitral stenosis); rheumatic fever; atrial myxoma

• rheumatic fever during childhood?

Valvular disease with subacute bacterial endocarditis

• a recent operation?

Postoperative abscess (postoperative fever is usually related to the surgical procedure, not to some unrelated disease)

• an intravascular graft?

May become infected and give rise to prolonged bacteremia

• a recent childbirth?

Pelvic thrombophlebitis in postpartum patients

8 Family Medical History Pertaining to the FUO

8.1 Does anyone else in your family have fever?

Tuberculosis; exposure to a common etiologic agent; familial Mediterranean fever

PHYSICAL SIGNS PERTAINING TO FEVER OF UNKNOWN ORIGIN

Possible significance

Tachycardia

The heart rate normally increases about 9 to 10 beats per minute for each degree (F) of temperature rise

Normal pulse

Relative bradycardia in typhoid or other enteric fever; psittacosis; *Mycoplasma pneumoniae* pneumonia; Legionnaire's disease; heart disease with AV block; factitious fever

Skin

• petechiae (also in conjunctivas); splinter hemorrhages (nailbeds)

Subacute bacterial endocarditis

• rash

Meningococcal infection; sarcoidosis; vasculitis; lymphoma; rheumatic fever; Rocky Mountain spotted fever

• nodules

Metastatic malignancy

Heart murmur	Subacute bacterial endocarditis; atrial myxoma
Lymphadenopathy	Malignancy; lymphoma; leukemia; sarcoidosis; infectious mononucleosis; toxoplasmosis; drug fever
Splenomegaly	Lymphoma; leukemia; infection; subacute bacterial endocarditis
Hepatosplenomegaly	Lymphoma; leukemia; chronic infection; liver cirrhosis
Hepatomegaly without splenomegaly	Liver abscess; metastatic cancer
Abdominal mass	Neoplastic disease; hypernephroma; intraabdominal abscess
Arthritis	Collagen-vascular disease; rheumatic fever; subacute bacterial endocarditis; atrial myxoma
Sternal tenderness	Chronic granulocytic leukemia; acute leukemia; metastatic tumor; multiple myeloma
Bone tenderness	Osteomyelitis; metastatic tumor
Inflamed, tender temporal artery	Giant cell arteritis
Abnormal testicles	Tumor; tuberculosis
Rectal and pelvic examination	May reveal: masses, abscesses, perirectal abscess; pelvic thrombophlebitis; prostatic disease
Funduscopic examination:	
• choroidal tubercles	Miliary tuberculosis
• flame-shaped hemorrhages	Subacute bacterial endocarditis

LABORATORY TESTS PERTAINING TO FEVER OF UNKNOWN ORIGIN[†]

Blood

- Complete blood cell count, erythrocyte sedimentation rate, biochemical screening
- Immunologic tests: helpful in the diagnosis of fever caused by collagen-vascular disorders, infectious endocarditis
- Serologic tests: antistreptolysin O titers; antinuclear antibodies; rheumatoid factor; febrile agglutinins
- Blood smears for: abnormal morphology, parasites, LE cells
- Cultures of blood (aerobically and anaerobically), urine, bone marrow, other body fluids, pus

[†]See the appendix on Laboratory Reference Values for the associated normal laboratory values.

Skin tests

Tuberculin, histoplasmin, coccidioidin, etc.: rarely helpful

Stool

Occult blood tests; ova, parasites; culture

LABORATORY PROCEDURES PERTAINING TO FEVER OF UNKNOWN ORIGIN

Procedure*	To Detect
Chest x-ray	Pulmonary tuberculosis
IV pyelogram; renal ultrasonography	Tumor; intrarenal or perinephric abscess; pyelonephritis
Sinus, bone films	Sinusitis; osteomyelitis; primary or metastatic tumor abscess
GI barium studies, upper GI x-rays, IV cholangiography; endoscopic retrograde cholangiopancreatography	Tumor, abscess, diverticulitis; inflammatory bowel disease; biliary tract disease
Liver-spleen scan	Hepatic abscess; tumor, cyst; vascular malformation
Perfusion and ventilatory lung scan	Pulmonary emboli
Bone scans	Primary or metastatic tumor; osteomyelitis
Computerized tomography (CT) and ultrasonography of the abdomen	Subphrenic, abdominal, and pelvic abscesses or tumors; retroperitoneal lymph nodes, tumors, abscesses; hematomas; space-occupying lesions in the liver
Biopsy of: liver (rarely helpful)	Primary or metastatic tumor; granulomas, tuberculosis, histoplasmosis, sarcoidosis, lymphoma, etc.
lymph node	Lymphomas, metastatic cancer; tuberculosis; mycotic infection
bone marrow	Metastatic carcinoma; granulomas; leukemias
muscle	Polyarteritis nodosa; dermatomyositis; sarcoidosis; trichinosis
temporal artery	Giant cell arteritis
Abdominal aortography and selective arteriography	Tumor of the kidneys, pancreas, liver: retroperitoneal mass lesions

*In selected patients if indicated

Procedure*	To Detect
Echocardiogram	Endocarditis; atrial myxoma
Peritoneoscopy	Tuberculous peritonitis; peritoneal carcinomatosis; cholecystitis; pelvic inflammatory disease

*In selected patients if indicated

SELECTED BIBLIOGRAPHY

Brush JL, Weinstein L: Fever of unknown origin. *Med Clin North Am* 72:1247–1261, 1988.

Cunha BA: Clinical implications of fever. *Postgrad Med* 85(5):188–200, 1989.

Larson EB, Featherstone HJ, Petersdorf RG: Fever of undetermined origin. Diagnosis and follow-up of 105 cases, 1970–1980. *Medicine* 61:269–292, 1982.

McGee ZA, Gorby GL: The diagnostic value of fever patterns. *Hosp Pract* 22(10A):103–110, 1987.

Nolan SM, Fitzgerald FT: Fever of unknown origin. *Postgrad Med* 81(5):190–205, 1987.

49
Hyperglycemia

INTRODUCTION

Hyperglycemia   A fasting plasma glucose concentration greater than some agreed-upon upper limit of normal (usually >110 to 120 mg/dL).

The principal determinants of the blood glucose level are the dietary intake of glucose, the rate of entry of glucose into the cells of muscles, adipose tissue, and other organs, and the regulatory activity of the liver, which takes up glucose and stores it as glycogen (glycogenesis) when the blood glucose is high, and discharges glucose into the circulation through glycogenolysis (breakdown of glycogen) when the blood glucose is low. The overall control of glucose homeostasis is affected by the action of numerous hormones. When carbohydrate is fed, the increase of blood glucose concentration provokes increased secretion of insulin. Insulin acts to decrease blood sugar by stimulating hepatic glycogenesis and decreasing hepatic gluconeogenesis (conversion of nonglucose molecules to glucose). In addition, insulin increases the entry of glucose into muscles and adipose tissue, and stimulates the synthesis of protein from amino acids and the synthesis of lipids from fatty acids. Carbohydrate metabolism is also regulated by other hormones. Glucagon stimulates hepatic glycogenolysis, thereby increasing blood glucose concentration, and increases gluconeogenesis in the liver. Epinephrine blocks insulin secretion, stimulates glucagon release, activates glycogen breakdown, and impairs insulin action in target tissues. Glucocorticoids increase gluconeogenesis, with resulting hyperglycemic effect. Growth hormone increases hepatic glucose output and decreases glucose uptake into some tissues.

   Insulin deficiency, either absolute or relative, causes diabetes mellitus. In type 1, insulin-dependent diabetes mellitus (IDDM), an environmental (viral?) event initiates in a genetically susceptible individual an inflammatory response in the pancreas called "insulitis." The beta cell is no longer recognized as "self" but is seen by the immune system as a foreign cell. Cell-mediated immune mechanisms acting in concert with cytotoxic islet-cell antibodies result in the destruction of the beta cell and the appearance of diabetes. Type 1 diabetics have little or no endogenous insulin. In type 2, non-insulin-dependent diabetes mellitus (NIDDM), impaired insulin secretion, increased hepatic glucose production, and resistance to insulin action in target tissues contribute to the hyperglycemia.

CLASSIFICATION OF DIABETES

Primary Diabetes

Insulin-dependent diabetes mellitus (IDDM, type 1)
Non-insulin-dependent diabetes mellitus (NIDDM, type 2)
   Nonobese; obese; maturity-onset diabetes of the young (MODY)

Secondary Diabetes

Pancreatic diseases: pancreatitis; pancreatectomy; cystic fibrosis; hemochromatosis
Hormonal abnormalities: pheochromocytoma; acromegaly; Cushing's syndrome,

steroid hormones; primary aldosteronism; somatostatinoma; glucagonoma; endogenous release of glucagon and catecholamines: "stress" hyperglycemia, severe burns, acute myocardial infarction

Drug- or chemical-induced

Insulin receptor abnormalities

Genetic syndromes: lipodystrophies; myotonic dystrophy, ataxia-telangiectasia

Impaired Glucose Tolerance

Gestational Diabetes

Iatrogenic Causes of Hyperglycemia

Corticosteroids; oral contraceptives; chlorthalidone, ethacrynic acid, thiazides, furosemide, diazoxide; growth hormone; phenytoin

HISTORY TAKING*

Possible meaning of a positive response

1   Mode of Onset and Duration

1.1 At what age were you found to have hyperglycemia?	Approximately ten times as many cases of diabetes are diagnosed in people over the age of 45 as in those under 45
• before the age of 40?	Insulin-dependent diabetes: in the U.S. peak incidence is around age 14
• in middle life or beyond?	Non-insulin-dependent diabetes
1.2 Under which circumstances was diabetes discovered?	
• during a routine examination?	NIDDM is frequently diagnosed when an asymptomatic person is found to have an elevated plasma glucose on routine laboratory examination
• because of an acute complication?	IDDM may be heralded by the appearance of ketoacidosis during an intercurrent illness or following surgery. The acute metabolic decompensation may be followed by a symptom-free interval (the "honeymoon" period in IDDM) during which no treatment is required. Patients with NIDDM do not develop ketoacidosis. Rarely, the initial event in elderly patients with decompensated NIDDM may be hyperosmolar nonketotic coma, precipitated by a stroke or infection

*In this section, items in *italics* are characteristic clinical features, and items in **boldface** are potentially life-threatening or urgent conditions.

- because you had any complaints?

Polyuria, polydipsia, polyphagia may be the first manifestations of diabetes. Occasionally, NIDDM is first diagnosed because of peripheral vascular insufficiency, diabetic neuropathy, or some other complication

1.2a Was the onset of symptoms
- abrupt? (days to weeks)

IDDM often has a rather abrupt onset of symptomatic hyperglycemia

- gradual? (weeks to months)

Symptoms begin more gradually in NIDDM than in IDDM. Many nonobese patients with NIDDM may have a slow autoimmune form of the disease

1.2b How long have you had these complaints?

2 Precipitating or Aggravating Factors

2.1 In case of rapid (days to weeks) development of symptoms: Did you have, prior to the appearance of your complaints
- an acute infection? mumps? hepatitis? infectious mononucleosis? coxsackievirus infection?

Viral infections of the pancreas could cause diabetes by direct inflammatory disruption of islets or induction of an immune response

- a trauma? an operation? an acute illness? a pregnancy?

Explosive onset of diabetes may be related to stresses which simultaneously increase the need for insulin and decrease the ability to secrete it

2.2 What is your usual weight?

Obesity is a major risk factor for the development of NIDDM. Most patients with type 2 diabetes are obese. Obesity-induced insulin resistance could lead to exhaustion of the beta cells; obesity increases insulin levels and decreases the concentration of insulin receptors in tissues, including muscle and fat

3 Accompanying Symptoms

3.1 Acute or subacute onset of diabetes

3.1a Do you
- *urinate more than usual?*

Polyuria: excretion of the osmotically active glucose molecules provokes an osmotic diuresis

- have excessive thirst? *ingest more fluids than usual?*

Polydipsia: the dehydrating osmotic diuresis activates the mechanisms regulating water intake

• have an increased appetite? increased food intake?

Polyphagia: (?)decreased activity of the hypothalamic satiety center (due to deficient glucose utilization in its cells) with unopposed activity of the feeding center

3.1b Do you have
• a loss of strength?

Neuropathy may be an initial manifestation of diabetes

• a loss of weight?

Type 1 patients vary from normal weight to wasted, depending on the length of time between onset of symptoms and start of treatment. In untreated diabetes, increased protein catabolism and diminished protein synthesis lead to protein depletion and wasting

• frequent skin or mouth infections? boils?

Cellulitis; furunculosis; gingival diseases. Infections in diabetics may not occur more frequently than in nondiabetics, but they tend to be more severe (? due to impaired leukocyte function)

• severe pain in the ear? drainage? fever?

Malignant external otitis, usually due to *Pseudomonas aeruginosa* (in older patients)

• episodes of pain in the flank? fever? chills? pain on urination?

Recurrent urinary tract infections with dysuria

• for the female patient: vulvar pruritus? vaginal discharge?

Associated with bacterial and *Candida albicans* infections of vulva and vagina

3.1c Do you have headaches? drowsiness? loss of appetite? nausea? vomiting? increased urination? abdominal pain?

Early phase of ketoacidosis. Digestive complaints may also result from delayed gastric emptying (diabetic autonomic neuropathy), a late complication of diabetes

3.2 Accompanying symptoms related to chronic or late complications of diabetes

On the average, late complications of diabetes develop 15 to 20 years following the appearance of overt hyperglycemia

3.2a Do you have
• pain in your calves when walking? disappearing when you stop walking?

Peripheral occlusive arterial disease, primarily due to premature atherosclerosis

• chest pain on exertion?

Atherosclerotic (macrovascular) coronary heart disease: 2 to 3 times more common among diabetics than nondiabetics

- fatigue? shortness of breath on exertion? when lying down? (orthopnea)

Left ventricular failure; may be due to a silent myocardial infarction (increased frequency in diabetics); cardiomyopathy, with angiographically normal coronary arteries

- numbness, tingling, burning, pain in your feet? hands? worse at night?

Symmetrical peripheral polyneuropathy ("glove-and-stocking" pattern). Pain at rest in the lower extremities may be due to ischemia

- a sudden wrist drop? foot drop? loss of movement of an eye? double vision?

Diabetic (asymmetrical) mononeuropathy: may involve the median, ulnar, femoral, or sciatic nerves. The third, fourth, or sixth cranial nerves may be affected unilaterally

- severe pain in the chest wall? or abdomen?

Radiculopathy: sensory syndrome with pain over the distribution of one or more spinal nerves

- difficulty swallowing? constipation? urinary retention?

Autonomic neuropathy with motility disturbances of the esophagus, intestine, bladder

- episodes of nausea? vomiting?

Diabetic gastroenteropathy: vagal neuropathy delays gastric emptying

- nocturnal diarrhea?

Autonomic neuropathy: in poorly controlled, longstanding insulin-requiring diabetes (anal sphincter dysfunction and fecal incontinence may mimic diabetic diarrhea)

- syncopal episodes?

Orthostatic hypotension (autonomic neuropathy)

- ulcers of the feet and lower extremities?

Due to abnormal pressure distribution secondary to diabetic neuropathy and atherosclerosis in the smaller arteries with diminished blood supply. All diabetics should be instructed about proper foot care in an attempt to prevent ulcers

- blurred vision?

Diabetic retinopathy, simple and proliferative. Some 10 to 18 percent of patients with simple retinopathy progress to proliferative disease in a ten-year period. About half of patients with proliferative disease progress to blindness within five years

- retrograde ejaculation? sexual impotence?

Retrograde ejaculation is caused by damage to the pelvic parasympathetic nerves with relaxation of the internal vesical sphincter during orgasm. Impotence ultimately occurs in approximately half of diabetic men; may be due to neuropathy or vascular disease

• swollen legs? facial edema?	Microvascular disease leading to diabetic nephropathy; nephrotic syndrome may occur prior to azotemia

4   Iatrogenic Factors   See Etiology

5   Personal and Social Profile

5.1   How do you control your disease?

5.1a Are you treated with
      • diet? insulin?: type? number of units? oral hypoglycemic agents?

5.1b How do you adapt your medication and diet to the results of urine tests? blood tests?	The plasma glucose should be maintained as near normal as possible

5.1c In a patient treated with insulin: Do you have

• episodes of sweating? nervousness? tremor? hunger?	Daytime episodes of hypoglycemia
• night sweats? unpleasant dreams? early-morning headache?	Nocturnal episodes of hypoglycemic reaction to evening insulin injection
5.2 How do you adapt to your diabetes?	The emotional response to diabetes often hampers treatment. Extensive education and emotional support of the patient are vital in the proper management of diabetic patients

6   Personal Antecedents Pertaining to the Hyperglycemia

6.1 Have you ever had episodes of unconsciousness?	Hypoglycemia; ketoacidotic coma; hyperglycemic hyperosmolar nonketotic coma; lactic acidosis; orthostatic hypotension with syncope due to autonomic neuropathy

6.2   Do you have any of the following conditions:

• recurrent episodes of abdominal pain? attacks of pancreatitis? a past operation on your pancreas?	Pancreatic disease (particularly chronic pancreatitis in alcoholics) is a common cause of secondary diabetes
• a heart disease?	Ischemic heart disease
• a kidney disease? proteinuria?	Diabetic nephropathy: diffuse and/or nodular
• urinary tract infections?	High frequency of acute and chronic pyelonephritis in diabetics: attributed to impaired immune responses, high levels of glucose in urine, renal microvascular disease, bladder paralysis

- a high blood pressure?

- an endocrine condition? anemia? a muscle or joint condition?

6.3 For female patients: What was the birth weight of your children?

Diabetics are particularly vulnerable to renal damage when hypertensive

Autoimmune disorders: Addison's disease, Hashimoto's thyroiditis, hyperthyroidism, pernicious anemia, vitiligo, myasthenia gravis, collagen-vascular disease frequently coexist with IDDM

Infants of diabetic mothers have a higher incidence of macrosomia (oversized fetus)

7 Family Medical History Pertaining to the Hyperglycemia

7.1 Are there any other members of your family who have hyperglycemia?

NIDDM runs in families. The presence of NIDDM in a parent increases the risk for IDDM in the offspring. Maturity-onset diabetes of the young (MODY, mild hyperglycemia in young persons resistant to ketosis) is transmitted as an autosomal dominant trait

PHYSICAL SIGNS PERTAINING TO HYPERGLYCEMIA

Possible significance

Obesity

80 to 90 percent of non-insulin-dependent diabetics are obese

Round, firm, brown to yellow plaques over the anterior surfaces of the legs

Necrobiosis lipoidica diabeticorum: may appear within the first year of the diabetes

Ulcers on the feet and lower extremities

Coexisting vascular insufficiency and neuropathy

Symmetrical sensory loss in the distal lower extremities, decreased vibratory sensation; decreased to absent deep-tendon reflexes in the legs

Peripheral diabetic polyneuropathy: loss of axons in peripheral nerves and segmental demyelinization

Orthostatic hypotension

Autonomic diabetic neuropathy

Round moon facies; truncal obesity; buffalo hump; purple striae

Cushing's syndrome

Skin pigmentation; hepatomegaly; cardiac failure

Hemochromatosis

Funduscopic examination

Simple retinopathy: increased vascular permeability, microaneurysms, hemorrhages, exudates
Proliferative retinopathy: new vessel formation and scarring, vitral hemorrhage, retinal detachment

LABORATORY TESTS PERTAINING TO HYPERGLYCEMIA

Diagnostic Criteria for Diabetes Mellitus

Presence of classic symptoms of diabetes with random plasma glucose ≥200 mg/dL
Fasting plasma glucose: ≥140 mg/dL on more than one occasion
Oral glucose tolerance test, following ingestion of 75 g of glucose: both the 2-hour
  plasma glucose and some other sample before 2 hours after glucose ≥200 mg/dL
Impaired glucose tolerance:
  Fasting plasma glucose <140 mg/dL
  Oral glucose tolerance test:
    2-hour plasma glucose: between 140 mg/dL and 200 mg/dL
    plasma glucose before 2 hours: 200 mg/dL or greater

SELECTED BIBLIOGRAPHY

Foster DW: Diabetes mellitus, in Wilson J, Braunwald E, Isselbacher KJ et al (eds). *Harrison's Principles of Internal Medicine,* 12th ed., chap. 327, New York: McGraw-Hill, 1991.

Raskin P, Rosenstock J: Blood glucose control and diabetic complications. *Ann Intern Med* 105:254–263, 1986.

Rizza RA, Greene DA (eds): Diabetes mellitus. *Med Clin North Am* 72(6):1271–1576, 1988.

50
Lymphadenopathy

INTRODUCTION

Lymphadenopathy Lymph node enlargement.

Lymph node enlargement may be due to an increase in the number of benign lymphocytes and macrophages during response to antigens or to in situ proliferation of malignant lymphocytes or macrophages. A lymph node can also be infiltrated by cells normally not present in it [inflammatory cells in infections involving the lymph nodes (lymphadenitis), metastatic malignant cells, metabolite-laden macrophages in lipid storage diseases]. Lymphadenopathy associated with malignant disease may be due to direct node involvement by tumor, lymphoid hyperplasia in response to tumor, or both.

ETIOLOGY

Infections
  Viral infections: infectious hepatitis, infectious mononucleosis syndromes, human immunodeficiency virus (acute infection, persistent generalized lymphadenopathy), rubella, varicella-herpes zoster
  Bacterial infections: streptococci, staphylococci, salmonella, brucella, *Francisella tularensis, Listeria monocytogenes, Yersinia pestis, Haemophilus ducreyi,* cat-scratch disease
  Fungal infections: coccidioidomycosis, histoplasmosis
  Chlamydial infections: lymphogranuloma venereum, trachoma
  Mycobacterial: tuberculosis, leprosy
  Parasitic: toxoplasmosis, trypanosomiasis, microfilariaris
  Spirochetal: syphilis, yaws, leptospirosis
Malignant diseases
  Hematologic: leukemias, Hodgkin's disease, non-Hodgkin's lymphomas, malignant histiocytosis
  Metastatic neoplasms: breast, prostate, kidney, head and neck, gastrointestinal tract, melanoma, Kaposi's sarcoma, neuroblastoma, seminoma
Immunologic diseases
  SLE; dermatomyositis; rheumatoid arthritis; hypersensitivity states: serum sickness, drug reactions; angioimmunoblastic lymphadenopathy; Sjögren's syndrome
Lipid storage diseases: Gaucher's disease; Niemann-Pick disease
Miscellaneous
  Sarcoidosis; amyloidosis; hyperthyroidism; adrenal insufficiency; sinus histiocytosis; mucocutaneous lymph node syndrome (Kawasaki's disease); lymphomatoid granulomatosis; dermatopathic lymphadenopathy

Iatrogenic Causes of Lymph Node Enlargement

Allopurinol; phenytoin; primidone; isoniazid; antithyroid agents; phenylbutazone; hydralazine

HISTORY TAKING*

Possible meaning of a positive response

1 Location of Lymphadenopathy

1.1 Have you noticed only one lump? several lumps?

1.2 Where have you noticed the swelling(s)? See "Location of lymphadenopathy", in "Physical Signs Pertaining to Lymphadenopathy"

2 Mode of Onset and Duration

2.1 When did you notice the swelling(s) for the first time? Patients with neoplastic nodes have a longer history (months) than patients with infectious or inflammatory adenopathy (days)

2.2 Has the onset of the mass(es) been
   • sudden? Nonneoplastic: acute infection; hypersensitivity state; drug reaction

   • gradual? (over several weeks) Malignant lymphoproliferative disease; tuberculosis; fungal infection

3 Character of the Lymphadenopathy

3.1 Is the swelling
   • tender? painful? Acute inflammation: cat-scratch disease (unilateral); syphilis (secondary stage, 2 to 10 weeks after infection); cancer of the salivary glands; acute lymphoblastic leukemia; malignant invasion of adjacent bone or nervous structures

   • painless? nontender? Lymphoma; leukemia; metastasis (in the neck: metastatic cancer from a primary lesion in the head and neck, until proved otherwise); tuberculosis; sarcoidosis

3.2 Has the mass grown rapidly, over a short time? Inflammatory process; rapid changes in size can be seen in malignant neoplasms owing to the adjacent inflammatory response around the tumor

4 Precipitating or Aggravating Factors

4.1 In case of a cervical mass with sudden onset: Have you recently had

*In this section, items in *italics* are characteristic clinical features.

• a sore throat? a dental abscess?	Tonsillitis, pharyngitis, or dental infections can cause cervical adenopathy. Dental infections account for 30 percent of all inflammatory neck masses
4.2 Have you recently had a sore throat with a skin rash?	In a young patient: infectious mononucleosis

5 Accompanying Symptoms

5.1 Do you have • fever? chills? malaise?	Infections: acute human immunodeficiency virus (HIV) infection, AIDS-related complex, infectious mononucleosis, toxoplasmosis, cytomegalovirus, parapharyngeal abscess, syphilis; sinus histiocytosis (with generalized lymphadenopathy); angioimmunoblastic lymphadenopathy; acute leukemia; Hodgkin's disease
• night sweats? weight loss?	Granulomatous disease (tuberculosis, fungal infection); malignancy; Hodgkin's disease
• a sore throat?	Infectious mononucleosis (in a young patient). Neck mass: primary intraoral syphilitic chancre
• cough? wheezing? increasing dyspnea?	Airway compression due to hilar or mediastinal node enlargement; laryngeal carcinoma (with cervical lymphadenopathy)
• hoarseness?	Recurrent laryngeal nerve compression (by enlarged mediastinal or hilar nodes); squamous cell carcinoma of the pharyngolaryngeal area
• difficulty swallowing?	Dysphagia due to esophageal compression (by enlarged hilar or mediastinal nodes) or a mass in the oropharynx, hypopharynx or esophagus
• diarrhea?	AIDS-related complex (ARC)
• a skin rash?	Maculopapular skin lesions involving the palms and soles in secondary stage of syphilis; acute HIV infection; herpes zoster in ARC; Kaposi's sarcoma; erythema nodosum; sarcoidosis
• easy bruising?	Leukemia with thrombocytopenia
• *pain in enlarged lymph nodes following alcohol ingestion?*	Hodgkin's disease
5.2 In case of a cervical mass: Do you have • a blockage in one of your nostrils? frequent bleeding from the nose? increased pain in a sinus? a sore in your mouth?	Metastatic lymph nodes from primary oral, nasal, or pharynx cancer

- a draining fistula from the neck mass?

Cervical adenitis due to any infectious process; tuberculous lymphadenitis; congenital branchial cleft cyst

6   Iatrogenic Factors   See Etiology

7   Personal and Social Profile

7.1   Age of the patient?

Lymphadenopathy in:
a young college student: infectious mononucleosis
a patient under 30 years of age: benign cause in approximately 80 percent of cases; infectious mononucleosis
a patient older than 50 years of age: tumor; benign cause in 40 percent of cases

7.2   Do you keep or handle pets? cats? rabbits?

Cat-scratch disease; toxoplasmosis (cats implicated); tularemia; sporotrichosis

7.3   What is (was) your occupation?

Brucellosis in a veterinarian, slaughterhouse worker. Leukemia due to benzene, ionizing radiation in: chemists, furniture refinishing, cleaning, degreasing, radiation workers

7.4   Have you sustained lacerations while gardening?

Sporotrichosis

7.5   Have you recently traveled abroad? nationwide?

Infectious process: histoplasmosis; tuberculosis; coccidioidomycosis; toxoplasmosis; plague; brucellosis

7.6   Do you use narcotics?

Persistent generalized lymphadenopathy (AIDS) in an intravenous drug user

7.7   Have you been exposed to a venereal sexual contact?

Lymphadenopathy associated with the secondary stage of syphilis, 2 to 10 weeks after infection; gonorrhea; genital herpes; lymphogranuloma

7.8   What are your sexual habits? preferences?

Extragenital inoculation of syphilis and gonorrhea can cause cervical adenopathy
Generalized node enlargement in a homosexual male: persistent generalized lymphadenopathy (AIDS); cytomegalovirus; secondary syphilis; lymphoma; Kaposi's sarcoma of lymph nodes; opportunistic infection involving lymph nodes. Inguinal lymphadenopathy in a homosexual male: primary syphilis; lymphogranuloma venereum; granuloma inguinale; fungal dermatitis; herpes simplex proctitis

8   Personal Antecedents Pertaining to the Lymphadenopathy

8.1   Do you have any of the following conditions: tuberculosis? a sexually transmissible disease? recurrent infections? recurrent sore throats? dental problems? previous lung, breast, gastrointestinal, renal, testicular, or pancreatic, carcinoma?

PHYSICAL SIGNS PERTAINING TO LYMPHADENOPATHY

	Possible significance
Tender, asymmetrically enlarged, soft, warm, erythematosous nodes (matted together)	Local infectious process
Firm, rubbery, nontender mobile nodes	Lymphoma
Very hard, painless nodes, fixed to underlying tissue	Metastatic carcinomatous nodes
Sinus tract in the neck	Tuberculosis; aspergillosis; actinomycosis
Location of lymphadenopathy	
• occipital	Infection (origin in the scalp); malignancy unlikely (lymphoma occasionally)
• posterior auricular	Rubella (occasionally in lymphoma)
• anterior auricular	Infection of eyelid and conjunctiva; scalp infection; may occur in lymphoma
• anterior cervical	Infection of the oral cavity and pharynx
• posterior cervical	Scalp infection; toxoplasmosis; rubella
• unilateral cervical or submandibular	Lymphadenitis (tuberculosis, catscratch disease); buccal cavity infection; dental abscess; parotitis; otitis externa; soft tissue infection of the face; pharyngitis; metastatic disease originating in the nasopharynx, thyroid, lung, breast, GI tract, pancreas; Hodgkin's disease; histiocytic or lymphocytic lymphoma. Warrants a careful ear, nose, and throat examination for malignancy
• left supraclavicular lymph node	Virchow's node: metastatic tumor usually from an occult abdominal neoplasm
• unilateral jugular (along the anterior border of the sternocleidomastoid muscle) or mandibular	Lymphoma; nonlymphoid head-and-neck malignancy
• near the angle of mandible and lobule of the external ear	Parotid gland tumor or infection

- bilateral cervical

Tuberculosis; coccidioidomycosis; infectious mononucleosis; toxoplasmosis; pharyngitis; sarcoidosis; lymphoma; leukemia. To be distinguished from bilateral parotid enlargement (mumps, sarcoidosis)

- supraclavicular (behind mid-portion of the clavicle) and scalene nodes

Of ominous significance: metastases from intrathoracic or intraabdominal malignancies; lymphoma; breast cancer; inflammatory process unlikely. Biopsy is usually indicated

- enlarged suppurative cervical nodes

Mycobacterial lymphadenitis (scrofula)

- unilateral axillary

Breast carcinoma; lymphomas; upper extremity infection; cat-scratch disease; staphylococcal infection; sporotrichosis; tularemia; brucellosis

- unilateral epitrochlear

Hand infection

- bilateral epitrochlear

Sarcoidosis; tularemia; secondary syphilis; repeated minor trauma and/or infections in manual laborers

- unilateral inguinal

Lower extremity or local infection; syphilis; lymphogranuloma venereum

- bilateral inguinal

Various venereal infections; malignancy; lymphoma; metastatic melanoma arising in the lower extremities; cellulitis of the lower extremities

- generalized

Serious systemic illness: malignant, infectious, or immunologic. Chronic lymphocytic leukemia; Hodgkin's disease; non-Hodgkin's lymphoma (uncommon in nonhematologic malignancies); HIV infection (acute infection, persistent generalized lymphadenopathy); Epstein-Barr virus-associated infectious mononucleosis; cytomegalovirus infection; histoplasmosis; toxoplasmosis; chronic mycobacterial, parasitic, and spirochetal diseases; brucellosis; sarcoidosis, collagen-vascular diseases; drug reaction

Nasopharyngeal examination

May reveal a primary tumor with cervical metastases

Dental caries; pharyngitis

Possible infectious origin of cervical lymphadenopathy

Fever

Infectious process; neoplasm

Skin rash

Viral infection

Ecchymoses; petechiae

Bleeding tendency: leukemia, lymphoma

Sternal tenderness	Leukemia
Hepatomegaly	Malignancy; hepatitis
Splenomegaly	Infectious mononucleosis; collagen-vascular disease; serum sickness syndrome; sarcoidosis; hematologic malignancies; leukemias, lymphomas, Hodgkin's lymphoma
Hepatosplenomegaly	Angioimmunoblastic lymphadenopathy; malignancy
Swelling of the neck, face, or arms	Superior vena cava or subclavian vein compression by hilar or mediastinal node enlargement

LABORATORY TESTS PERTAINING TO LYMPHADENOPATHY[†]

Test	Finding	Diagnostic Possibilities
Blood		
WBCs	Lymphocytosis, atypical lymphocytosis	Infectious mononucleosis; other viral infections; toxoplasmosis; chronic lymphocytic leukemia, lymphomas
	Lymphocytopenia	AIDS
	Granulocytosis	Pyogenic infection
	Eosinophilia	Hypersensitivity state; Hodgkin's disease
RBCs	Anemia	Malignancy

Serologic evaluation for HIV, Epstein-Barr virus, cytomegalovirus, toxoplasmosis infection, syphilis

Intermediate strength tuberculin PPD skin test

Chest x-ray	Bilateral mediastinal adenopathy	Lymphoma (especially the nodular sclerosing type of Hodgkin's disease)
	Hilar adenopathy	Sarcoidosis; tuberculosis; systemic fungal infections; lymphoma; Hodgkin's disease. Unilateral hilar adenopathy: metastatic carcinoma (usually lung)
Biopsy of lymph node or accessible mass		To detect lymphoma; sarcoidosis; tumor; carcinoma; granuloma; tuberculosis; etc.

[†]See the appendix on Laboratory Reference Values for the associated normal laboratory values.

SELECTED BIBLIOGRAPHY

Abrams DI: Lymphadenopathy related to the acquired immunodeficiency syndrome in homosexual men. *Med Clin North Am* 70:693–705, 1986.

Damion J, Hybels RL: The neck mass. 1. General concepts and congenital causes. 2. Inflammatory and neoplastic causes. *Postgrad Med* 81(6):75–93; 97–107, 1987.

Haynes BF: Enlargement of lymph nodes and spleen, in Wilson J, Braunwald E, Isselbacher KJ et al (eds). *Harrison's Principles of Internal Medicine,* 12th ed., pp. 353–359, New York: McGraw-Hill, 1991.

Williams WJ: Lymph node enlargement, in Williams WJ, Beutler E, Erslev AJ et al (eds). *Hematology,* 4th ed., pp. 954–955, New York: McGraw-Hill, 1990.

51
Obesity

INTRODUCTION

Obesity Any degree of excess adiposity that imparts a health risk. A person is considered obese if his or her weight exceeds by 9 to 10 kg the ideal weight; obesity implies an excess of adipose tissue.

Obesity occurs when the caloric intake exceeds the caloric expenditure of the body for basal metabolism and physical activity. Caloric intake is controlled by a satiety center in the hypothalamic ventromedial nucleus (destruction of this center causes overeating and obesity) and a feeding center in the ventrolateral nucleus of the hypothalamus (destruction of this center results in decreased food intake). Pituitary, thyroid, adrenal, and sex hormones influence the regulation of fat deposition.

Obesity due to hypothalamic or endocrine disorders is rare. Excess caloric intake is the cause of obesity in the majority of cases. In most cases of obesity various developmental, psychological, social, and genetic factors play critical roles. Major metabolic abnormalities have not been detected in obese individuals. There is no evidence that obese patients have an intrinsic abnormality of energy expenditure or a greater efficacy in their ability to digest, absorb, and utilize food. It has been suggested that individuals who develop obesity in early or late childhood have an increased number of adipocytes with variable degrees of enlargement of fat cells (hyperplastic hypertrophic obesity), whereas in those who develop obesity in adult years, the adipocytes are increased in size but not in number (normocellular hypertrophic obesity). However, the number of fat cells can increase at any age.

ETIOLOGY

Energy intake in excess of energy output
    Psychological, social, cultural factors
    Diminished physical activity
Hypothalamic damage (rare): tumor, inflammatory lesion, trauma to the head
Endocrine
    Cushing's syndrome; hypothyroidism; insulinoma; hypogonadism; polycystic ovary syndrome
Congenital diseases
    Unusual syndromes associated with obesity: Prader-Willi syndrome; Laurence-Moon-Biedl syndrome; Alström syndrome

Iatrogenic Causes of Obesity

Anabolic steroids; oral contraceptives; glucocorticoids; insulin excess; phenothiazines and other tranquilizers; cyproheptadine; sulfonylureas

445

HISTORY TAKING*

Possible meaning of a positive response

1   Mode of Onset and Chronology

1.1   At what age did obesity appear?
    • early in life? during childhood?

Predominantly adipocyte hyperplasia: there are periods during childhood and adolescence when overnutrition has an enhanced ability to induce the development of new adipocytes; congenital disease (rare): Prader-Willi syndrome, Laurence-Moon-Biedl syndrome

    • in adult life?

Predominantly adipocyte hypertrophy. Patients with adult-onset obesity are more amenable to treatment than patients with lifelong obesity

1.2   Do you know your weight
    • at birth?

Generally normal in both adipocyte hyperplasia and adipocyte hypertrophy types of obesity

    • during childhood?

Heavy children usually become heavy adults

    • at age 25?

For the lowest mortality, the pattern of body weight should be leanness in the twenties followed by a very moderate weight gain as one gets older

    • during military service? at marriage? at age 40?

If thin or of average weight until age 20 or 40: adult-onset obesity, associated with environmental factors

1.2a For female patients: What was your weight before your first pregnancy? after each pregnancy?

There exists a relationship between parity and obesity

1.3   Do you have serial photographs of yourself?

The patient with Cushing's syndrome is sometimes unrecognizable in earlier photographs, whereas the appearance of the obese patient has not changed much during adult life

2   Severity of Obesity

2.1   What has been your highest weight? lowest weight?

Variations possibly related to stressful events in patient's life history

2.2   What is your present weight?

In severe obesity: increased adipocyte size and number. In mild to moderate obesity: predominantly adipocyte hypertrophy

*In this section, items in *italics* are characteristic clinical features.

2.3 Is your weight still increasing?

A 20 percent excess over desirable weight imparts a health risk (e.g., skin infections, osteoarthritis, diabetes mellitus, hypertension). Significant health risks at lower levels of obesity can occur in the presence of diabetes, hypertension, heart disease, or other associated risk factors

2.3a Has your weight gain occurred
• rapidly? over a several-day period?

Increase in body fluid content rather than in tissue mass. Weight gain in excess of 1 kg/day almost invariably implies excess fluid retention (edema)

• over a period of weeks or months?

Change in tissue mass

3 Location of Obesity   See "Physical Signs Pertaining to Obesity"

4 Precipitating or Aggravating Factors

4.1 How many meals a day do you eat? at home? in restaurants? on your job?

May reveal peculiar eating habits, usually with high carbohydrate and low protein intake. Economic considerations may lead to low-protein, high-carbohydrate and high-fat meals

4.2 Please describe your present daily intake at breakfast, at lunch, at dinner

Overeating is the usual cause of obesity. Obese patients often deny overeating and underestimate the calories they consume. The true situation can be assessed by interviewing the patient's family and friends

4.3 What did you eat for breakfast today? lunch today? supper yesterday?

The questions about the patient's diet must be specific; the major caloric intake of the very obese subject usually occurs during late afternoon and evening

4.4 Do you skip breakfast? lunch? supper?

Frequent in teenagers or in obese patients on a self-reducing diet

4.5 Do you eat between meals?

Many obese patients do not regard a midmeal or bedtime snack as food and do not report it as part of their daily food intake

4.6 How much and/or how many times a day do you eat any of the following items:

Gives an estimate of the total ingested foods with respect to both type and amount; the amounts of sugar and starch foods, and of fats, readily show the main sources of calories

• sugar and starches:	Carbohydrate yields 4 kcal/g
• bread?	1 slice = 80 kcal
• potatoes?	1 medium = 113 kcal
• fruit?	1 apple = 100 kcal
• candy bars? crackers? pie? cake?	pancake with syrup = 124 kcal
• fats:	Pure fat yields 9 kcal/g
• butter?	1 pat butter = 90 kcal
• margarine? gravy?	
• mayonnaise?	1 tbsp = 92 kcal
• fried foods? sauces?	
• cheese, cottage?	1 tbsp = 27 kcal
• nuts? peanuts?	
• proteins:	Protein gives 4 kcal/g
• meat? fish? poultry?	4 oz = 285 kcal
• chicken, fried?	½ breast = 232 kcal
• milk? cheese? eggs?	1 egg = 75 kcal; egg, fried = 110 kcal
• side dishes of: rice? potatoes?	
• spaghetti?	(1 serving) = 400 kcal

4.7 How many times a day (a week) do you eat any of the following snack foods?

"Snack foods" have usually a high-calorie, low-protein content

• whole milk? (white)	8 oz = 161 kcal
• milk shake?	1 glass = 421 kcal
• carbonated beverage?	1 glass = 106 kcal
• ice cream?	⅙ qt = 193 kcal
• popcorn?	1 cup = 54 kcal
• potato chips?	1 serving = 108 kcal
• plain doughnut?	1 = 125 kcal
• sandwich, hamburger?	1 = 350 kcal
• pizza, cheese?	¼ = 180 kcal

4.8 What is your intake of beer? alcohol? wine? a day? a week?

Use and abuse of alcohol contribute to obesity; alcohol has significant caloric value: 1 glass beer = 114 kcal, 1 martini = 24 oz beer = ± 200 kcal

4.9 Please describe your eating patterns: time of day? length of eating period? place of ingestion? simultaneous activities (reading, watching television)? companions or alone?

May reveal abnormal (and treatable) eating behavior

4.10 Do you often attend meetings? celebrations? cocktail parties?

Social contributing factors: calorie-rich refreshments. Obese subjects usually overrespond to external signals such as times of day, social setting, food abundance, food attractiveness, and smell or taste of food, to a greater extent than do persons of normal weight

4.11 Do you snack frequently? (from re-frigerators, cookie jars, etc.)

Recurring eating patterns which can be disrupted or aborted by behavior mod-ification techniques

4.12 Do you have any psychologic prob-lems?

Weight gain with emotional stress is a common characteristic of obese patients

4.13 Did you recently stop smoking?

May contribute to weight increase

4.14 Have you recently had an illness? an injury?

May lead to chronic restricted activity and predispose to weight gain unless caloric intake is appropriately curtailed

5   Ameliorating Factors

5.1 Do you lose weight on a strict diet?

5.1a Do you regain weight when you discontinue the diet?

The major problem in the treatment of obesity is not weight reduction but maintenance of the reduced weight. Ex-cessive levels of adipose tissue lipopro-tein lipase (ATLPL) could induce obe-sity by causing preferential deposition of fat calories in adipose tissue. ATLPL levels are increased in obese patients and do not return to normal following weight reduction (could explain the propensity of obese patients to regain lost weight)

6   Accompanying Symptoms

6.1 Do you have
  • pain in your knees? hips? spine?

Osteoarthritis (especially the hips): me-chanical and physical stress of gross obesity

  • skin lesions? axillae? perineal re-gion? under the breasts?

Moist folds with fungal lesions

  • varicose veins?

Often present in obese persons, with in-creased propensity for vein thrombosis and thromboembolism

  • *somnolence?*

Obesity-hypoventilation (Pickwickian) syndrome with sleep apnea. Upper air-way obstruction during sleep results in hypoxemia and hypercapnia with many arousals leading to chronic sleep dep-rivation and daytime somnolence. The obese habitus plus sleep-induced relax-ation of the pharyngeal musculature is believed to be the cause of the in-termittent upper airway obstruction

- headaches? a (partial) loss of vision? vomiting?

  Hypothalamic disorder; craniopharyngioma

- fatigability? muscular weakness? easy bruising?

  Cushing's syndrome (with centripetal obesity)

- intolerance to cold? constipation?

  Hypothyroidism

- episodes of hunger? sweating? palpitations? trembling?

  Hypoglycemia leading to frequent feedings with resulting obesity

  - after a prolonged fast?

    Insulinoma

  - 1 to 2 h after eating?

    "Reactive" hypoglycemia

6.2 For the female patient: Do you have absent or scanty menstruations?

Obesity and polycystic ovarian syndrome often coexist; Cushing's syndrome

7 Iatrogenic Factors   See Etiology

8 Personal and Social Profile

8.1 What is (was) your present (past) profession?

Sedentary work contributes to obesity; patients who have previously been physically active may fail to reduce their caloric intake when they suddenly change to a sedentary occupation. Obesity is 7 to 12 times more prevalent in lower socioeconomic groups than in upper socioeconomic groups

8.2 What is your daily activity pattern?

Most of obese persons are less active, both in engaging in physical activities and in moving about once engaged. The obese adult patient may continue previous alimentary habits despite less physical activity

8.3 What is (was) your relationship with your parents? school? friends? society?

A cause for overeating may be found in a maladjustment problem

8.4 Does your obesity cause you any problem: personal? psychological? social? sexual?

Obesity makes the satisfaction of social and sexual desires less likely. There is a strong prejudice and discrimination against the obese, particularly women, adolescent girls, and the morbidly obese. There is no evidence, however, of any particular neurotic or psychotic character in obese individuals

8.5 Do you have any reason—social, economic, medical—for undertaking a weight reduction program? Do you want to lose weight?

Motivation is the single most important factor in weight reduction

9 Personal Antecedents Pertaining to the Obesity

9.1 Have you ever attempted to lose weight
   • by adhering to a diet? by increased exercise? by group therapy? with Weight Watchers? with medications? Specify

A high percentage of persons in the juvenile obese group show poor response to therapy

9.1a Have you ever had any depression after a weight-reducing treatment?

Severe psychologic reaction to treatment may occur in juvenile type of obesity, in obese patients whose increased food intake was a manifestation of anxiety or depression. Prolonged dietary restriction may increase both the risk of negative emotional reactions and the risk of bulimia

9.2 Do you have
   • diabetes?

Diabetes mellitus is three times more common in obese than in lean adults. Women with android (central) obesity are more prone to diabetes than women with gynecoid (lower abdominal and femoral area) obesity

   • an elevated blood pressure?

The prevalence of hypertension is approximately three times higher for the overweight than for the nonoverweight

   • high blood lipids?

Hypertriglyceridemia is more prevalent in obese persons

   • gallstones?

Cholesterol gallstones are more prevalent in obesity; can lead to cholecystitis

   • a thyroid condition?

Hypothyroidism (the weight gain in hypothyroidism is actually edema and usually only moderate)

   • depression? anxiety?

Situational rather than endogenous; often improved if obesity is ameliorated

10 Family Medical History Pertaining to the Obesity

10.1 Do you know the weight of your
   • parents? siblings?

Obesity tends to run in families: genetic and/or environmental factors. Genetic diseases associated with obesity (Prader-Willi syndrome, etc.): rare

   • twin, if any?

If obese: genetic factor(?); the variability in body weight between identical twins is much less than that observed in fraternal twins

10.2 Is there any member of your family who has (had) obesity? diabetes?

Genetic and/or environmental influences

PHYSICAL SIGNS PERTAINING TO OBESITY

Indices Used to Express Obesity

Body mass index (BMI): body weight in kg/(height in meters)^2. The mean BMI is 22.4 for men and 22.5 for women. A BMI of 30 is considered "obesity."

Skin-fold thickness (subscapular or triceps): correlates rather well with total body fat. Obesity is diagnosed when the triceps skin-fold thickness is greater than 20 mm in men or 30 mm in women between the ages of 20 and 50.

	Possible significance
Fat deposition distributed	
• In the upper body above the waist	Android (male) fatness: occurs primarily by hypertrophy of the existing fat cells; carries a greater risk for hypertension, cardiovascular disease, diabetes mellitus
• In the lower body: lower abdomen, buttocks, hips, thighs	Gynecoid (female) pattern: occurs by differentiation of new fat cells (hyperplasia): more resistent to weight reduction
• *About the waist and flank* with ratio of waist to hip circumference > 0.7 to 0.8	Associated with a greater health risk than fat deposition at the hips
Osteoarthritis; flat feet; varicose veins; intertriginous dermatitis; ventral hernias	Mechanical trauma of excessive body weight
Hypertension	More common among the obese; Cushing's syndrome
Moon facies; truncal obesity; "buffalo hump" (cervical or supraclavicular fat deposits)	Cushing's syndrome
Purple striae over abdomen, shoulders, hips, elsewhere	Cushing's syndrome; also observed with rapid weight gain
Nonviolaceous striae over breasts, abdomen, upper arms, hips, thighs	Frequently observed in obese adolescents with normal adrenal function
Dry, coarse, cool skin; prolonged tendon reflex relaxation time	Hypothyroidism
In a female patient: hirsutism	Stein-Leventhal syndrome (with polycystic ovaries, infertility)

LABORATORY TESTS PERTAINING TO OBESITY

Note: In the absence of clues pointing to an endocrine or hypothalamic disorder, laboratory and radiologic screening are unnecessary

Test	To Detect

Blood

Glucose tolerance test; cholesterol, fasting triglycerides	Diabetes mellitus; hyperlipoproteinemia
Thyroid function tests*	Myxedema
Cortisol diurnal variation*	Absence in Cushing's syndrome
Arterial blood gases;* pulmonary function tests*	Elevated PCO_2, depressed PO_2, reduced lung volumes in obesity-hypoventilation syndrome
Skull films*	Cushing's disease
Psychologic evaluation*	Psychologic problems, depression, anxiety, associated with obesity

*When indicated

SELECTED BIBLIOGRAPHY

Bray GA (ed): Obesity: Basic aspects and clinical applications. *Med Clin North Am* 73(1):1–269, 1989.

Foster DW: Eating disorders: Obesity and anorexia nervosa, in Wilson JD, Foster DW (eds). *Williams Textbook of Endocrinology,* 7th ed., pp. 1081–1107, Philadelphia: Saunders, 1985.

National Institutes of Health Consensus Development Conference Statement: Health implications of obesity. *Ann Intern Med* 103:1073–1077, 1985.

52
Weight Loss and/or Eating Disorders

INTRODUCTION

Anorexia   Loss of the desire to eat.
Bulimia   Compulsive episodes of overeating (binges) followed by acts to "undo" the possible weight gain.

Anorexia is common in patients with gastrointestinal, extraintestinal, and psychologic disorders and therefore is an important but nonspecific symptom. Anorexia may be due to toxic products released by microorganisms, the "tumor neurosis factor" in cancer, or retention of metabolic end products in late-stage renal and hepatic disease. Anorexia with decreased food intake results in undernutrition and weight loss.

Mechanisms of weight loss include decreased appetite, accelerated metabolism, and loss of calories in urine or stools, acting singly or in combination.

Anorexia nervosa and bulimia are different clinical expressions of a primary psychologic disturbance focused on the intense fear of becoming fat coupled with a perceptual disturbance that causes overestimation of body size.

ETIOLOGY

Weight Loss with Anorexia

Malignancy
Psychiatric disorders: depression; anorexia nervosa; alcoholism
Uremia; liver disease; chronic lung disease; chronic congestive heart failure
Chronic infection; chronic inflammatory disease
Addison's disease; hypercalcemia

Weight Loss without Anorexia

Insulin-dependent diabetes mellitus; thyrotoxicosis; pheochromocytoma; carcinoid syndrome
Malabsorption; intestinal parasite infection
Decreased food intake secondary to painful oral lesions; poor dentition; esophageal disease; duodenal ulcer with outlet obstruction; postgastrectomy syndrome; inflammatory bowel disease; food faddism

Iatrogenic Causes of Anorexia

Any medication, particularly: amphetamines; digitalis; propranolol; broad-spectrum oral antibiotics; fenfluramine; salicylates; methylphenidate; antimetabolic drugs; codeine; opiates; (x-ray treatment)

HISTORY TAKING

Possible meaning of a positive response

1   Mode of Onset and Duration

1.1   How long have you been losing weight?

(In a female patient): the anorexia nervosa syndrome usually begins before age 25** or shortly after puberty, rarely later than the middle twenties

1.2   How many pounds have you lost?

The magnitude of weight loss reflects either the seriousness or the duration of the underlying disorder. Profound weight loss in anorexia nervosa (patients deny thinness); edema in the legs (and parotid enlargement, which gives a fullness to the face) may mask the true state of emaciation when the patient is fully dressed. Weight is near normal in bulimia

• at least 25 percent of the original body weight?**

A diagnostic criterion for anorexia nervosa; anorectics refuse to maintain normal body weight

1.3   Has your weight loss occurred
• rapidly? over several days?

Body fluid loss rather than alteration in tissue mass

• gradually? over a period of weeks or months?

Suggests a loss of tissue mass

1.4   Are you still losing weight?

Underlying process still present. Occasionally true loss of tissue mass is obscured by fluid retention (e.g., the cirrhotic patient who develops ascites or the patient with anorexia nervosa who has significant edema). Patients with anorexia nervosa have an intense fear of becoming obese, which does not diminish as weight loss progresses**

1.5   What was your average weight? maximum weight? minimum weight?

Comparison with prior measurements documents the reliability of the patient's history concerning the importance and duration of weight loss

1.6   Does your weight fluctuate?

Cyclical gains and losses are common in bulimia: due to alternating binges and fasts

**Diagnostic criteria for anorexia nervosa

2   Character of the Eating Disorder

2.1   How is your appetite?

Patients with anorexia nervosa deny hunger; true loss of appetite does not occur until late in the illness

2.2   Has your appetite (food intake) remained the same or increased?

Weight loss without anorexia or with increased appetite: thyrotoxicosis; diabetes mellitus; malabsorption; painful oropharyngeal lesions

2.3   Has your appetite decreased?

Anorexia with reduced food intake: medical or psychiatric disorder

2.4   Do you have
  • episodes of rapid and uncontrollable consumption of large amounts of foods?

Bulimia with binge eating (may occur in anorexia nervosa**). The drive to eat in bulimic patients is overwhelming

2.4a   Are the eating binges followed by induced vomiting? ingestion of large quantities of diuretics? use of laxatives? fasting? overactivity?

Attempts to get rid of the excess calories consumed

2.4b   Do you eat sensibly around other people? and then "pig out" when you are alone?

Overeating is ordinarily carried out secretly and alone, generally in the afternoon and evening

2.4c   Do you eat when you are not hungry? when you are anxious? depressed?

The binge-vomit or binge-purge cycle occurs secretly and at times of frustration, loneliness, or psychological distress

2.4d   Do you feel guilty, depressed, after an eating binge?

Unlike anorectic patients, bulimics experience a deep sense of shame and are aware of the possible consequences of their behavior but also fear not being able to stop voluntarily

2.5   Do you have an intense fear of becoming obese?**

Bulimics and anorectics share an obsessive concern about body size and fear of fatness

2.5a   Do you "feel fat"?

Patients with anorexia nervosa have a disturbance of body image, insisting that they are too fat, despite profound weight loss**

2.6   Are you aware that your eating pattern is abnormal?

Patients with bulimia recognize that their behavior is maladaptive. Patients with anorexia nervosa may deny any disturbance of appetite or emaciation; they refuse to maintain body weight over minimal normal weight for age and height**

3 Precipitating or Aggravating Factors

3.1 Please describe your present daily intake: at breakfast? at lunch? at supper?	May reveal nutritional deficiencies (in alcoholics, addicts, elderly, or poor people) or the presence of unusual eating habits, either extreme dieting or gorging/regurgitation. The overall eating pattern is usually quite disrupted in bulimia and routine mealtimes are rarely observed
3.1a Please describe your daily diet at your previous normal weight	
3.2 Do you avoid eating certain foods?	Food faddism or aversion to certain foods may produce malnutrition
3.2a What happens if you eat them?	Allergy to certain foods may produce abdominal discomfort and result in avoidance of these foods
3.2b Do you observe • a reducing diet? a therapeutic diet?	May initiate or perpetuate weight loss, or inadvertently cause malnutrition
3.3 Do you have • any dental problems?	Ill-fitting dentures, or lack of dentures, may interfere with mastication, resulting in a decreased intake of food
• painful lesions in your mouth?	May be caused by vitamin B group or C deficiencies; oral candidiasis
3.4 Has any recent personal or familial problem occurred in your life?	Onset of anorexia nervosa frequently follows a stressful event in the patient's life

4 Accompanying Symptoms

4.1 Has your food intake decreased? Do you eat less than usual • because eating produces abdominal discomfort?	Sitophobia: fear of eating because of subsequent or associated discomfort. In anxiety, postgastrectomy dumping syndrome, carcinoma of stomach or pancreas, regional enteritis with partial obstruction, abdominal angina
• because of a loss of appetite?	Anorexia: malignancy, infection, renal disease, endocrine deficiency; psychiatric syndrome
4.2 Do you have • a change in your bowel habits? • chronic diarrhea?	Gastrointestinal carcinoma Malabsorption syndrome; Crohn's disease; ulcerative colitis

• constipation?	Tumor of bowel; anorexia nervosa
• black, tarry stools?	Melena: gastrointestinal carcinoma
• pain in the abdomen?	Neoplasm; pancreatic carcinoma
• difficulty swallowing?	Obstructive esophageal lesion; neuro-muscular disorder impairing swallowing and resulting in an insufficient caloric intake
• nausea? vomiting?**	Uremia; anorexia nervosa (vomiting may be self-induced); increased intracranial pressure (brain tumor)
• excessive thirst? an increased intake of fluid? increased volumes of urine?	Polydipsia, polyuria: diabetes mellitus
• fever?	Tuberculosis; chronic infection; fever by itself can cause weight loss
• cold intolerance?	In anorexia nervosa: attributed to a defect in regulatory thermogenesis secondary to hypothalamic dysfunction
• heat intolerance? palpitations?	Thyrotoxicosis (weight loss with normal or increased appetite)
• fatigue?	Organic disease; depression. Patients with anorexia nervosa deny fatigue
• amenorrhea?**	Nearly always present in anorexia nervosa; it usually accompanies or follows weight loss. Half of bulimic patients continue to menstruate
4.3 Do you feel depressed? anxious?	Depression plays a significant role in the eating disorders. Patients with anorexia nervosa fail to recognize anger, anxiety, depression. Depressed mood and self-deprecating thoughts follow eating binges. Depression is common and suicide is a definitive risk in bulimia

5   Iatrogenic Factors   See Etiology

6   Personal and Social Profile

	Anorexia nervosa and bulimia occur most often among young (age less than 25), well-educated, white females of at least normal intelligence, from middle-class or upper-middle-class families
6.1 Where do you usually eat?	Unfavorable environmental factors may adversely influence appetite
6.1a For the single male patient: Who prepares your meals?	Adequate food may be made unpalatable because of the way it is prepared or served

6.2	What is your occupation?	Athletes (runners, jockeys, wrestlers, gymnasts), models, ballet dancers, actors, actresses, are vulnerable to the eating disorders
6.3	Do you engage in sports? exercise vigorously?**	Patients with anorexia nervosa are often physically active and ritualized exercise programs are common; frenzied calisthenics or running may follow food intake
6.4	What is your daily consumption of	
	• cigarettes?	Extremely heavy tobacco abuse is a cause of anorexia and weight loss
	• alcohol?	Alcoholics often drink instead of eating; alcohol produces anorexia. High rate of alcohol abuse in bulimia
6.5	Do you use street drugs?	Drug abuse, kleptomania, and impulsive or antisocial behavior are common in bulimia
6.6	What is your sexual orientation?	Unexplained weight loss in a homosexual man: AIDS-related condition, lymphoma. Sexual promiscuity is common in bulimia

7 Personal Antecedents Pertaining to the Eating Disorder

7.1	Have you ever had a chest x-ray? an x-ray of your stomach? intestine? When? With what results?	
7.2	Have you ever had any GI surgery?	Some weight loss is common after subtotal gastrectomy; it may be due to fear of eating because of the dumping syndrome, reduced caloric intake because of early satiety, or mild steatorrhea following surgery. In case of intestinal resection: decreased absorptive surface
7.3	Do you have any of the following conditions:	
	• a thyroid condition? a renal disease? a liver disease? chronic bronchitis? emphysema? tuberculosis?	
	• a cardiac condition?	Anorexia due to congestion of the liver and GI tract in right-sided failure

• diabetes mellitus?

Initial weight loss (with the onset of diabetes) is due to the osmotic diuresis induced by hyperglycemia; subsequently, loss of tissue mass in the insulin-dependent diabetes results from caloric wastage (the consequence of glycosuria), and accelerated proteolysis and lipolysis due to insulin deficiency and glucagon excess

• a known psychiatric or physical illness that could account for the weight loss?

Absent in anorexia nervosa** and in bulimia

8   Family Medical History Pertaining to the Eating Disorder

8.1   Are there alcoholics or drug abusers in your family?

High incidence of affective disorders, alcoholism, and illicit drug use in families of patients with bulimia

PHYSICAL SIGNS PERTAINING TO WEIGHT LOSS AND/OR EATING DISORDERS

	Possible significance
Fever	Chronic infection; tuberculosis
Enlarged thyroid; tremor; warm, moist skin; tachycardia	Thyrotoxicosis
Lymphadenopathy; splenomegaly	Malignancy: leukemia; lymphoma
Abnormal abdominal examination	Malignancy; gastrointestinal obstruction
Hepatomegaly	Cirrhosis; chronic hepatitis
Hypotension; bradycardia;** hypothermia; dry skin; lanugo-type hair;** retained breast tissue, and pubic and axillary hair	Anorexia nervosa
Examination of the mouth and pharynx	May reveal local causes of decreased intake of food: lack of dentures, ulcerations of tongue or oral mucosa; candidiasis
Skin changes over the dorsum of the hand	In bulimia, secondary to the trauma of the skin caused by using the hand as an instrument to stimulate the gag reflex
Hypertrophy of the parotid glands	May occur in bulimia, anorexia nervosa, and other forms of starvation

**Diagnostic criteria for anorexia nervosa

Dental erosions	In bulimia: the frequent presence of vomitus and stomach acid in the mouth causes tooth enamel to dissolve
Neurologic abnormalities	Neuromuscular disorders may interfere with mastication: stroke, brainstem lesions, amyotrophic lateral sclerosis, muscular dystrophy

LABORATORY TESTS PERTAINING TO WEIGHT LOSS AND/OR EATING DISORDERS[†]

Test	To Detect
Blood	
Complete blood cell count	Anemia; leukemia (anemia and leucopenia in anorexia nervosa)
Erythrocyte sedimentation rate	Not specific: infection, malignancy, collagen-vascular diseases, etc.; normal in anorexia nervosa
Beta-carotene level	Elevated in anorexia nervosa
BUN, creatinine	Chronic renal failure; prerenal azotemia may occur in anorexia nervosa
Fasting glucose	Uncontrolled diabetes mellitus; glucose tolerance may be abnormal in anorexia nervosa as in other forms of starvation
Electrolytes	Endocrinopathies: Addison's disease; hypercalcemia; hypokalemia in anorexia nervosa, bulimia (hypokalemia with metabolic alkalosis in bulimia secondary to vomiting and laxative use)
Total protein, albumin	Hypoproteinemic states; moderate hypoalbuminemia in anorexia nervosa
Thyroid function tests	Thyrotoxicosis; normal free T4, reduced T3, increased reverse T3 levels in anorexia nervosa and other wasting diseases

[†]See the appendix on Laboratory Reference Values for the associated normal laboratory values.

Test	To Detect
Stool	
Occult blood tests	Gastrointestinal tumor
Ova, parasites	Parasitic diseases
Fat	Malabsorption syndromes
Skin tests	Tuberculosis; histoplasmosis; etc.
Chest x-ray; complete GI series*	Tuberculosis; bronchogenic carcinoma; GI lesion
Psychologic evaluation*	Anxiety; depression; anorexia nervosa; bulimia

*When indicated

SELECTED BIBLIOGRAPHY

Balaa MA, Drossman DA: Anorexia nervosa and bulimia: The eating disorders. *DM* 31(6):1–52, 1985.
Fitzgerald BA, Wright JH, Atala KD: Bulimia nervosa. *Postgrad Med* 84(2):119–123, 1988.
Health and Public Policy Committee, American College of Physicians: Eating disorders: Anorexia nervosa and bulimia. *Ann Intern Med* 105:790–794, 1986.
Herzog DB, Copeland PM: Eating disorders. *N Engl J Med* 313:295–303, 1985.
Herzog DB, Copeland PM: Bulimia nervosa—Psyche and Satiety. *N Engl J Med* 319:716–718, 1988.

PART TWO

Obtaining General Information

53
Obtaining an Occupational and Environmental History

Symptoms of hazardous exposure may appear as nondiagnostic complaints involving any body system. Therefore screening occupational questions should be incorporated into the routine history taking. A comprehensive occupational history should be taken in cases of acute or chronic respiratory disease, acute or chronic skin disease, and neurologic conditions with no clear-cut cause; back and musculoskeletal problems; liver disorders; any form of cancer; reproductive system problems; hearing impairment; any illness of unknown cause. The occupational history is the key to correctly diagnosing work-related disease.

1 Routine Survey Related to Present Illness

1.1 What is your occupation? (present, past; title and nature)
1.2 Are symptoms associated with work?
1.3 Are your complaints improved during weekends? vacations?
1.4 Are other workers similarly affected?
1.5 Are you currently exposed to any dust, fumes, chemicals, loud noise, radiation?
1.6 Was a first report of work injury filed by a physician?

2 Work History

2.1 List in chronological order all jobs. Describe in detail the work site. Describe a typical work day.
2.2 Was protective equipment issued? Do you have knowledge of safety programs given on the job?
2.3 Is ventilation in your workplace appropriate?
2.4 Was a preemployment examination done?
2.5 Is any specialized periodic testing or medical surveillance done on current or prior jobs?
2.6 Are you aware of industrial hygiene sampling of the workplace?
2.7 Have you ever been off work for more than a day because of an illness or injury related to work?
2.8 Has a worker compensation claim ever been filed in your behalf? If so, list the specifics.
2.9 Have there been special health and safety issues presented by your labor union?
2.10 In addition to your regular work, have you ever moonlighted? List additional jobs.

3 Review of Systems

3.1 Do you have any allergic conditions?
3.2 Have you ever worked at a job which caused you
  • trouble breathing? cough? wheezing?

- a rash?
- lower back pain?

3.3 What are your working hours?

3.4 Has your job schedule required major changes of shift work that have disturbed your sleep?

3.5 Reproductive history: Record the number of miscarriages, children, stillbirths, prior pregnancies, difficulties conceiving.

3.5a Have you noted any change in libido or menses?

4 Past History

4.1 Have you regularly been exposed to loud noises, excessive vibration, or heat?

4.2 Have you ever been exposed to asbestos?

4.3 Have you ever been exposed to radioactive chemicals? excessive radiation? chemicals?

4.4 During military service what were your duties? Did you have any exposure to potentially toxic agents?

5 Environmental Health History

5.1 Are there any industrial plants? new factories located in your neighborhood?

5.2 Have you been exposed to any hazardous waste sites or toxic spills?

5.3 Does your spouse or any other household member have contact with dusts or chemicals at work or during leisure?

5.4 Is there commonly air pollution in your environment?

5.5 Do you have a hobby or craft which you do at home?

5.5a Do you work with painting, sculpting, welding, or woodworking? If so, what is the location and ventilation?

5.6 What is the insulation and heating in your current and past living areas?

5.7 What agents are used to clean your home and workplace?

5.8 Do you use insecticides, pesticides in your home or garden?

5.9 Do you maintain firearms in your home or workplace?

5.10 Do you wear seat belts?

5.11 Do you smoke?

SELECTED BIBLIOGRAPHY

Becker CE: Key elements of the occupational history for the general physician. *West J Med* 137:581–582, 1982.

Goldman RH, Peters JM: The occupational and environmental health history. *JAMA* 246:2831–2836, 1981.

Levy BS, Wegman DH: The occupational history in medical practice. *Postgrad Med* 79(8):301–311, 1986.

The Occupational and Environmental Health Committee of the American Lung Association of San Diego and Imperial Counties: Taking the occupational history. *Ann Intern Med* 99:641–651, 1983.

54
Obtaining an Alcohol-Use History

1 How much drinking have you been having? during (periods)?
2 Do you feel you are a normal drinker? drink no more than average?
3 Do you have to drink to feel good? to relax? to sleep?
4 Do you ever drink in the morning?
5 Have you ever awakened the morning after some drinking the night before and found that you could not remember a part of the evening?
6 Are you always able to stop drinking when you want to?
7 Was there ever a period in your life when you drank too much?
8 Have you gotten into physical fights when drinking?
9 Have you ever been arrested because of driving while intoxicated?
10 Has anyone in your family or anyone else ever objected to your drinking?
11 What effect does your drinking have on your family, work, health?
12 Have you ever lost friendships because of your drinking?
13 Have you ever lost a job because of drinking?
14 Have you ever gone to anyone for help about your drinking?
15 Have you ever been in a hospital because of drinking?
16 Have you ever been told by a doctor to stop drinking?

The CAGE questionnaire has proved useful in helping to make a diagnosis of alcoholism.

1 Have you ever felt you ought to Cut down on your drinking?
2 Have people Annoyed you by criticizing your drinking?
3 Have you ever felt bad or Guilty about your drinking?
4 Have you ever had a drink first thing in the morning to steady your nerves or get rid of a hangover? (Eye-opener)?

SELECTED BIBLIOGRAPHY

Ewing JA: Detecting alcoholism. The CAGE questionnaire. *JAMA* 252:1905–1907, 1984.
Hurt RD, Morse RM, Swenson WM: Diagnosis of alcoholism with a self-administered alcoholism screening test. *Mayo Clin Proc* 55:365–370, 1980.
Schuckit MA, Irwin M: Diagnosis of alcoholism. *Med Clin North Am* 72:1133–1153, 1988.
Schulz JE, Mersy DJ: Chemical dependency. *Postgrad Med* 85(5): 89–96, 1989.

55
Obtaining a Sexual History

INTRODUCTION

Sexual problems are common in the general population. However, many patients find it difficult to mention sexual concerns. The inclusion of routine screening questions in the review of systems ensures that the area is not overlooked. The physician must also initiate a discussion of sexuality when coexisting medical problems are likely to affect sexual function. Sexual problems can be brought up after questions about menstrual function in women or questions about urinary function in men. When a sexual complaint is elicited or volunteered, a detailed history of the manifestations and associated symptoms should be obtained.

When taking a sexual history, it is good practice to supply reasons to justify your questions. Begin with general questions that allow the patient to speak about him/herself. Then focus the patient into areas that might be ambiguous or omitted. Do not be too general in probing patients about their sexuality. If there is a question that has not been addressed, ask it. However, do not press inquiries on a reluctant patient. The history of a sexual complaint necessarily includes information about relationships with partners. Never assume the sexual preference of any patient. Refer to all sexual partners as partners and not by gender. Statements should be phrased as nonspecifically as possible. It is important to ask open-ended questions that do not probe for a specific answer. "Tell me about your sexual activity" is preferable to "Do you have sex anonymously?"

Questions should indicate that your concern is informational and not judgmental. Treat the patient with consideration, regardless of your own sexual preferences. To respect the dignity of the patient, it is best to use scientific words for sexual parts and sexual activities, unless the patient is more comfortable with vernacular or informal expressions. Reassurances about confidentiality may be necessary during the discussion of sexual matters. Use as little recording of interview as possible.

Patients are often grateful when they are interviewed about their sexual function. As in other areas of medicine, diagnosis of sexual problems begins with the history.

Screening Questions

1 Are you sexually active?
2 Have there been any recent changes in your level of sexual desire?
3 Is intercourse satisfactory?
4 Does your partner have any problem with sex?
5 Has your present illness affected your sexual functioning?
6 Do you have any questions or concerns about your sexual functioning?
For the male patient
7 Do you have any problems having or maintaining an erection?
   • If so, in what situations?
8 Do you have any problems ejaculating? having an orgasm?
   • If so, in what situations?
For the female patient
7 Do you have any discomfort during intercourse?

8   Do you have any difficulty coming to orgasm?
    • If so, in what situations?

Female Sexual Dysfunction

1   Do you have difficulty becoming
    or staying sexually aroused?

1a   Are you able to reach a climax?

Failures of satisfaction from sexual contact are the most common female sexual disorders. Inhibited sexual arousal most commonly has psychological causes; may be due to omission of foreplay or coitus severely shortened by premature ejaculation

2   Does your vagina seem too dry
    during intercourse?

Decreased vaginal lubrication may be due to: psychological causes; estrogen deprivation (surgical or natural menopause); impaired neurological function (diabetes mellitus); decreased vascular supply (atherosclerosis)

3   Do you have pain on penetration?

Dyspareunia: a common sexual dysfunction. Most commonly due to an organic disorder: vaginitis; atrophic vaginitis; inadequate lubrication; pelvic infection; pressure on a normal ovary; pelvic growth. Functional dyspareunia is a diagnosis of exclusion

4   Do you have an involuntary contraction of the muscles surrounding the vaginal orifice making intercourse difficult or impossible?

Vaginismus: a conditioned (psychological) response to fear of vaginal penetration; may be induced by a painful pelvic lesion

5   Do you have the same complaint(s) with all partners at all times?

Primary dysfunction likely to be related to inner conflicts about the patient's sexuality

6   Do you have the same complaints occasionally? with some partners but not with others?

Secondary dysfunction; may be due to interpersonal problems

7   Have you maintained an interest in sex?

Failure of sexual desire may be due to incompatibility with partner

8   When was the last time you had sexual contact?

9   Are you satisfied with your sex life as it is now?

10   How satisfied do you think your partner is?

Male Sexual Dysfunction   See Chapter 29 "Impotence"

Assessing the Risk for AIDS

With the current epidemic of the acquired immunodeficiency syndrome (AIDS), it is especially important for the physician to identify patients at high risk for human immunodeficiency virus (HIV) infection: homosexual men, bisexual men, intravenous drug abusers, recipients of blood products or organ transplants, hemophiliacs, persons with multiple sexual partners, prostitutes (male or female), sexual partners of persons in the foregoing groups, children born to HIV-infected women.

Before eliciting a history of risk behavior for HIV infection, it is useful to give a brief introductory explanation: "Certain conditions, like AIDS, may be related to a person's sexual practices." A nonjudgmental attitude is essential when questioning a patient about his sexual preferences, sex with prostitutes, extramarital affairs, or use of intravenous drugs. Do not stigmatize the patient. Avoid negatively phrased questions ("You don't have homosexual contacts, do you?"). Ask direct, detailed questions about the risk behavior of the patient and his or her sexual partners with sensitivity, empathy, and understanding.

Questions to Identify Persons at Risk for HIV Infection

For the male patient
1   Do you prefer to have sex with men, women, or both?
2   Have you ever had sex with a woman who used intravenous drugs?
3   Have you ever had sex with a prostitute (male or female)?
For the female patient
1   Have you ever had sex with a man whom you know or suspect is bisexual?
2   Have you ever had sex with a man who used intravenous drugs?
For both sexes:
1   Have you ever used intravenous drugs?
2   Have you ever had a blood transfusion?
3   How many sexual partners would you estimate you have had per year in the past five years?
4   Have you ever had genital herpes? gonorrhea? syphilis? *Chlamydia* infection? pelvic infections? (Indirect evidence of possible sexual relations with multiple partners or with partners that the patient does not know well)
5   Have you ever had sex with someone who developed AIDS?
6   Have you ever paid money or received money for sex?
7   Have you taken any precautions such as "safe sex" to avoid AIDS?
8   Do you have any concerns or questions about AIDS?

SELECTED BIBLIOGRAPHY

Antoniskis D, Sattler FR, Leedom JM: Importance of assessing risk behavior for AIDS. *Postgrad Med* 83(5):138–152, 1988.

Ende J, Rockwell S, Glasgow M: The sexual history in general medicine practice. *Arch Intern Med* 144:558–561, 1984.

Felman YM, Nikitas JA: Obtaining history of patient's sexual activities. *NY State J Med* 79:1879–1881, 1979.

Owen WF Jr: The clinical approach to the male homosexual patient. *Med Clin North Am* 70:499–535, 1986.

56
Evolution of the Illness

1   Have you ever had the same complaints before? When?

1.1   Were you in good health during the symptom-free period(s)?

1.2   How long has it been since you were perfectly well?

2   Do you know someone (relative, friend, acquaintance) who has the same complaint as you?

3   Have you visited other physicians since the beginning of your troubles? Name(s)? When?

3.1   Have they ordered blood tests? x-rays? other examinations? Date of tests? Results?

3.2   What was their diagnosis?

3.3   Did they give you any treatment? When? Result? Any side effect(s)?

4   Did you take any medication for your trouble? On your own? Prescribed by a physician? Which ones? Dosage? Results? Any side effects?

5   Has your trouble caused you
- to stop working?
- to stay in bed?

For how long?

6   Is your trouble getting worse? better? Spontaneously? Due to treatment? Since when?

6.1   Has your illness remained stationary since its beginning?

7   Do you suspect any factors which could possibly be playing a role in your illness?

8   What illness do you think you are suffering from?

8.1   What do you think is causing your trouble?

9   What prompted you to consult a physician at this time?

57
Personal Past Medical History

1   Have you ever been sick before? What did you have? When?
1.1   What were the symptoms of the illness?
1.2   What kind of treatment did you receive?
1.3   Do you have any aftereffects of the illness? Of the treatment?
2   Have you ever been confined to bed at home? Why? When?
2.1   For how long? For more than 2 weeks?
2.2   Did you call for a physician?
2.3   What was his diagnosis? Treatment?
2.4   What were the results of the treatment?
3   Have you ever been hospitalized? When? Where? For how long?
3.1   What was the diagnosis made by the physicians?
3.2   What kind of treatment did you receive?
3.3   What were the results of the treatment?
4   Have you ever been operated on? Why? When? Where? Name of hospital, city, state? Surname of surgeon(s)?
4.1   What kind of operation was it?
4.2   What was the result of the operation? Any aftereffects?
5   Have you ever had an accident? When?
5.1   Under which circumstances?
5.2   Was it followed by a period of unconsciousness?
5.3   Did you have any fractures?
5.4   Were you hospitalized?
5.5   What was the treatment given?
5.6   Did it necessitate blood transfusion(s)?
5.7   Do you have any aftereffects?
5.8   Are you currently seeking compensation for your injury?
6   For the female patient:
6.1   Have you ever had miscarriages? abortions? stillbirths? curettages? cesarian deliveries?
6.2   Have you ever used contraceptives?
7   Were you a full-term baby?
7.1   Were you delivered spontaneously (normally)? With forceps?
7.2   Did you have any abnormalities at birth?
7.3   How was the health of your mother during pregnancy?
8   Did you have during your childhood: chickenpox? measles? German measles? scarlet fever? mumps? pertussis? diphtheria? rheumatic fever?
8.1   Were you excused from participating in sports in school? Why?
9   Allergic disorders: Have you ever had asthma? allergy? hives? hay fever? eczema?
9.1   Are you allergic to any foods? animals? feathers? paints? soaps? ointments? hair colorants? chemical products? drugs?
9.1a   Are you allergic to aspirin? penicillin? other antibiotics? sulfonamides? sedatives? laxatives? others?
9.2   Are there any drugs which have adversely affected you?

9.2a What happened when you took these drugs?

9.3 Have you ever received injections of immune serums, antitoxins? Why? Without any side effects?

10 Have you ever received blood transfusions? Why? When? Any side effects?

10.1 Do you know your blood group?

11 Have you been immunized against poliomyelitis? tetanus? rubella? diphtheria? measles? tuberculosis (BCG)? influenza? pertussis? mumps?

11.1 Date of last immunization?

12 Have you ever lived in, or traveled to, foreign countries? Where? When? Were you ever sick while there?

13 Have you ever been treated for a sexually transmitted disease? Diagnosis? When? Treatment received? With what results?

14 Have you ever been treated for emotional problems? your nerves? When? At home? Hospitalized? Treatment received? With what results?

15 Have you ever had to stop working because of health problems? When? How often? For how long? Why?

16 Have you ever had a medical examination for life insurance? Employment purposes? Military service? When? With what results? Date of last thorough medical examination?

16.1 Have you ever been turned down because of health problems?

17 When did you last consult a physician? Why?

17.1 Did he or she prescribe any treatment?

18 Have you ever had any blood tests done? Urine tests? Pap smears? ECG? X-rays? Isotopic examinations? CT scans? Eye (ocular fundus) examinations? EEG? Endoscopic examinations?

18.1 When were these tests performed? Why? Results?

18.2 Do you possess any report of these tests?

Family Medical History

1   Is your mother (father) still living? Age?
1.1   Is she/he well? in good health?
1.1a   If not: What disease is she/he suffering from?
1.2   If deceased: Age at death? Cause of death? How did she/he die?
2   Do you have any brothers? sisters? twins? Age?
2.1   State of health? Diseases, if any?
2.2   If deceased: Age at death? Cause of death?
3   Is your wife (husband) in good health? Age?
3.1   If not: What disease is she (he) suffering from?
3.2   If deceased: Age at death? Cause of death?
4   If any children: Age and state of health?
5   Do you know of any diseases running in your family?
6   Have any of your relatives suffered from:

Diabetes?	Coronary artery disease?	High cholesterol?
Arterial hypertension?	Stroke?	Gout?
Tuberculosis?	Obesity?	Anemia?
Migraine?	Allergy?	Bleeding tendency?
Depression?	Asthma?	Cancer?
Mental disease?	Hay fever?	Goiter?
Epilepsy?	Renal disease?	Arthritis?

6.1   Have any of your relatives committed suicide?

Review of Systems

1   General Information

1.1   Have you recently noticed any change in weight? How many pounds? Since
       when?
1.2   Do you have fever?
1.3   Do you feel tired?

2   Head

2.1   Do you have headache or pain anywhere in the head?

3   Eyes

3.1   Do you need glasses to see things at a distance? to read?
3.2   Do you ever see double?
3.3   Do you ever see halos about light?
3.4   Do you have any blurring, loss of vision? Recent? Old?
3.5   Are your eyes often red or inflamed?
3.6   Does light hurt your eyes?
3.7   Do you have a cataract?

4   Ears

4.1   Do you have difficulty hearing?
4.2   Do you have any earaches?
4.3   Do you have any ear discharge?
4.4   Do you have constant buzzing in your ears?

5   Nose

5.1   Do you have nasal obstruction when you do not have a cold?
5.2   Does your nose run constantly?
5.3   Do you have sinus trouble?
5.4   Do you ever have excessive bleeding from the nose?
5.5   Can you smell coffee, flowers, perfumes, as usual?

6   Mouth

6.1   Do you have any problems with your teeth?
6.2   Do you wear dentures? Do they fit comfortably? Can you chew well with
       them?
6.3   Do you have bleeding gums?
6.4   Do you have any sore swellings on your gums?
6.5   Do you have any pain or burning of the tongue or mouth?
6.6   Has your sense of taste changed lately?

7   Throat

7.1   Do you have frequent or severe sore throats?
7.2   Has your voice become hoarse lately?

8   Neck

8.1   Do you have pain, stiffness in the neck?
8.2   Does twisting your neck cause pain?
8.3   Have you noticed a swelling or lumps in your neck?

9   Breasts (female patient)

9.1   Do you have any bleeding, discharge from the nipples?
9.2   Have you felt any lump, or tenderness, in the breasts?

10   Respiratory System

10.1   Are you troubled by constant coughing?
10.2   Are you troubled by expectorations? Amount? Character?
10.3   Have you ever coughed up blood?
10.4   Do you have shortness of breath?
10.5   Do you ever have wheezing in your chest when you breathe?
10.6   Do you have chest pain?
10.7   Do you have night sweats?
10.8   Do you have bronchitis more than once a month?

11   Cardiovascular System

11.1   Do you know your blood pressure?
11.2   Do you have palpitations?
11.3   Do you have pain, or tightness, in your chest when sitting still? On exertion?
11.4   Do you have difficulty in breathing on exertion? When lying down? Just
        sitting still?
11.5   Do you have to rest during or after climbing two flights of stairs?
11.6   Do your ankles or feet swell?
11.7   Do you have cramps in your legs when walking?
11.8   Do you have varicose veins? Cold or blue feet?

12   Gastrointestinal System

12.1   Is your appetite good? poor? as usual?
12.1a   Have you lost your interest in eating lately?
12.2   Do you have any difficulty swallowing?
12.3   Do you have heartburn?
12.4   Do you feel bloated after eating?
12.5   Do you have excessive belching?
12.6   Do you have nausea? vomiting?
12.7   Have you ever vomited blood?
12.8   Do you have pain in your stomach? After eating?
12.9   Do you have pain elsewhere in your abdomen?
12.10   Do you have abdominal pain when you move your bowels?
12.11   What is the frequency, consistency, color, of your stools?

12.11a Are you constipated more than twice a month?
12.11b Do you have diarrhea?
12.11c Are your bowel movements ever black?
12.11d Have you ever seen fresh blood in your feces?
12.12   Do you have hemorrhoids?

13   Genitourinary System

13.1   Do you have burning when you urinate?
13.2   Do you urinate more than five or six times a day?
13.3   Do you have to get up at night to urinate? How many times?
13.4   Do you have a constant feeling that you have to urinate?
13.5   Do you sometimes lose control of your urine?
13.6   What is the color of your urine?
13.6a   Have you ever seen blood, pus, in your urine?
13.7   Have you ever passed a stone?
13.8   For the female patient:
13.8a   At what age did your menstruation begin?
13.8b   What is the interval between periods? The regularity, the duration of your periods?
13.8c   Is the flow normal? excessive? slight? How many pads do you use per day? per period?
13.8d   Are the menstruations associated with pain? For how many days?
13.8e   Do you feel bloated and irritable before your periods?
13.8f   Do you bleed between your menstruations?
13.8g   What was the date when your last menstrual period began?
13.8h   Do you use birth control pills? other contraceptive methods?
13.8i   Do you have any excessive discharge from your vagina?
13.8j   If the patient is menopausual: When did your periods cease? Have you had any vaginal bleeding since your menopause? Do you have hot flushes?
13.8k   Are you satisfied with your sex life as it is now? (See Chapter 55 "Obtaining a Sexual History")
13.9   For the male patient:
13.9a   Do you have any difficulty in starting your urine flow?
13.9b   Have you noticed that your urine stream is weak and slow?
13.9c   Do you have any burning or discharge from your penis?
13.9d   Are there any swellings or lumps on your testicles?
13.9e   Are your genitals painful or sore?
13.9f   Are you satisfied with your sex life as it is now? (See Chapters 55 and 29 "Obtaining a Sexual History" and "Impotence")

14   Musculoskeletal System

14.1   Do you have stiff or painful joints? back? muscles? arms or legs?
14.2   Are your joints ever swollen?

15   Skin

15.1   Do you have any skin problem? Itching? rash? eczema?
15.2   Have you noticed any changes in coloration of your skin?
15.3   Have you noticed any lumps under your arms? In your groins?
15.4   Do you have excessive perspiration?

15.5   Do you bruise easily? Do you have difficulty in stopping a small cut from bleeding?

16   Neurologic System

16.1   Do you have vertigo? drowsiness?

16.2   Do you ever faint or feel faint?

16.3   Have you ever had convulsions?

16.4   Do you have any muscular weakness? paralysis?

16.5   Do you have any loss of sensation, tingling, numbness, in your fingers, toes, limbs?

16.6   Have you noticed any tremor, clumsiness, or awkwardness of your hands or feet?

16.7   Has your handwriting changed lately?

16.8   Do you consider yourself nervous?

60
Personal and Social Profile

1 Marital History

1.1 Are you single? married?
  - At what age were you married?
  - How old is your husband (wife)?
  - Is he (she) in good health?
  - Have you been married more than once?
  - divorced?
  - separated?
  - widowed? Since when? What was the cause of the death of your husband (wife)?

1.2 Do you have children? How many? Age(s)?

1.2a Are they in good health?

1.2b Were complications encountered at birth?

1.2c What were your children's weights at birth?

1.2d If remarried: Do you have children by second or subsequent marriage?

1.2e Do you have children who live with you?

1.2f Do you have any particular problems with them?

1.3 If no pregnancies: why?

1.3a Have you used contraceptive measures? Which one(s)? Do you still use them?

2 Home Conditions

2.1 Are you satisfied with your present housing?

2.2 Have you changed domicile recently? How often? Why?

2.3 How many people are living in your house, your apartment?

2.4 Besides your husband (wife) and children, are there other persons living with you?

3 Education

3.1 How far did you get in school? Elementary school? high school? college? business or trade school?

3.2 Did you have to interrupt your education? Why?

4 Employment

4.1 What is your present occupation? Since when?

4.2 Are you satisfied with it? If not: Why?

4.3 Is the physical activity you have on your job heavy? limited?

4.4 How many hours a day do you work?

4.5 How long have you been with your present company?

4.6 What were your past occupations? What kind of work have you done?

4.6a Why did you take different jobs?

4.6b Do you have any difficulty in holding an occupation?

4.7   In case of unemployment: how long have you been unemployed? For what reason?

4.8   If retired: Since when?

4.9   Do you think you are being (have been) exposed to occupational hazards? (See Chapter 53 "Obtaining an Occupational and Environmental History")

5   Military Service

5.1   Have you ever served in the armed forces? When? Where? How long?

5.2   Were you rejected? deferred? For what reasons?

5.3   During the military, what were your duties?

5.4   Were you ever sick while in the service? What kind of disease? sexually transmitted disease?

5.5   Have you been exposed to excessive noise, ionizing radiation, hazardous chemicals?

5.6   If served: Honorably discharged? If not: why?

6   Travels

6.1   Have you ever lived or traveled in foreign countries? In tropics? When? For how long?

6.2   Did you contract any disease while there? What kind of disease?

7   Dietary Habits

7.1   What is your usual weight?

7.1a When did you weigh yourself last?

7.1b What was your weight at age 25? Your maximum adult weight? Minimum adult weight? When?

7.2   Do you follow a weight-reducing diet? On your own? Prescribed by a physician?

7.3   Do you avoid eating certain foods? Which ones? Why?

7.3a What happens if you eat these foods?

7.4   Do you skip any meals? Why?

7.5   Do you have snacks between meals? before retiring? during the night?

7.6   Do you drink coffee? tea? How many cups daily?

7.7   Do you drink beer? alcohol? wine? How much a day? For how long? (See Chapter 54 "Obtaining an Alcohol-Use History")

8   Tobacco, Medication, and Drugs

8.1   Have you ever smoked cigarettes?

8.1a How old were you when you started smoking?

8.1b On average, how many packs have you smoked a day?

8.1c Do you currently smoke? If not: how old were you when you stopped smoking?

8.2   Do you use any medications? Rarely? frequently? regularly?
   • On your own? prescribed?
   • How long? Why? How many a day?

8.2a Specifically, do you take tranquilizers? sleeping pills? aspirin? other analgesics? pep pills? vitamins? laxatives? contraceptive pills? ulcer remedies? antihypertensive drugs? insulin? corticosteroids? anticoagulants?

8.3   Have you ever used marijuana? heroin? "crack"? similar drugs? For how long?

9 General and Psychologic Information

9.1 How many hours do you sleep on the average?
9.1a Do you have difficulty falling asleep? staying asleep?
9.1b Do you wake up very early in the morning?
9.1c Do you take sleeping pills?
9.2 Do you take vacations? How many weeks a year? Where?
9.2a When did you last have at least 2 weeks' vacation?
9.3 Do you exercise regularly? If not: Why?
9.3a Are you actively engaged in sports? Which ones?
9.4 What do you do with your spare time?
9.4a Do you have any special interests or hobbies?
9.4b How much time do you give to them?
9.5 Do you have any pets? dogs? cats? birds?
9.5a Do they look healthy?
9.6 Do you generally feel better at your job? at home?
9.7 Have you ever sought (or wanted) psychiatric advice or care? Why?
9.7a Do you have periods of excessive depression?
9.7b Do you have any anxieties regarding personal, marital, sexual, familial, professional, financial matters?
9.8 Do you have any problem you would like to discuss?

Laboratory Reference Values

Laboratory values are given in conventional and international (SI, système international d'unités) units. SI units appear in parentheses.

Blood

Acetoacetate: <1.0 mg/dL (<0.1 mmol/L)

Adrenocorticotropin (ACTH) 8 A.M.: 25–100 pg/mL (25–100 ng/L)

Aldolase: 0–8 U/L (0–8 U/L)

Aldosterone, 8 A.M. (100 meq Na and 60 to 100 meq K intake, patient supine): <8.5 ng/dL (<0.24 nmol/L)

Alpha-1-antitrypsin: 85–213 mg/dL (0.85–2.13 g/L)

Alpha fetoprotein (adult): <30 ng/mL (<30 μg/L)

Aminotransferases:

   Alanine (ALT, SGPT): 0–35 U/L (0–35 U/L)

   Aspartate (AST, SGOT): 0–35 U/L (0–35 U/L)

Ammonia: 80–110 μg/dL (47–65 μmol/L)

Amylase: 0–130 U/L (0–130 U/L)

Bicarbonate, arterial: 21–28 meq/L (21–28 mmol/L)

Bilirubin, direct (conjugated): 0.1–0.3 mg/dL (2–5 μmol/L)

Bilirubin, total: 0.1–1.0 mg/dL (2–17 μmol/L)

C-reactive protein: 7–820 μg/dL (70–8200 μg/L)

Calcium: 9.0–10.5 mg/dL (2.2–2.6 mmol/L)

Carbon dioxide content: 21–30 meq/L (21–30 mmol/L)

Carbon dioxide tension, arterial: 35–45 mmHg (4.7–6.0 kPa)

Carbon monoxide: <5% of total hemoglobin

Carcinoembryonic antigen (CEA), in healthy nonsmokers: <2.5 ng/mL (<2.5 μg/L)

Carotenoids: 50–300 μg/dL (0.9–5.6 μmol/L)

Catecholamines:

   Epinephrine: <88 pg/mL (<480 pmol/L)

   Norepinephrine: 104–548 pg/mL (615–3240 pmol/L)

Ceruloplasmin: 27–37 mg/dL (1.8–2.5 μmol/L)

Chloride: 98–106 meq/L (98–106 mmol/L)

Cholesterol, total (desirable level): <200 mg/dL (<5.17 mmol/L)

Complement:

   Total hemolytic (CH$_{50}$): 75–160 U/mL (75–160 kU/L)

   C3: 80–155 mg/dL (0.80–1.55 g/L)

Copper: 70–140 μg/dL (11.0–22.0 μmol/L)

Cortisol:

   8 A.M.: 5–25 μg/dL (138–691 nmol/L)

   4 P.M.: 3–12 μg/dL (82–331 nmol/L)

Creatine kinase (CK): 0–130 U/L (0–130 U/L)

Creatine kinase, isoenzyme MB: <5% of total

Creatinine: 0.6–1.5 mg/dL (53–133 μmol/L)

Estradiol:

   Women: Adult: 23–361 pg/mL (84–1325 pmol/L)

    Postmenopausal: <30 pg/mL (<110 pmol/L)

  Men: <50 pg/mL (<184 pmol/L)

Ethanol:

  Mild to moderate intoxication: 80–200 mg/dL (17–43 mmol/L)

  Marked intoxication: 250–400 mg/dL (54–87 mmol/L)

  Severe intoxication: >400 mg/dL (>87 mmol/L)

Ferritin: 15–200 ng/mL (15–200 μg/L)

Fibrinogen: 200–400 mg/dL (2.0–4.0 g/L)

Folic acid

  Serum: 6–15 ng/mL (14–34 nmol/L)

  Erythrocytes: 150–450 ng/mL packed cells (340–1020 nmol/L packed cells)

Follicle-stimulating hormone (FSH):

  Women: 2.0–15.0 mU/mL (2–15 U/L)

    Midcycle peak: 20–50 mU/mL (20–50 U/L)

    Postmenopausal: >50 mU/mL (>50 U/L)

  Men: 4–25 mU/mL (4–25 U/L)

Gamma glutamyltransferase (GGT): 0–30 U/L (0–30 U/L)

Gastrin: 40–200 pg/mL (40–200 ng/L)

Glucose, fasting: 70–110 mg/dL (3.9–6.1 mmol/L)

Haptoglobin: 100–300 mg/dL (1.0–3.0 g/L)

Hemoglobin A_{1c}: 5.6–7.5% of total hemoglobin

Human chorionic gonadotropin, beta subunit:

  Men and nonpregnant women: <3 mU/mL (<3 U/L)

Immunoglobulins:

  IgA: 90–325 mg/dL (0.90–3.25 g/L)

  IgD: 0–8 mg/dL (0–0.08 g/L)

  IgE: <0.025 mg/dL (<0.00025 g/L)

  IgG: 800–1500 mg/dL (8.00–15.00 g/L)

  IgM: 30–230 mg/dL (0.30–2.30 g/L)

Insulin, fasting: 6–26 μU/mL (43–186 pmol/L)

Iron: 60–180 μg/dL (11–32 μmol/L)

Iron-binding capacity: 250–410 μg/dL (45–73 μmol/L)

Ketones, total: 0.5–1.5 mg/dL (5.0–15.0 mg/dL)

Lactate dehydrogenase (LDH): 50–150 U/L (50–150 U/L)

Lactic acid: 5–15 mg/dL (0.6–1.7 mmol/L)

LDL-cholesterol (desirable level): <130 mg/dL (<3.36 mmol/L)

Lead: <40 μg/dL (<1.93 μmol/L)

Lipids, total: 450–850 mg/dL (4.5–8.5 g/L)

Luteinizing hormone (LH):

  Women: Pre- or postovulatory: 5–25 mU/mL (5–25 U/L)

    Midcycle peak: 75–150 mU/L (75–150 U/L)

    Postmenopausal: >50 mU/mL (>50 U/L)

  Men: 5–20 mU/mL (5–20 U/L)

Magnesium: 1.8–3.0 mg/dL (0.80–1.20 mmol/L)

Osmolality: 275–295 mOsmol/kg water (275–295 mmol/kg water)

Oxygen saturation, arterial: 96–100% (0.96–1.00)

Oxygen tension: 80–100 mmHg (11–14.4 kPA)

Parathyroid hormone: <25 pg/mL (<2.94 pmol/L)

pH, arterial: 7.35–7.45

Phosphatase, acid: 0–3 King-Armstrong units/dL (0–5.5 U/L)

Phosphatase, alkaline: 30–120 U/L (30–120 U/L)

Phosphorus, inorganic: 3.0–4.5 mg/dL (1.0–1.5 mmol/L)

Potassium: 3.5–5.0 meq/L (3.5–5.0 mmol/L)

Progesterone:
  Women: Follicular phase and postmenopausal: <2 ng/mL (<6 nmol/L)
    Luteal phase: 2–20 ng/mL (6–64 nmol/L)
  Men: <2 ng/mL (<6 nmol/L)

Prolactin: 2–15 ng/mL (2–15 μg/L)

Protein, total: 6.0–8.0 g/dL (60–80 g/L)
  Albumin: 3.5–5.5 g/dL (35–55 g/L)
  Globulin: 2.0–3.5 g/dL (20–35 g/L)
    Alpha$_1$: 0.2–0.4 g/dL (2–4 g/L)
    Alpha$_2$: 0.5–0.9 g/dL (5–9 g/L)
    Beta: 0.6–1.1 g/dL (6–11 g/L)
    Gamma: 0.7–1.7 g/dL (7–17 g/L)

Renin (normal diet), supine: 1–2.5 ng/mL/h (1–2.5 μg/L/h)

Sodium: 136–145 meq/L (136–145 mmol/L)

Testosterone:
  Men: 300–1000 ng/dL (10–35 nmol/L)
  Women: <100 ng/dL (<3.5 nmol/L)

Thyroid hormones:
  Free thyroxine index (FT$_4$I): 1.2–5.0
  Resin T$_3$ uptake: 25–35 percent (0.25–0.35)
  Thyroid-stimulating hormone (TSH): <5 μU/mL (<5 mU/L)
  Thyroxine, free (FT$_4$): 0.8–2.4 ng/dL (10–31 pmol/L)
  Thyroxine (T$_4$), total: 5–12 μg/dL (64–154 nmol/L)
  Thyroxine-binding globulin: 15.0–34.0 μg/mL (15.0–34.0 mg/L)
  Triiodothyronine (T$_3$), total: 70–190 ng/dL (1.1–2.9 nmol/L)

Triglycerides: 40–150 mg/dL (0.4–1.5 g/L)

Urea nitrogen, serum: 8–18 mg/dL (3.0–6.5 mmol/L)

Uric acid: 3.0–7.0 mg/dL (0.18–0.42 mmol/L)

Vitamin B$_{12}$: 200–700 pg/mL (148–516 pmol/L)

Pancreatic Exocrine Function

Secretin test (1 unit/kg of body weight, intravenously):
  Volume (pancreatic juice): >2.0 mL/kg in 80 min
  Bicarbonate concentration: >80 meq/L (>80 mmol/L)
  Bicarbonate output: >10 meq in 30 min (>10 mmol in 30 min)

Hematology

Bleeding time:
  Duke: <4 min
  Simplate: <8 min

Clot lysis, 37°C: 48–72 h

Clotting time, Lee-White: 5–8 min

Erythrocyte count: 4.2–5.9 million/mm^3 (4.2–5.9 × 10^{12}/L)

Erythrocyte sedimentation rate (Wintrobe):
  Males: 0–9 mm/h; Females: 0–20 mm/h

Euglobulin lysis time: >2 h

Fibrin degradation products: <10 μg/mL (<10 mg/L)

Hematocrit:
  Females: 36–46% (0.36–0.46)
  Males: 42–52% (0.42–0.52)
Hemoglobin:
  Females: 12.0–16.0 g/dL (120–160 g/L)
  Males: 14.0–18.0 g/dL (140–180 g/L)
Hemoglobin A_2: 1.5–3.5 percent of total hemoglobin (0.015–0.035)
Hemoglobin, fetal: <2 percent (<0.02)
Leukocyte count, total: 4,500–11,000/mm^3 (4.5–11.0 × 10^9/L)
  Differential count:
      Band neutrophils: 150–450/mm^3 (150–450 × 10^6/L); 3–5 percent
      Segmented neutrophils: 3000–5800/mm^3 (3000–5000 × 10^6/L); 54–62 percent
      Lymphocytes: 1500–3000/mm^3 (1500–3000 × 10^6/L); 25–33 percent
      Monocytes: 300–500/mm^3 (300–500 × 10^6/L); 3–7 percent
      Eosinophils: 50–250/mm^3 (50–250 × 10^6/L); 1–3 percent
      Basophils: 15–50/mm^3 (15–50 × 10^6/L); 0–0.75 percent
Leukocyte alkaline phosphatase: 30–188 U (30–188 U)
Mean corpuscular hemoglobin (MCH): 27–32 pg/cell (27–32 pg/cell)
Mean corpuscular hemoglobin concentration (MCHC): 32–36 g/dL RBC (320–360 g/L
  RBC)
Mean corpuscular volume (MCV): 80–100 μm^3 (80–100 fL)
Osmotic fragility of erythrocytes: slight hemolysis in 0.45–0.39 percent NaCl; com-
  plete hemolysis in 0.33–0.30 percent NaCl
Partial thromboplastin time (activated): 25–38 s
Platelet count: 150,000–400,000/mm^3 (150–400 × 10^9/L)
Prothrombin time: less than 2-s deviation from control
Reticulocyte count: 10,000–75,000/mm^3 (10–75 × 10^9/L); 0.5–1.5% of erythrocytes
Schilling test: excretion in urine of orally administered radioactive vitamin B_{12}: 7–40
  percent
Thrombin time: control ± 3 s

Urine

Aldosterone: 5–19 μg/24 h (14–53 nmol/day)
Amylase: 1–17 U/h (1–17 U/h)
Calcium:
  Normal diet: <250 mg/24 h (<6.2 mmol/day)
Catecholamines:
  Epinephrine: <20 μg/24 h (<109 nmol/day)
  Norepinephrine: <100 μg/24 h (<590 nmol/day)
Creatinine: 15–25 mg/kg/24 h (130–220 μmol/kg/day)
Creatinine clearance: 88–137 mL/min/1.73 m^2 (0.85–1.32 mL/s/m^2)
17-Hydroxycorticosteroids: 2–10 mg/24 h (5.4–28 μmol/day)
5-Hydroxyindoleacetic acid (5-HIAA): 2–9 mg/24 h (10–47 μmol/day)
17-Ketosteroids:
  Men: 7–25 mg/24 h (24–88 μmol/day)
  Women: 4–15 mg/24 h (14–52 μmol/day)
Lead: <0.08 μg/mL (<0.39 μmol/L)
Osmolality: 40–1400 mOsmol/kg (40–1400 mmol/kg)
pH: 5–7
Potassium (varies with intake): 25–100 meq/24 h (25–100 mmol/day)

Protein: <150 mg/24 h (<0.15 g/day)
Sodium (varies with intake): 40–220 meq/24 h (40–220 mmol/day)
Specific gravity, random: 1.002–1.030
   Concentration and dilution test:
      After 12-h fluid restriction: 1.025 or more
      After 12-h deliberate water intake: 1.003 or less
Urea nitrogen: 12–20 g/24 h (430–700 mmol/day)
Urea clearance: 60–100 mL/min (1.0–1.7 mL/s)
Urobilinogen: 0–4.0 mg/24 h (0.0–6.8 μmol/day)
Vanillylmandelic acid: <8 mg/24 h (<40 μmol/day)
D-Xylose excretion: 5–8 g within 5 h after ingestion of 25 g (33–53 mmol in 5 h)

Cerebrospinal Fluid

Cells: 0–5 mononuclear cells/mm^3 (0–5 × 10^6 cells)/L)
Chloride: 116–122 meq/L (116–122 mmol/L)
Glucose: 40–70 mg/dL (2.2–3.9 mmol/L)
Pressure: 50–180 mm H$_2$O (50–180 arbitrary units)
Protein, total (lumbar): 15–45 mg/dL (0.15–0.45 g/L), predominantly albumin

Stool

Bulk:
   Wet weight: <197.5 g/24 h
   Dry weight: <66.4 g/24 h
Fat (on diet containing at least 50 g fat): <7 g/24 h
Nitrogen: <2 g/24 h (<2 g/day)
Water: approximately 65 percent

Pulmonary Function Tests

Spirometry:
Forced vital capacity (FVC): Men: ≥4.0 L; Women: ≥3.0 L
Forced expiratory volume in 1 s (FEV$_1$): Men: >3.0 L; Women: >2.0 L
FEV$_1$/FVC (FEV$_1$%): Men: >60%; Women: >70%
Lung volumes:
Total lung capacity (TLC): Men: 6–7 L; Women: 5–6 L
Functional residual capacity (FRC): Men: 2–3 L; Women: 2–3 L
Residual volume (RV): Men: 1–2 L; Women: 1–2 L
Inspiratory capacity (IC): Men: 2–4 L; Women: 2–4 L
Expiratory reserve volume (ERV): Men: 1–2 L; Women: 1–2 L
Vital capacity (VC): Men: 4–5 L; Women: 3–4 L

SELECTED BIBLIOGRAPHY

Laboratory values of clinical importance, in Wilson J, Braunwald E, Isselbacher KJ et al (eds). *Harrison's Principles of Internal Medicine,* 12th ed., Appendix, New York: McGraw-Hill, 1991.
Normal reference laboratory values. *N Engl J Med* 314:39–49, 1986.

Glossary of Clinical Manifestations

The following is a list of the main symptoms and signs of frequently occurring diseases and syndromes.

AIDS (acquired immunodeficiency syndrome)
acute infection: mononucleosis-like syndrome
asymptomatic infection
persistent generalized lymphadeno-pathy
fever; weight loss; diarrhea
neurologic disease: dementia, myelo-pathy, peripheral neuropathy
secondary infections: *Pneumocystis carinii* pneumonia, cryptosporidio-sis, toxoplasmosis, mycobacterial infection, etc.
secondary cancers: Kaposi's sarcoma, lymphomas
autoimmune manifestations

Aldosteronism, primary
hypertension
potassium depletion
hypokalemic alkalosis
muscular weakness
polyuria
ECG: U waves

Ankylosing spondylitis
low back pain
sciatica
hip involvement
anterior uveitis
aortic regurgitation
cardiac conduction abnormalities
peripheral arthritis

Aortic regurgitation
palpitations
exertional dyspnea
orthopnea
paroxysmal nocturnal dyspnea
exertional chest pain

Aortic regurgitation *(continued)*
diaphoresis
congestive heart failure

Aortic stenosis
exertional dyspnea
angina pectoris
exertional syncope
orthopnea
paroxysmal nocturnal dyspnea
pulmonary edema

Bronchiectasis
chronic cough
expectorations
hemoptysis
recurrent pneumonia
sinusitis
cor pulmonale

Carcinoid syndrome
flushing
diarrhea
abdominal cramping
bronchoconstriction
pulmonic stenosis
tricuspid regurgitation
ectopic hormone production syn-dromes

Cirrhosis of the liver
fatigue
anorexia
jaundice
spider angiomas
in men: gynecomastia
testicular atrophy
palmar erythema
hepatomegaly
splenomegaly
ascites
esophageal varices

Colitis, ulcerative
bloody diarrhea
abdominal pain
fever
weight loss
arthritis
ankylosing spondylitis
uveitis, iritis
erythema nodosum
pyoderma gangrenosum
intestinal perforation
toxic dilatation of the colon
carcinoma of colon
hepatobiliary disease
venous thrombosis, thromboembolism

Colorectal cancer
rectal bleeding
change in bowel habits
abdominal pain
weight loss
iron deficiency anemia
progressive constipation
tenesmus

Crohn's disease
diarrhea
abdominal pain
fever
anorectal complications: fistulas, fissures, perirectal abscess
arthritis
skin lesions
episcleritis, uveitis, iritis
intestinal obstruction
fistula formation
hepatobiliary disease
small bowel and colonic malignancy

Cushing's syndrome
truncal obesity
"buffalo" hump
"moon" facies
weakness
hypertension
hirsutism
amenorrhea
cutaneous striae
bruising
edema
emotional changes

Cushing's syndrome (continued)
carbohydrate intolerance
polyuria, polydipsia
osteoporosis

Cystitis
dysuria
frequency
urgency
suprapubic pain

Diabetes insipidus
polyuria
excessive thirst
polydipsia

Diabetes mellitus
polyuria
polydipsia
polyphagia
late complications
  coronary artery disease
  stroke
  intermittent claudication
  in men: organic impotence
  neuropathy
  retinopathy
  nephropathy
  foot ulcers

Endocarditis, subacute infective
fatigue
fever
weight loss
arthralgia
embolic phenomena
petechiae
splinter hemorrhages
Osler's nodes
clubbing
cardiac murmurs
splenomegaly

Felty's syndrome
chronic rheumatoid arthritis
splenomegaly
neutropenia
anemia, thrombocytopenia

Folic acid deficiency
diarrhea
cheilosis

Folic acid deficiency (*continued*)
glossitis
wasting

Glomerulonephritis, acute
hematuria, proteinuria
oligoanuria
edema
arterial diastolic hypertension
congestive heart failure

Goodpasture's syndrome
pulmonary hemorrhage
glomerulonephritis
antibody to basement membrane
antigens

Gout
(hyperuricemia)
arthritis: acute, chronic
tophi
urate nephropathy
uric acid nephrolithiasis

Graves' disease
thyrotoxicosis
diffuse goiter
exophthalmos
pretibial myxedema

Heart failure
dyspnea
orthopnea
paroxysmal nocturnal dyspnea
acute pulmonary edema
Cheyne-Stokes respiration
fatigue
congestive hepatomegaly
edema
hydrothorax, ascites
jaundice
oliguria
cardiac cachexia

Hemochromatosis
skin pigmentation
diabetes mellitus
hepatomegaly
arthropathy
palmar erythema
cardiac involvement
loss of libido
testicular atrophy

Hepatitis, viral
fever
anorexia, nausea, vomiting
malaise
arthralgias, myalgias
dark urine
clay-colored stools
right upper quadrant pain
jaundice
hepatomegaly

Huntington's disease
(dominant autosomal)
choreoathetotic movements
progressive dementia

Hyperkalemia
cardiac arrhythmias
ECG: high-peaked T waves
muscular weakness
flaccid quadriplegia
respiratory paralysis

Hyperparathyroidism
(hypercalcemia)
renal stones
anorexia, nausea, vomiting
polyuria, polydipsia
weight loss
bone disease
personality disturbance
proximal muscle weakness
pruritus
duodenal ulcer
pseudogout
multiple endocrine neoplasia (MEN):
Men I: hyperparathyroidism,
tumors of the pituitary and
pancreatic islet cells, peptic
ulcer, gastric hypersecretion
Men II: hyperparathyroidism,
pheochromocytoma, medullary
carcinoma of the thyroid

Hypoglycemia
acute epinephrine release
sweating
tachycardia
tremor
anxiety
hunger
central glucopenia
faintness
headache

Hypoglycemia *(continued)*
  mental confusion
  convulsions
  coma

Hypokalemia
  muscle weakness
  flaccid paralysis
  hyporeflexia
  paralytic ileus
  rhabdomyolysis
  ECG abnormalities
  decreased renal concentrating ability
    polyuria, polydipsia

Hypoparathyroidism
  (hypocalcemia)
  tetany
  seizures
  mental confusion
  papilledema
  cataracts
  extraneous calcification
  skin, hair, fingernail abnormalities
  cutaneous candidiasis

Hypopituitarism
  oligomenorrhea or amenorrhea
  decreased libido
  loss of axillary, pubic hair
  fatigue
  cold intolerance
  hypoglycemic episodes
  hypotension
  decreased skin pigmentation
  weight loss

Hypothyroidism
  cold intolerance
  dry skin
  brittle, sparse hair
  constipation
  slow speech
  lethargy
  hoarseness
  periorbital puffiness
  bradycardia
  menorrhagia
  diminished hearing
  obstructive sleep apnea
  "hung up" reflexes

Intracranial mass lesions
  headache
  mental changes

Intracranial mass lesions *(continued)*
  vomiting
  papilledema
  diplopia, hemianopsia
  ataxia, hemiplegia
  convulsions
  arterial hypertension
  bradycardia

Irritable bowel syndrome
  intermittent watery diarrhea
  chronic constipation
  alternating constipation and diarrhea
  chronic abdominal pain
  excessive bloating

Leriche syndrome
  occlusion of terminal aorta
  hip, thigh, buttock claudication
  impotence

Lung, cancer
  cough
  hemoptysis
  dyspnea
  chest pain
  atelectasis
  pleural effusion
  hoarseness
  dysphagia
  superior vena cava syndrome
  pericardial effusion
  Pancoast's (superior sulcus tumor)
    syndrome
  Horner's syndrome
  paraneoplastic syndromes
    clubbing, hypertrophic pulmonary
      osteoarthropathy
    neurologic-myopathic syndromes
    adrenal hyperfunction
    inappropriate antidiuresis
    hypercalcemia

Malabsorption
  diarrhea
  steatorrhea
  weight loss
  malnutrition
  abdominal distention
  peripheral neuropathy
  glossitis
  tetany
  bone pain

Malabsorption *(continued)*
anemia
bleeding tendency

Mediterranean fever, familial
attacks of
fever
peritonitis
pleuritis
arthritis
skin lesions

Ménière's disease
paroxysmal vertigo
tinnitus
progressive hearing loss

Mitral regurgitation
fatigue
exertional dyspnea
orthopnea
right-sided heart failure

Mitral stenosis
dyspnea
pulmonary edema
atrial arrhythmias
hemoptysis
pulmonary and peripheral emboli
pulmonary infections
infective endocarditis

Mitral valve prolapse
mitral regurgitation
arrhythmias: palpitations, syncope
atypical chest pain
mid- or late systolic click
late systolic murmur
thoracic skeletal abnormalities

Myasthenia gravis
diplopia, ptosis
facial weakness
difficulty in chewing
dysarthria
dysphagia
generalized weakness
easy fatigability

Myocardial infarction, complications
pulmonary edema
arrhythmias
cardiogenic shock
heart failure

Myocardial infarction, complications *(continued)*
thromboembolism
septal perforation
mitral regurgitation
aneurysm of left ventricle
pericarditis
Dressler's syndrome
fever, pericarditis, pleuritis
cardiac rupture

Nephrotic syndrome
heavy proteinuria
hypoalbuminemia
edema
hyperlipidemia
thromboembolic complications

Pancreas, carcinoma
anorexia
weight loss
abdominal pain
obstructive jaundice
migrating thrombophlebitis
depression, anxiety

Pericarditis, acute
chest pain
pericardial friction rub
ECG changes

Pericarditis, chronic constrictive
peripheral edema
ascites
exertional dyspnea
distended cervical veins
hepatomegaly
paradoxical pulse
normal-sized heart
pericardial calcification
protein-losing enteropathy
nephrotic syndrome

Pheochromocytoma
paroxysmal or permanent hypertension
attacks of
headache
excessive perspiration
palpitations
apprehension
impaired glucose tolerance
weight loss
orthostatic hypotension

Polyarteritis nodosa
fever
weakness
weight loss
myalgia
arthralgia, arthritis
peripheral neuropathy
mononeuritis multiplex
pericarditis, heart failure
abdominal pain
renal involvement
hypertension
cutaneous involvement

Prostate, hypertrophy
slowing of the stream
frequency
hesitancy
postvoiding dribbling
dysuria, frequency, urgency
urinary retention

Pulmonary embolism
sudden dyspnea
substernal discomfort
tachycardia
syncope
ECG changes

Pulmonary infarction
pleuritic chest pain
hemoptysis
dyspnea
pleural friction rub
pleural effusion
tachycardia
fever
chest x-ray densities

Reiter's syndrome
arthritis
urethritis
conjunctivitis
mucocutaneous lesions

Rheumatoid arthritis, extraar-ticular manifestations
subcutaneous nodules
episcleritis, scleritis
pericarditis
pleuritis
interstitial lung disease

Rheumatoid arthritis, extraar-ticular manifestations *(continued)*
nodular pulmonary lesions
vasculitis

Sjögren's syndrome
keratoconjunctivitis sicca
xerostomia
interstitial nephritis
vasculitis
polyneuropathy
interstitial pneumonitis
lymphadenopathy
Hashimoto's thyroiditis

Systemic lupus erythematosus
arthralgia, arthritis
fever
skin eruptions
protenuria, cylindruria, hematuria
nephritic picture
nephrotic syndrome
pericarditis
myocarditis
pleurisy
myalgia
anorexia, nausea, vomiting
abdominal pain
psychosis, seizures
lymphadenopathy
venous or arterial thrombosis

Thoracic outlet syndrome
pain, numbness, parasthesies in arm
weakness of the small hand muscles

Thyrotoxicosis
emotional lability
excessive sweating
heat intolerance
lid lag, infrequent blinking
tremor
hyperdefecation
palpitations, sinus tachycardia, atrial fibrillation
weight loss
well-maintained or increased appetite
thyrotoxic myopathy
oligomenorrhea or amenorrhea

Vitamin B$_{12}$ deficiency

fatigability, weakness
sore tongue
anorexia
diarrhea
palpitations
dyspnea
distal paresthesias
subacute combined degeneration
mental changes

Wegener's granulomatosis

purulent or bloody nasal discharge
paranasal sinus pain, drainage
serous otitis media
cough
hemoptysis
dyspnea
pulmonary infiltrates

Wegener's granulomatosis *(continued)*

glomerulonephritis
eye involvement
skin lesions
nervous system manifestions

Wolff-Parkinson-White (preexcitation) syndrome

ECG: short P$-$R interval ($<$ 0.12 s)
    slurred upstroke of the QRS complex (delta wave)
    wide QRS complex
arrhythmias

Zollinger-Ellison syndrome

gastrinoma of pancreas
intractable ulcer disease
gastric acid hypersecretion
diarrhea

INDEX

Entries with an asterisk (*) also appear in the Glossary of Clinical Manifestations.